AN INTRODUCTION TO HAEMATOLOGY

AN INTRODUCTION TO HAEMATOLOGY

Dr Nandini Mukherjee

Visiting Professor
Medical College, Odisha
Former
Professor Dept. of Medicine
RG Kar and NRS
Medical College Kolkata

Publishing Globally

NEW AGE INTERNATIONAL (P) LIMITED, PUBLISHERS

New Delhi • Bangalore • Chennai • Cochin • Guwahati
Hyderabad • Kolkata • Lucknow • Mumbai
Visit us at **www.newagepublishers.com**

Published by New Age International (P) Ltd., Publishers
First Edition: 2014

BRANCHES

- **Bangalore** 37/10, 8th Cross (Near Hanuman Temple), Azad Nagar, Chamarajpet Bangalore-560 018 Tel.: (080) 26756823, Telefax: 26756820 **E-mail: bangalore@newagepublishers.com**
- **Chennai** 26, Damodaran Street, T. Nagar, Chennai-600 017, Tel.: (044) 24353401 Telefax: 24351463, **E-mail: chennai@newagepublishers.com**
- **Cochin** CC-39/1016, Carrier Station Road, Ernakulam South, Cochin-682 016 Tel.: (0484) 2377004, Telefax: 4051303 **E-mail: cochin@newagepublishers.com**
- **Guwahati** Hemsen Complex, Mohd. Shah Road, Paltan Bazar, Near Starline Hotel, Guwahati-781 008 Tel.: (0361) 2513881, Telefax: 2543669 **E-mail: guwahati@newagepublishers.com**
- **Hyderabad** 105, 1st Floor, Madhiray Kaveri Tower, 3-2-19, Azam Jahi Road Nimboliadda, Hyderabad-500 027 Tel.: (040) 24652456 Telefax: 24652457, **E-mail: hyderabad@newagepublishers.com**
- **Kolkata** RDB Chambers (Formerly Lotus Cinema) 106A, 1st Floor S.N. Banerjee Road, Kolkata-700 014 Tel.: (033) 22273773 Telefax: 22275247, **E-mail: kolkata@newagepublishers.com**
- **Lucknow** 16-A, Jopling Road, Lucknow-226 001, Tel.: (0522) 2209578, 4045297 Telefax: 2204098, **E-mail: lucknow@newagepublishers.com**
- **Mumbai** 142C, Victor House, Ground Floor, N.M. Joshi Marg, Lower Parel Mumbai-400 013 Tel.: (022) 24927869, Telefax: 24915415, **E-mail: mumbai@newagepublishers.com**
- **New Delhi** 22, Golden House, Daryaganj, New Delhi-110 002 Tel.: (011) 23262368, 23262370 Telefax: 43551305 **E-mail: sales@newagepublishers.com**

ISBN: 978-81-224-3589-4

₹ 200.00

C-13-03-6836

Printed in India at Glorious Printers, Delhi.
Typeset at Aakriti Graphics, Delhi.

PUBLISHING FOR ONE WORLD
NEW AGE INTERNATIONAL (P) LIMITED, PUBLISHERS
7/30 A, Daryaganj, New Delhi - 110002
Visit us at **www.newagepublishers.com**

Dedicated to

My parents who helped me to become what I am today

and

My patients who are continuous sources of aspiration

Devoted to

My students who are interested to learn more
and
My teachers who created interest in me to learn more

Compiled and Released

in

Loving Memory of My Late Husband Prof. Debidas Mukhopadhyay (18.3.43–12.11.08)

(Former Prof. and Head, Electronics and Telecommunication Dept. J.U.)

My Friend, Philosopher and Guide

Ph: 0413-2272380-2272390; Tele-fax: 2272066, 2272067, 2272735 E-mail: jipmer@jipmer.edu.in; Website: www.jipmer.edu

JAWAHARLAL INSTITUTE OF POSTGRADUATE MEDICAL EDUCATION & RESEARCH (JIPMER)

Dhanvantari Nagar, Puducherry-605006

(An Institution of National Importance under the Ministry of Health & FW, Govt. of India)

Dr. ASHOK KUMAR DAS,

MD, PhD, FICP, FACP, FAIID, FAMS, FRCP

Senior Professor of Medicine &
Medical Superintendent.

FOREWORD

Haematology is one of the most important contemporary, ever advancing and challenging branch of medicine and the scope of the speciality is ever expanding. Globally or more so in our country, between one-third to one-fourth patients have haematological problems. This branch of Haematology is very aptly blended to Internal Medicine, Obstetrics and Gynaecology, Haepatology and Nephrology because many of the problems manifest as bleeding. A myriad tropical diseases including viral fever, and a common health hazard snake-bite induce haematological disorders, which are extremely important facet of medicine. Further, anaemia in all age groups and in either sex is an important entity. Needless to mention, there is an imperative need of a good monogram on important areas in haematology. Dr. Nandini Mukherjee is an adept in the field of haematology and her entire academic teaching and research is focused on haematology and her contribution of various chapters and monograms have contributed immensely in the field of haematology in our country.

This book on Haematology is centered round the chapters under various headings. Part I and Part II encompass introduction to haematological diagnosis and management of all major types of anaemia. In Part III, the author has addressed the issue of haematological oncology and the chapters are very well written. Part IV and Part V addresses the coagulation and the platelet disorders forwarded by the miscellaneous chapter containing the chapter on Transfusion Medicine etc. All these chapters are written very simply, beautifully and with easy reading. The tables and charts are important assets of this book.

I congratulate Dr. Nandini Mukherjee for this Herculean task of bringing out this book so beautifully.

I am sure the book will fill the void of lack of haematological books and go a long way as a wonderful treatise on common haematological disorders and their management with special reference to our country.

(Dr. ASHOK KUMAR DAS)

Acknowledgements

I am greatly indebted to my senior teachers and colleagues, as well as, my students and junior colleagues, who always encouraged me in all my academic activity, and appreciated my academic achievements. I am grateful to the personnel working in the library and laboratory of my working place, for their constant, meticulous co-operation.

I am grateful to the New Age Publication, and its Printers and Binders, without the help of whom, it would have been impossible to bring out the book in the present form. I am personally grateful to Mr T. K. Chatterjee and the photographer Mr Kanu Das, for their unstinted support to my difficult task.

It is my honour and pleasure, to express my gratitude to Prof. Ashok Das, The Director, JIPMER, Pondicherry, who didn't hesitate to spare his worthy moments of the busy schedule, to write the introductory notes for release of this book.

I am thankful to my son and daughter Koustuv and Poulomi, who rendered their valuable technical assistance during the preparation of the book.

Finally, the acknowledgement will be incomplete, without expressing my immense gratitude to my late husband, Prof. Debidas Mukhopadhyay, who trained me with knowledge of computer, technical skill for writing scientific article, and continuously inspired me, and spared me for academic activity. Incidentally I am writing this page, on the very date of his sad demise, i.e. 12th November, 2008.

Nandini Mukherjee

Prologue

Haematology is an ever increasing wide field of Medicine, be in clinical practice or be in researches. Particularly it is of special interest in molecular biology, as blood cells, in different stages of development can be directly visualized in the peripheral blood. About one-fourth of total patients, attended in indoor or OPD of a general hospital, are affected by some haematological disorder. Among the rest of the patients, about half may suffer from haematological consequences of some systemic diseases. Any internist, hepatologist, nephrologist or cardiothoracic surgeon, or even obstetrician must face haematological problem in day-to-day clinical practice, like bleeding, thrombosis, anaemia due to different reasons or specific haematological problems like disseminated intravascular coagulation or microangiopathic haemolytic anaemia. Blood transfusion in any form may be needed at any stage of treatment of systemic diseases, for several reasons, apart from combating anaemia or bleeding. In the tropical country like ours, anaemia is often a problem to the clinician, as it is often difficult to solve, due to mixed etiology.

Considering importance of studying haematology, at least knowing some important facts and facets, in every specialty of Medicine, the present book is designed aiming at students, house staff, postgraduate trainees and practitioners of Internal Medicine. The book is divided into eighteen chapters and six parts to include some of the important haematological diseases, commonly met in the wards of our hospital. Some chapters are intended to be included in the revised edition.

Two chapters, "Glucose-6-phosphate dehydrogenase deficiency" and "Anaemia of chronic disease" are depicted in this book. These are not usually included in the textbook of Medicine, but are quite common in this part of the world, and need to be mentioned especially.

The present book is not a textbook in the truest sense, but it retains the purpose. The book elaborates, in every chapter, modern methods of diagnosis and recent advances in therapy, as far as practicable, as well as pathogenesis in detail.

If this book is found to be useful to the people, for whom it is intended, and creates interest to study more in the subject, I will feel my endeavour has been successful. Finally at the beginning of this very difficult task I feel bound to utter the great oath of Hippocrates, "I swear by Apollo Physician, Asclepiads, by Health, by Heal-all and by all the gods and goddesses, making them witness, that I will carry out according to my ability and judgment, this indenture."

Author

Contents

Part I

Introductory Notes

CHAPTER 1

Introduction

Haematology is the study of blood and blood forming organs. Blood is the connective tissue in the real sense, as it flows through different organs, connecting them structurally and functionally. It is unique in composition and function. Formed elements of blood are suspended in fluid medium, called plasma, having some peculiar physicochemical properties. It contains some electrolytes, sodium and chloride being the major component, as well as, some proteins, albumin, globulin and fibrinogen. Each component, along with, fluidity of the plasma plays some important role in maintaining milieu interne of the body. Plasma maintains the temperature and electrolyte balance and serves as acid base buffer of the body. It carries oxygen and other nutrients to different tissues, collects and carries waste products of metabolism to organs of excretion, like lungs, liver, kidney, carries hormonal substances to different organs for signaling their function. Plasma proteins are mainly of three types, albumin, globulin and fibrinogen Albumin maintains osmotic pressure of blood and retains fluid in the intravascular compartment. Globulin, rather immunoglobulin, gives rise to protective antibodies. Fibrinogen helps in clotting of blood and repair of damaged endothelium.

Formed elements of blood are of three types, namely, red cells, white cells and platelets. Red cells carry oxygen to different vital tissues, through its haemoglobin content. White blood cells are defensive in function, neutrophils produce defense against acute infection, lymphocytes act against chronic infection and eosinophils and basophils are active in hypersensitivity reaction to foreign antigen. Platelets help in haemostasis and thrombus formation.

In addition to nutritive, excretory, and defensive function, blood carries different antigens to the target organ, triggers formation of both protective and damaging antibodies at the cellular level, and mediates antigen-antibody reaction.

The peculiarity of blood is that it is the tissue, which can be most easily transplanted (blood transfusion). Transplantation of blood forming tissue, bone marrow, or its component, stem cell, is one of the most recent advances in medicine. The procedure not only corrects malignant proliferation of haemopoietic cells but also causes arrest of some genetic disorders like thalassaemia or non-haematological disorders like Alzeheimer disease or degenerative neurological disease.

Different haemopoietic growth hormones e.g. erythropoietin, granulocyte macrophage colony stimulating factors, are in current use to combat anaemia and infection, when they arise from defective haemopoietic tissue or as a result of chemotherapy for malignancy.

Haematology is one of the widest field of researches of molecular biology, as blood cells, in different stages of development can be directly visualized in the peripheral blood.

About one-fourth of total patients, attended in indoor or OPD of a general hospital, are affected by haematological disorder. Among the rest of the patients, about half may suffer from haematological complications e.g. vascular thrombosis, disseminated intravascular coagulation, microangiopathic haemolytic anaemia, as seen in hepatic disease, renal parenchymal disease or in obstetric patients with complications like abruptio placentae or eclampsia.

Any internist, hepatologist, nephrologist or even obstetrician must face haematological problem in day-to-day clinical practice.

1.1 DEVELOPMENT OF HAEMATOLOGY

Haematology in Ancient Medicine

Since ancient time, blood has been recognized as the essential component of life. In the Holy Bible, a universal truth about blood was mentioned that heart is the seat of the soul and blood is the source of energy for life. Ancient Romans hope to acquire vigor by drinking blood of the defendants at the end of the victory.

Before the invention of laboratory methods, **Hippocrates** formulated that four essential fluids of life are blood, black bile, yellow bile, phlegm and held the idea was that health is maintained by a balance of these four fluids. Thus in the days of Hippocrates, blood was thought to be one component of four essential "humours". In the days of Galen haematopoiesis was presumed to be a process maintained by proper balance of body's nutrients and body heat.

Examination of excavated skull in order to assess changes as a result of marrow hyperplasia is an essential component of modern haematology. Thalassaemia and Malaria are parts of Archeological diagnosis from ancient Greece.

At Lyndex Glecenstrshire, remains of a Roman temple of fourth century A.D. were excavated and remains of a unique arm and hand show kolionychia or spoon shaped nail, a condition caused by severe issue iron deficiency.

Development of New Concept

Thomas Sydenham (1624–1689) was known as English Hippocrates, for his study on clinical cases. For the treatment of iron deficiency anaemia, oral medication containing iron, was first prescribed by him. This recommendation was made 32 years before, Limzcy and Geffy demonstrated presence of iron in the ash of blood and 151 years before Paedlsch demonstrated deficiency of iron in chlorotic blood (1832). Sydenham did this unaided by laboratory. This is the first therapy suggested for world's most common form of anaemia in ancient and even in modern time. **Sydenham deserves the designation as the father of Modern Haematology.**

Pythagorus and his followers realized that use of beans should be forbidden for maintaining health in certain parts of world. Today residents of southern Italy show the highest incidence of Mediterranean type of G6PD deficiency. It is probable the same genetic trait was present in ancient time which gives rise to favism i.e. explosive haemolytic anaemia, following ingestion of particular type of beans.

In the eighteenth century, blood was recommended for treatment of fits, depression, palsy, but not for pallor or bleeding.

Further Developments

Following renaissance, many physicians attempted various methods of administering blood directly or indirectly into circulation. Louis K Diamond (1780) made many unsuccessful attempts at transfusion.

In 1901–02 Karl Landsteiner identified in the laboratory, four basic human blood groups, and this marked beginning of era of modern transfusion medicine.

Faharacus (1921), a Swedish physician, who devised the **erythrocyte sedimentation rate,** observed the phenomenon of **clotting of blood** in a transparent container. This showed separation of blood into homogenous red fluid, dark red clot at the bottom with a thin layer of red cells above it. **The concept of plasma** as essential constituent of blood thus arises.

Leeuwhoak (1632–1723) was able to describe **the red corpuscles or erythrocytes.** Improved methods for microscopy of blood in 1920s, and an increased knowledge of blood physiology and blood forming organs in the 1930s, subsequently gave rise to the concept of a number of blood disorders.

1.2 WOMEN PIONEERS IN THE DEVELOPMENT OF HAEMATOLOGY

An outstanding feature in the history of Haematology is that women pioneered a number of commendable studies in this subject. Some of them were research workers in Anatomy. Physiology or Community Medicine, while others were laboratory workers, technicians, or science graduates, rather than medical graduates only. Haematology is the product of endless intellectual attempts of people of different categories and women contribute a significant proportion in this respect.

When greater perils men environ, then women show a front of iron, and gentle in their manner, they do hold things in a quiet way.

—Thomas Dawn English (1819-1902)

Some of these researches are detailed below.

Wilfred Ashy (1879–1975) introduced serological method for estimating **red cell life span in 1919.** Born in London, graduated as a bachelor of science from Washington, this lady worked in the Rush Medical School of Chicago. *She found that if a person is in good health the lifespan of transfused red cells is in excess of 120 days whereas in sick patients, it is shortened to one-half to one-third.* Her findings resulted in serious debate, as some authorities argued that lifespan of a non-nucleated cell with little capability of metabolic activity (as then thought), should not be more than 2-3 weeks.

Florence Rena Sabin (1871–1953), granddaughter of a physician and daughter of a marine engineer, enrolled herself in New Medical Franklin School of John Hoffkins University, which offered a number of seats to women students at that time. She soon fell under the influence of Franklin P Mall, professor of anatomy. During internship she was attracted towards laboratory medicine rather than to clinical medicine and professor Mall readily offered her such a position. Sabin worked on developmental anatomy of lymphatic system. She demonstrated first that **lymphatic system developed as a network derived from venous system.** Then she commenced studies on **development of blood cells,** conducting studies on chick blastoderm, by initiating supravital staining and using early tissue culture methods. ***Morphology of cellular elements of blood as well as development of monocyte and its involvement in phagocytosis became thus evident.*** **Dorothy Reed** was another woman who graduated in 1900, the same year as Sabin. *She later became famous for her description of Reed Sternberg cells classically present in Hodgkin disease.*

Lucy Wills (1888–1964) studied Botany in Newham College of Cambridge University in 1911. She travelled to South Africa as lecturer of Botany, returned to England, where she enrolled in London School of Medicine for Women. Graduated in 1929, she became more interested in biological aspect of Medicine and joined the department of chemical pathology at Royal Free Hospital. From late 1920 to 1930, she visited India on a number of occasions, where **she worked on nutritional anaemia,** supported by **Lady Tata Fund** of John Hopkins University. **Lucy Hills discovered that macrocytic anaemia in pregnancy differed from pernicious anaemia** because they do not have achlorhydria and responded to crude liver extract but not the pure liver extract. She postulated that there must be another factor responsible for macrocytic anaemia, other than vitamin B_{12}. **For some years this was called Willis factor and later shown up to be folic acid.** Thus *a cheap remedy for macrocytic anaemia in pregnancy in the tropics has been found. In 1938 she published the classical paper on " Tropical Macrocytic Anaemia: its relation to Pernicious Anaemia"* and in 1939, at the end of the World War she established the first Haematology Department in Royal Free Hospital.

It is doubtful whether any haematologist could lay several foundations in haematological studies like **Jennet Vaughan (1839–1993)**. At the London Hospital, the lady worked on ***Anatomy of Bone Marrow and its involvement in leucoerythrblastic anaemia.*** In 1934 she published a monograph on Anaemia. **At Hammersmith she developed transfusion technique.**

Virginia Minnich (1910–95) was a technician in the department of haematology of Ohio State University. Virginia's knowledge of **morphology of blood cells** grew to legendary of proportion but she took part in early studies on ***iron deficiency anaemia,*** *initially involving the variations in iron load,* ***in women during pregnancy and menstrual cycle.***

Virginia became essential component for training of technicians and medical students, evolved new tests, which led to ***eventual discovery of thalassaemia, caused by HbE.***

She established haematological laboratory in Havana and Thailand.

Judith Pool (1919–75) was born in New York and gained her PhD in University of Chicago in 1946. She moved to Stanford University in California, where she became a member of Haematology Department in 1953. She first published a paper on **blood coagulation.** Her discovery was published in Nature in 1964, about high potency **antihaemophilic factor concentrate** prepared from supernatant portion of plasma, after a single process of freezing and thawing.

These are few examples of leading women figures in haematology. They contributed towards its advancement at every level.

1.3 MODERN HAEMATOLOGY

Leukaemia

Robert Virchow (1858), a 24 year old graduate of Berlin Army School, studying pathology of phlebitis, confirmed the findings of D Hughes Bernnet, a physician, physiologist and teacher, who first described a case of chronic myeloid leukaemia and suggested the term thirty years before invention of staining methods, Virchow proposed two varieties of chronic leukaemia, splenic and lymphatic types. In 1995,

Leukaemia Research Fund and Royal College of Physicians held a symposium in Edinburgh, to commemorate the achievements in studies on leukaemia.

Since 1940, attempts to detect chromosomal abnormalities in leukaemic cells began. In 1960, **Peter Norwell from University of Pennsylvania and David Hungerford, from Fox Chase Cancer Center Institute** working on phlebothrombosis, described a minute acrocentric chromosome in cells cultured from blood of seven patients of CML. With consent of all the workers in this field this chromosome was named as "Philadelphia chromosome", after the place where major work was conducted. The chromosome was also found in erythroid and megakaryocytic cells also. In 1995, a symposium on leukaemia was organized in Edinburgh by joint effort of Leukaemia Research Fund and Royal College of Physicians. In 1973, the chromosome was identified, as deleted portion of chromosome 9, translocated on chromosome 22, by **Janet Rowby of Chicago University.** In 1980s consequence of genetic material between two chromosomes was found to be production of protooncogene BCR-ABL, the fusion protein. "Abl" stands for Ablson, a leukaemia virus that carries a similar protein.

Targeted Therapy

A drug discovery programme started aimed at developing a drug to shut down the activity of BCR-ABL protooncogene i.e. signalling the proliferation of malignant cells. The compound Imatinib was developed in 1992. Studies show that this compound inhibits tyrosine kinase-mediated activity. In 1998 the drug was tested in patients suffering from CML. In clinical trials blood counts come down to normal. Imatinib is approved by US FDA in 2001. Unfortunately resistance to Imatinib appeared soon. This is due to mutation of BCR-ABL gene. The gene acts as the lock and the drug acts as the key. The lock changes, so the key doesn't fit. Dasatrinib and Nilotinib have been developed that can shut down the mutated form of gene.

Multiple Myeloma

In 1845, a patient, treated by **Dr. Watson,** for lumbar pain in the set up of extreme weakness, anaemia and albuminuria, was reported.

Dalrymple (1846) observed that cancellous parts of bones of such patients become filled up with gelatinous material, which was postulated as degenerated material excreted in urine as abnormal protein. **Dr. Macintyre (1850),** when consulted, found, in urine of this patient, a peculiar type of protein of specific gravity 1.035. This protein had peculiar property of developing haziness, when heated, and this disappears on addition of nitric acid, though precipitate appears after an hour of standing.

Henry Bence Jones, at about same time, confirmed the peculiar nature of protein, that it forms precipitate on cooling, which dissolves on heating, and clears on addition of nitric acid. He further corroborated that the precipitate was made up of hydrated detruxide of albumin. The protein was named after him.

The term "Multiple Myeloma was first introduced by **J. von Rustizky (1873)**, while he was working in the Institute of Professor E. D. von Recklinghausen and studying a case of temple mass in a 47 year old man developing quadriplegia.

The first reported case of multiple myeloma in USA possibly was that published by **Herriec** and **Hketoen (1894)** and they reviewed 412 cases in the literature since 1848. They estimated that multiple myeloma accounted for 0-3% of all malignancies and peak incidence is 55%.

Dr. Christian Roger (1898) made first antimortem diagnosis of multiple myeloma, 18 months after onset of symptoms. In this patient right clavicle enlarged and fractured without trauma. Microscopical examination of tumor shows that it consists of round lymphoid cells with large nuclei.

The term plasma cell introduced by **Waldeyer (1875).** He described large cells with granular cytoplasm.

Marschalkv (1895) described characteristic features i.e. eccentric position of nuclei, perinuclear pale zone and spherical or irregular cytoplasm. Diagnosis of multiple myeloma was facilitated by reports of bone marrow aspiration by **Arnium (1929), Rosenthal Vogel (1938).**

Longsworth (1939) first applied electrophoresis to identify the monoclonal protein i.e. the protein with homogeneity. Later on with improved method of immuno-electrophoresis and immunofixation, it was possible to identify even small amount of monoclonal protein, to differentiate inflammatory (giving rise to polyclonal protein) and malignant disease.

Bone Marrow Transplantation

In early part of 20th century work of **Alexis Carrel and others** showed that allografts of skin or kidney would function for a time. **Medawer and colleaugues (1940)** explained immunological basis of allograft rejection. Studies of **Jacobson et al. (1949)** showed shielding of spleen of the mice exposed to lethal irradiation permitted survival of the animal. This is the beginning of era of transplantation.

Immune rejection of grafted lymphoid cells (**Bilingham and Brent 1959)** marks the understanding of graftversus host disease.

Development of concept of histocompatibility antigens came from demonstration of antibodies induced by transfusion or pregnancy, which reacted with antigens in human white blood cells. **(Miescher and Faucomet 1954)**.

Galli et al. (1968) reported first successful allogenic marrow graft in a patient with severe immunodeficiency. In 1969 Seattle marrow transplant team began a series using HLA-matched sibling donors for patients of leukaemia and aplastic anaemia. The first patient was in blast stage of CML. In 1970 stem cell therapy was accepted as a treatment of malignant disease. During the years 1970–1986 long -term survival was attempted by ablating the malignant disease with chemotherapy. For treatment of haematological malignancy and solid tumour, autologous HCT (stem cell therapy) after high dose chemotherapy and / or irradiation was tried by **Harowitz (1999).**

Marrow transplant for non-malignant haematological diseases were attempted in thalassaemia (Thomas et al. 1982; Lucacelli et al. 1984) and in sickle cell disease (Johnson et al. 1984).

With progress of improved methods of blood banking, advent of newer antibiotics, understanding of chemotherapeutic agents, 5 year survival rate, after marrow transplant, gradually increases 10 to 20% per year after first successful transplant in late 1960s.

Dr. Edward Donall Thomas was awarded Nobel Prize for his pioneering work on bone marrow transplant.

Nobel prize in Physiology or Medicine was awarded jointly to Joseph E Murray and E Donall Thomas in 1990, for their discoveries concerning "organ and cell transplantation in the treatment of human disease". Dr. Edward Donall Thomas was an American physician, who was an emeritus professor of Medicine in Washington, USA. Born in 1920, he studied chemistry and chemical engineering from University of Texas and obtained MD from Harvard Medical School in 1946. He also received National Medal of Science in 1990.

Haematology has developed step by step to modern era. It involves all the fields of science like biochemistry, pathology, physiology, molecular biology, and genetics.

Various forms of therapy e.g. targeted therapy and stem cell therapy and bone marrow transplant thus evolved. Today, most of the haematological, even some non-haematological diseases are amenable to treatment, at least symptom-free survival or arrest of the disease process. Estimates suggest that, about 30,000 to 40,000 of transplants are performed yearly all over the world. Many more people are benefited by targeted therapy. More than 20,000 people have survived 5 years or more after a haemopoietic stem cell transplant. March of haematology is never complete, but will go forever to conquer the suffering of human being. It is difficult to think of such a subject in which so many advancements have been made in a century. It is wonderful to think that from an abnormal biochemical finding in urine, an malignant clone of cells and its secretion are found out, and finding of an abnormal chromosome in cells led to the discovery of targeted therapy.

History of discoveries in haematolgy is so vast that it can't be covered in such a short span. This is only to create an interest in learning such an everdeveloping subject and also a humble tribute to the men and women who devoted their wholehearted attempts in the development of the subject.

REFERENCES

1. Descriptions of blood and blood disorders before the advent of laboratory studies. G. Hart, B J H (2001); 115: 71917281.
2. Some women pioneers in haematology. BG Frakin, B J H (2000); 108:6–12.
3. Brief historical review from ancient time. G J Pillar, B J H (2001); 112:282–292.
4. Multiple myeloma, an odessey of discovery. RA Kyle, B J H (2000); 111:1035–1044.
5. 50 years of haematology research that revolutionized patient care. Brian Druker, Special ASH anniversary brochure, (Dec. 2008).
6. A history of haemopoietic cell transplantation. E Donall Thomas, B J H (1999); 105:330-339.

CHAPTER

2 Diagnostic Approaches in Case of Anaemia

2.1 INTRODUCTION

Pallor, as a sign of disease, is perhaps recognized from the ancient times. It is the clinical counterpart of anaemia, which means less blood in the body. Anaemia is defined as a clinical condition resulting from a significant decrease in total body erythrocyte mass, reducing the oxygen carrying capacity of the blood. Free oxygen, the plant's unique gift to mankind, is highly reactive and dangerous on one hand, and the only security to free flow of all ATP for all intermediary metabolism of the body, on the other. All pathological damage due to anaemia is caused by hypoxia. The ultimate goal of all specialities is to prevent hypoxia; for cardiologists and pulmonologists this is at the gross mechanical level and for haematologists this at the molecular level. Hypoxia arises at the physicochemical level of haemoglobin or at the biochemical level of housekeeping erythrocyte membrane and its protective enzyme content.

2.2 POINTS TO REMEMBER IN EVALUATION OF ANAEMIA

1. Anaemia is a common clinical problem, which is very simple to detect but difficult to solve. For radical cure the condition requires etiological diagnosis, but this is a hard task. This is due to the fact that anaemia arises from pathological processes involving different organ-system of the body, like kidney, endocrine, G.I. System, apart from the haematological system.
2. Anaemia may exist as a simple laboratory finding, in a subjectively healthy individual, because there is compensatory mechanism which ensures adequate oxygen delivery to tissues, in the face of gradually diminishing red cell mass. This is effected by
   - (*i*) Decreased oxygen affinity of haemoglobin due to stimulation of 2, 3 DPG production [1].
   - (*ii*) Redistribution of blood flow to vital organs from the periphery.
   - (*iii*) Increased cardiac output by compensatory tachycardia, decreased peripheral resistance, decreased blood viscosity (thereby reducing B.P.) [2].
3. Depletion of whole blood volume produces symptoms when 20% of red cell mass is depleted in an acute episode, but it is not uncommon that the patient does not report till red cell mass is depleted up to 70% when depletion occurs gradually.
4. Symptoms of anaemia are very much non-specific, like fatigue, lethargy or breathlessness, or ankle oedema, which may simulate different diseases.

2.3 CLINICAL EVALUATION

1. Age of onset

   Early childhood: Genetic disorder of red cells or haemoglobin producing haemolysis.

   Prepubertal age: Nutritional deficiency as nutrition often lags behind growth spurt.

   Young people: Chronic infection, chronic inflammation, malignancy of lymphoreticular system, inflammatory bowel disease.

   Elderly people: Chronic renal failure, malignancy of G.I. tract, multiple myeloma.

2. Sex of the person concerned

   Female of reproductive age: Nutritional deficiency due to extra demand put by menstruation, pregnancy, lactation.

   Middle aged female: Hypothyroidism, chronic inflammatory disease *e.g.*, rheumatoid arthritis.

   Elderly female: Malignancy of genital tract, chronic renal failure.

   Elderly male: Malignancy of G.I. tract, chronic renal failure, aplastic anaemia, deficiency of folic acid, vitamin B_{12} or iron due to failure of procuring proper food stuff.

3. Any source of bleeding: Bleeding piles, bleeding peptic ulcers, haematuria, menorrhagia, (occult blood loss in stool to be excluded).
4. History of medication: Analgesic abuse (erosive gastritis), use of methotrexate for rheumatoid arthritis (antifolate action), use of cytotoxic anti-neoplastic agents (bone marrow suppression).
5. History of fever: Chronic infection, chronic inflammatory state, occult malignancy.
6. Multiple sexual exposure, weight loss, chronic diarrhoea: possibility of HIV infection.
7. History of jaundice: Hepatitis induced aplastic anaemia or chronic liver disease.
8. History of recurrent oliguria, paedal oedema: nephrotic syndrome leading to chronic kidney disease.
9. History of persistent dyspeptic syndrome along with anorexia in previously healthy individual: gastric malignancy.
10. History of gastrointestinal surgery: Deficiency of intrinsic factor, vitamin B_{12}.
11. Occupational exposure to lead (interference of haem synthesis or red cell damage), or napthelene (haemolysis) to be excluded.

2.4 PHYSICAL EXAMINATION

1. **Examination for anaemia:** Pallor on dorsum of tongue or lower bulbar conjunctiva, are not always reliable sites for confirmation of anaemia. Glossitis is very much common in avitaminossis, which is often associated with anemia. The surest sign of anaemia is the pallor found on palmar creases, when the hand is hyperextended. This usually occurs if haemoglobin level is below 8 gm%. [3]
2. Exclusion of cause of relative polycythaemia (which may mask pallor) *e.g.*, COPD must be sought for, by examining respiratory system.
3. Evidence of portal hypertension *e.g.*, splenomegaly, prominence of abdominal veins may indicate occult blood loss from oesophageal varices.

Chapter 2

4. Measurement of B.P. and assessment of kidney size and texture (by USG) are important for excluding kidney disease.
5. Petechiae, purpura, lymphadenopathy, hepatosplenomegaly may give important clue to the diagnosis of haematological malignancy.
6. Careful palpation of thyroid gland, relaxation of ankle jerk must be tested in patients presenting with lethargy, poverty of thought (which may be also symptoms of anaemia), to exclude hypothyroidism.

2.5 INVESTIGATIONS

The haematological investigations must follow preliminary routine testing like stool and urine examination for exclusion of occult blood loss, parasitic infection or evidence of nephritis, chest X-ray to exclude chronic infection like tuberculosis or mediastinal lymphoadenopathy.

Haematological investigations are planned under three categories:

Cytometric: Three red cell indices (MCV, MCH, MCHC).

Erythrokinetic: Evidence of haemolysis (Reticulocyte count, indirect serum bilirubin).

Biochemical/Molecular:

(*i*) Amino acid substitution produced by DNA point mutation in haemoglobin beta chain or red cell membrane enzyme tested by electrophoresis.

(*ii*) Serum iron, transferrin, TIBC to test metabolic status of the iron and its deficiency.

Before these specific tests to be performed, simple bedside test is peripheral blood smear examination, which may give some important clues.

2.6 PERIPHERAL BLOOD SMEAR EXAMINATION

Some of important features, in a Romanowsky stained blood film, which give important information about typing and etiological diagnosis of anaemia are mentioned below.

1. Hypochromia: The intensity of orange pink colour of haemoglobin gradually decreases from periphery to center, and the central pallor occupies more than one third of the diameter. It indicates poor haemoglobinization of red cells, as occurs in iron deficiency or haemoglobinopathy.
2. Polychromasia: This refers to the diffuse basophilic hue in red cells and correlates well with reticulocyte count. This occurs in myelodysplastic syndrome and megaloblastic anaemia when red cell DNA synthesis is poor.
3. Spherocytes have abnormally increased central staining, as found in hereditary spherocytosis, which is an important cause of haemolytic anaemia.
4. Target cells have a small normally stained centre surrounded by a hypochromic ring, finally a normally stained rim, which is found in thalassaemia, iron deficiency, liver disease as well as after splenectomy.
5. Howell Jolly bodies are purple black, usually round, chromatin fragments, more deeply staining than basophilic stippling, (found as discrete dots in lead poisoning). H-J bodies are found in haemolytic anaemia or after splenectomy.

6. Macrocytes are immature erythroid precursors sometimes they are blast like with Chromatin in large nuclei. They are formed due to defect in DNA synthesis and asynchronous nuclear-cytoplasmic maturation.
7. Presence of hypersegmented neutrophils with more than five lobes in the nuclei may be the first indication of megaloblastic anaemia.
8. Burr cells are fragmented erythrocytes formed in renal failure due to microangiopathy.
9. Myelodysplastic anaemia should be suspected if dimorphic anaemia is present *i.e.*, a mixture of normochromic cells with hypochromic microcytes.
10. Ring sideroblasts *i.e.*, erythroblasts with iron pigment deposited on the periphery of the cytoplasm as a ring, may be seen in some of the cases of myelodysplastic syndrome.

I. Erythrokinetic Studies

Reticulocyte count and indices

Reticulocytes are stained by supravital staining. Typical normal range is 0.5–1.5%. The count depends on total RBC count, the index is the corrected value in relation to total red cell mass and haemoglobin percentage. Increased count indicates increased red cell turnover, as seen in haemolytic anaemia. [4] Normal reticulocyte count is 0.5–2.5%.

Other evidences of haemolysis

If reticulocyte count is high, other evidences of haemolysis should be searched for. Serum unconjugated bilirubin and urine uribilinogen concentrations should be also measured. Unconjugated hyperbilirubinaemia in absence of urobilinogen in the urine is indicative of haemolysis. Serum haptoglobin and serum haemopexin are degraded haemoglobin, which form bound complexes. They become untraceable in acute intravascular haemolysis.

Complete blood count

This is the next step in the evaluation of anaemia. This test detects lymphocytosis (evidence of chronic infection), grossly diminished count of all formed elements (Neutrophils < 500/µl, platelets > 20,000/µl, reticulocytes < 1%), white blood cells in the leukaemic range *i.e.*, 50,000–1,00,000/µl with10% immature forms may indicate leukaemia, as cause of anaemia. Therefore, in most of the cases, this test prompts bone marrow examination.

II. Cytometric Tests

The mean cell volume (MCV) is measured in automated cell counter (by mean height or a selected span of the heights of pulses generated during the red cell count). Haemoglobin is measured by standard cyanide test. Packed cell volume (PCV) is deduced from MCV and red cell count. MCH is calculated from haemoglobin concentration and red cell counts.

MCV= PCV/ Red cell count per litre = 90 fentolitre (fl)

MCH- Hb in gm per litre /Red cell count per litre = 30 picograms

MCHC- Hb in gm per litre/ PCV = 32 – 38 per cent

Typing of anaemia is done by cytometric tests.

In macrocytic anaemia

MCV may be increased up to 150 fl

MCH may be increased up to 50 pg
MCHC normal or diminished
In microcytic hypochromic anaemia
MCV is diminished to 50 fl
MCH is diminished to 15 pg
MCHC is diminished to 22 per cent

Red cell distribution width (RDW)

This is a sensitive measurement of red cell anisocytosis, with potential value for discriminating between different causes of anaemia. It is expressed either as the SD(fl) or CV (%) of the MCV, after excluding the tail of the size distribution curve. In the Coulter counter, the normal range is 11.5%–14.5%. Nevertheless, measurement of RDW is useful in distinguishing between iron deficiency (high RDW) and thalassaemia (normal RDW). [5]

Discriminant function

DF = [MCV- (5 × Hb conc)-RBC-K], where K is constant (3.4), with haematocrit reading corrected for plasma trapping. The value may be greater than 1.0 in iron deficiency anaemia and less than 1.0 in thalassaemia. [6]

III. Biochemical Tests

Serum iron, ferritin, Total Iron Binding Capacity (TIBC)

Normal range of serum iron is 13–32 μmol/l (70–180 μg/dl) in the plasma, iron is bound to a beta globulin, called transferrin and TIBC depends on its concentration. The serum iron, not bound to transferrin, is the unsaturated part of the binding capacity. Serum iron + unsaturated binding capacity give the value of TIBC.Serum Transferrin is normally 2–3g/l and 1 mg of transferrin binds to 1.4 μg of iron. The serum ferritin value varies with age and sex and is normally 15 to 300 μg/l in adult male. The serum iron concentration is slightly lower in female and it has got a diurnal variation of up to 30% with the lower level at night. [7]

TIBC is 45 to 70 μmol/l (250 to 400 μg/dl), with 33% saturation. Immunoassay of transferrin is done by a method using an antibody as a ligand. Measurement of TIBC is done by a method using iron as a ligand. The principal advantage of transferrin measurement is that volume of sample required is small.

The serum iron is very low in iron deficiency anaemia and in infections, it is high in haemochromatosis, after multiple transfusions, siderooblastic anaemia *i.e.*, myelodysplasia and megaloblastic anaemia, when the erythropoiesis is ineffective.

TIBC is reduced in patients with anaemia of chronic disease but it is raised in iron deficiency anaemia.

Plotting of serum ferritin (SF) value against C-reactive protein (CRP), show that rate of rise is much less in iron deficiency than in anaemia of chronic disease, though values are raised in both the cases. [8]

Erythrocyte zinc protoporphyrin level

It helps to differentiate causes of microcytic anaemia. In iron deficiency anaemia it is increased, it is normal in thalassaemia. The value is also raised in lead poisoning. [9]

Serum soluble transferrin receptors (sTfR)

This factor is typically increased in iron deficiency anaemia, thalassaemia, myelodysplasia and secondary polycythaemia, in which conditions, erythropoiesis is increased. It is decreased in anaemia of chronic disease and aplastic anaemia. According to some authors this is also increased in rheumatoid arthritis without iron deficiency and in some malignant conditions, so more work is needed to establish its value as diagnostic tests. [10]

Haemoglobin electrophoresis

This is helpful in establishing diagnosis of haemoglobinopathy as a cause of hypochromic microcytic anaema, as well as confirming the type of haemoglobinopathy.

Red cell folate, serum folate and serum Vitamin B_{12} estimation and absorption tests are essential for evaluation of macrocytic anaemia.

IV. Aetiological Diagnosis

This may have to be established by function tests of different organs, as follows, of course, if dictated by results of clinical examination.

Kidney disease: Serum urea, creatinine, kidney size (USG).

Thyroid disease: Serum T3, T4, TSH.

Liver disease: Liver function tests, upper GI endoscopy.

Fresh bleeding per rectum: Colonoscopy.

Bone marrow examination

Microscopic examination of a specimen of bone marrow, stained by Pearl's Prussian blue stain, is the most reliable test for iron deficiency. Absence of iron in more abundant marrow particles is diagnostic sign of iron deficiency. Most of the iron which is stained, is haemosiderin, ferritin, being water soluble, is lost during fixation. The haemosiderin appears in irregular clumps either in histiocytes or lying free as a consequence of rupture of histiocytes during preparation of the slide. Globular or string like structures which stains blue are artifacts.

Besides the haemosiderin iron, tiny blue siderotic granules are seen in the cytoplasm of a fraction of normoblasts (20%). These siderotic granules are ferritin, lysosomes which contain them are called siderosomes. In iron deficiency, both haemosiderin and sideroblasts are absent.

Bone marrow smear examination gives confirmatory diagnosis in haematological malignancy, aplastic anaemia, megaloblastic anaemia and differentiates iron deficiency anaemia from anaemia of chronic disease. Decreased sideroblastic iron in the face of increased histiocytic iron shows impaired iron transport in anaemia of chronic disease.

Diagnostic approaches to anaemia entirely depend upon physician's skill and knowledge in planning the investigations.

REFERENCES

1. Zaroluis Cg, Kourides IA, Valeri Cr (1978): Red cell 2, 3-diphosphoglycerate and oxygen affinity of haemoglobin in patients with thyroidisorders. Blood 52:181–185.
2. Bainton DF, Finch CA (1964): *The diagnosis of iron deficiency anaemia.* Am J Med 37:62-70.

Chapter 2

3. Dallman PR (1982): *Manifestations of iron deficiency*. Seminar Haematol 19:19–30.
4. Brugnara C, Zurakowski D, Dicanzio J et al., (1999):*Reticulocyte haemoglobin content to diagnose iron deficiency in children*. JAMA 281:2225–2230.
5. Cesana BM, Maolo AT, Gidulli R, et al., (1999): *Relevance of Red Cell Distribution Width (RDW) in the differential diagnosis of microcytic anaemias*. Clinical Lab Haematol 13:141–151.
6. Johnson CS, Tegos C, Beutler E (1983): *Thalassaemia minor: routine erythrocyte measurements and differentiation from iron deficiency*. Am J clin Pathol 80:31–36.
7. Coenen JL, van Diejien-Visser MP, van Pelt J, et al., (1991): *Measurement of serum ferritin used to predict concentrations of iron in bone marrow in anaemia of chronic disease*. Clin Chem 37:560–563.
8. Vreugdenhil G, Ballus CA, van Ejik HG, et al., (1982): *Anaemia of chronic disease:diagnostic significance of erythrocyte and serological parameters in iron deficienct rheumatoid patients*. Brit J Rheumatica 29: 105–119.
9. Meloni T, Gallisai D, Demontis M, et al., (1982): *Free erythrocyte porphyrin (FFP) in the diagnosis of beta-thalassaemia trait and iron deficiency anaemia*. Haematologica (Pavia) 67:341–348.
10. Punnocen K, et al., (1997): *Serum transferrin receptor and its ratio to serum ferritin in the diagnosis of iron deficiency*. Blood 89:1052–1057.

Part II

Anaemia of Clinical Importance

CHAPTER

3 Anaemia in Tropics

3.1 INTRODUCTION

Anaemia is probably the second important cause of morbidity and mortality in individuals living in tropical countries, the infection being the first one. Anaemia is not a single disease entity, but a clinical condition produced by a number of diseases of diverse aetiology. The final outcome is chiefly determined by the type of the disease in the background multiplied by the effect of anaemia on different organ system of the body. Maximum morbidity and mortality of anaemia are found in preschool children and pregnant ladies, especially of underdeveloped rural communities. Anaemia is less commonly encountered in adult male, non-pregnant women and school children, though still it is a major heath problem also in these groups, as it is often associated with tuberculosis or any other chronic infection. Similarly in school girls, often anaemia is produced by blood loss due to menorrhagia. In recent days, HIV infection is the most common cause of anaemia both in adult male and female as well as in children, as seen in reports of hospital admission in sub-Saharan countries. [1]

3.2 DEFINITION OF ANAEMIA

Anaemia is defined by haemoglobin concentration in the peripheral blood, which must be lower than normal value for age, sex, and pregnancy state of the subject. Haemoglobin concentration also varies with altitude, residence in geographical areas, should, therefore, be considered. Usually the haemoglobin concentration is directly proportional to red cell volume, except some special situations. [2] Exceptions are the following:

1. In first few hours of life, there is haemo-concentration in the capillaries therefore, capillary blood samples underestimate anaemia. This is specially so in premature infants, who are acidotic, hypotensive, and are suffering from hypovolaemia. [3]
2. Immediately after acute haemorrhage, the haemoglobin remains unchanged until there is compensatory expansion of plasma volume over following 48 hours.
3. With splenomegaly there is both expansion of plasma volume and sequestration of cells, so that, patients having splenomegaly may have a Hb level of 8.0 gm/dl, while the total red cell mass is normal.

TABLE 3.1: Hb conc. matched with age, sex, pregnancy state in female at sea level below which anaemia produces a pathological condition. [4]

Individual	Hb (gm/dl)
New born infants	14.0
6 months-6 years	11.0
6-14 years	12.0
Adult males	13.0
Adult non-pregnant female	12.0
Adult pregnant female	11.0

For each increment of 1000 m above sea level, 2.5 g/l (2 g/l per 2500 ft) rise of Hb concentration is usually seen.

3.3 AETIOLOGY OF ANAEMIA IN TROPICS

Anaemia due to, all three basic causes, is seen in the tropics.

1. Blood Loss

Heavy loss in young females due to menorrhagia or during labour as well as in cases of repeated pregnancy, when not replenished properly, gives rise to anaemia. This is prevalent commonly in less privileged community, where diet is also deficient.

Occult or evident blood loss from G.I. tract is common due to hookworm infestation, bleeding peptic ulcer, bleeding piles, and congestive gastropathy due to portal hypertension.

2. Deficient Formation

A. Decreased red cell production due to

(*i*) Nutritional deficiency of iron, folate, B12.

(*ii*) Protein energy malnutrition.

(*iii*) Deficiency of vitamin A, C, E, riboflavin, pyridoxine, copper.

B. Depressed bone marrow function

(*a*) Depression due to chronic infection like tuberculosis, Chronic Kala-azar, HIV/AIDS, a sequela to viral hepatitis.

(*b*) Depression due to deficiency of haemopoietic growth factors:

- (*i*) Chronic hepatic disease — Deficiency of hepatocyte derived growth factor.
- (*ii*) Chronic renal failure — Deficiency of Erythropoietin.
- (*iii*) Thyroid disorder — Deficiency of thyroxine.

(*c*) Chronic inflammatory disorder — Transport block of essential element.

(*d*) Depression due to infiltration by malignant tissue:

- (*i*) Leukaemia
- (*ii*) Lymphomatosis
- (*iii*) Myelomatosis
- (*iv*) Carcinomatosis

(*e*) Depression due to drugs and chemicals, which are commonly used in tropical countries, for therapy and in domestic or agricultural products. Drugs are usually the anti-infective agents like chloramphenicol, sulphonamide, isoniazid, antidiabetic drugs like tolbutamide, chlorpropamide. Due to less expense, these are often used to treat diseases prevalent in tropical countries, like enteric fever, urinary tract infection or tuberculosis, and diabetes mellitus. Chemicals which produce bone marrow suppression are benzene and its products, used as an all purpose solvent in cleaning agents in household products and hobbies. Another notorious agent is lindane (gamma benzene hexachloride), used in insecticide, sprayed on plantations in agricultural farm.

3. Increased Red Cell Destruction

(*a*) Intrinsic defect of red cells:

(*i*) Genetic defect of Haemoglobin- Thalassaemia, Sickle cell disease.

(*ii*) Genetic defect of Protective Enzyme of red cell membrane-Glucose 6 phosphate dehydrogenase deficiency.

(*iii*) Abnormalities of cell membrane-Elliptocytosis, spherocytosis.

(*b*) Haemolysis due to extrinsic factors:

(*i*) Immune Haemolysis- Rh incompatibility, autoimmune disease like SLE.

(*ii*) Non-Immune Haemolysis;

Infection- Malaria

Toxin- Snake venom

Hypersplenism- Chronic Kala-azar, tropical splenomegaly

Drugs-Sulphonamides

Chemicals- Napthelene (used as preservative in clothes)

*Only the diseases and toxic effects of drugs relevant in pathogenesis of anaemia in Tropics are mentioned.

TABLE 3.2: Estimated Prevalence of Anaemia in Tropical Countries in Comparison to World Population (Modified from WHO data) [5]

Geographic Region	Children (0–4 years)	Children (5–15 years)	Adult male (15–59 years)	Adult female (non-pregnant)
World (excluding China)	43%	37%	18%	35%
Africa	56%	49%	20%	44%
Latin America	26%	26%	13%	17%
South Asia	56%	50%	32%	35%
Developed Regions	12%	7%	3%	11%
Developing Regions	51%	46%	26%	47%

• % means p.c. of anaemic individuals in total population

3.4 POSSIBLE FACTORS FOR PREVALENCE OF ANAEMIA IN TROPICAL COUNTRIES

1. In tropical countries, where heat and humidity prevail, food habits are different from those of temperate countries. Process of cooking and preservation techniques are also different as economic condition in under privileged community debars from procurement of costly preservative machine. Greater proportion of carbohydrate in relation to protein in the diet provides excess phytate and fibre which interfere with absorption of iron, the essential element for formation of haemoglobin. Excess frying and boiling are often practiced during cooking to prevent deterioration of cooked food, but this process causes denaturation of protein and removal of essential water soluble nutrients.
2. Infection of G.I. tract with bacteria and parasite is very much common in tropical countries, which give rise often to malabsorption and minute chronic blood loss as in hookworm infestation. Many associated chronic infection like tuberculosis may aggravate or perpetuate the anaemia. Incidence of HIV disease often goes unnoticed and gives rise to unexplained anaemia.
3. As agriculture is the mainstay of earning living in most of the countries, often persons have to work barefooted in the field and observe irregular dietary habit, the first one predisposing to hookworm infestation and the second one giving rise to peptic ulcer; both of these are potential sources of occult blood loss.
4. Women of child bearing age often suffer from menorrhagia, due to various reasons, but seldom seek medical help due to social prejudice. Women in rural poor communities often do not have proper nutrition during pregnancy so that blood loss during delivery may be detrimental. Repeated pregnancy at short interval may be an added factor. Increased demand for the growing foetus, pregnancy induced hypervolaemia, in the background of depleted iron store, and dietary deficiency all contribute to the development of anaemia.[6] Lack of knowledge about diet, low affordability due to poor economic condition coupled with anorexia, lead to dietary deficiency.
5. Regular medical check up in underprivileged community in remote parts of village is far from reality, in spite of serious attempt by the Health authority.

3.5 WHY DIAGNOSIS IS DIFFICULT?

Symptoms of anaemia at early stage are very much non-specific like fatigue, insomnia, lethargy or leg cramp. People rarely seek proper medical help at this stage. When breathlessness on exertion or ankle oedema interferes with daily activities, usually the patient first reports for medical advice. Diagnosis is often masked in black colored individuals in whom pallor is evident on palm and sole only when anaemia is severe. Pallor is rarely evident on dorsum of tongue due to associated avitaminosis and glossitis. Haematocrit values are sometimes misleading due to splenomegaly, so prevalent as a result of chronic malaria, chronic Kala-azar, or portal hypertension, as stated earlier.

3.6 PATHOPHYSIOLOGY OF ANAEMIA

Anaemia reduces oxygen carrying capacity of the blood. The body compensates for this by: (1) increasing the release of oxygen from the haemoglobin to the tissues (2) increasing the cardiac output (3) increasing the blood flow to the vital tissues with high oxygen requirements, while reducing flow to other organs

(4) increasing the respiration. The severity of anaemia is best considered as passing through the three stages: (1) stage of compensation (2) stage of decompensation (3) stage of life threatening complications. The severity of anaemia does not depend on the haemoglobin concentration alone, so that cut off points of haemoglobin of 7.0 g/dl and 3.0 g/dl for when decompensation and cardiac failure respectively are likely, must be taken as very approximate. Older patients are more likely to progress to decompensation or heart failure than the young; infants and young children are able to tolerate extremely low haemoglobin concentrations with few complaints. Patients who develop anaemia acutely have less time to compensate than patients with chronic anaemia such as sickle cell disease or aplastic anaemia. Patients who are suffering from hypervolaemia due to pregnancy, especially multiple pregnancy or splenomegaly are more liable to progress as far as congestive cardiac failure, as are patients with underlying cardiac, vascular, respiratory diseases. In contrast, patients with low level of activity, including the bedridden, are less likely to become de-compensated.

3.7 STAGE OF COMPENSATION

The major compensatory mechanism in mild to moderate anaemia is the increase of 2,3-diphosphoglycerate (2,3- DPG) concentration in red cells; this binds to deoxyhaemoglobin, shifts the oxygen dissociation curve of Hb to the right (decreased oxygen affinity) and increases oxygen release to the tissues by up to 40%. [7] Cardiac output is raised by an increase in stroke volume at rest; and on exertion, there is both an exaggerated tachycardia and further rise in stroke volume. Vasodilatation enhances the blood flow to the myocardium, skeletal muscle and brain, while there is vasoconstriction in the skin and kidneys. The plasma volume expands, but the total blood volume remains normal.

Patients complain of breathlessness on exertion only, but there are no physical signs except pallor, unless there are symptoms and signs from the underlying cause of anaemia.

3.8 IMPACT OF ANAEMIA ON PERSON AND ON THE SOCIETY

Maximal work capacity, as measured by the Harvard Step Test (HST), correlates directly with Hb at all levels, and is reduced by even mild anaemia; the average HST Guetamalan laborers was 65 at Hb 13.0-15.0 g/dl and 30 at 7.0-9.0 g/d. [8]

Productivity and earning of anaemic male manual workers are seriously reduced. The earnings of anaemic women performing less strenuous factory work are also reduced. Anaemia in either parent has an adverse effect on family through low food production, low income, poor care for the children; village life suffers from there being less ground under cultivation, and the national economy declines from overall low productivity. [9]

The incidence of low birth weight and perinatal mortality rise rapidly when the maternal haematocrit (Hct) falls below 0.30. [10]

In childhood, anaemia is associated with slow growth, delayed development and poor cognitive abilities.

Anaemia predisposes to any sort of infection. Infection easily thrives and spreads in tropical climate. This increases absences from schools and colleges, factories, and agricultural fields; thus hampers educational and economic progress of the country as a whole.

3.9 DE-COMPENSATED STAGE OF ANAEMIA

When Hb level is below 7.0 g/dl, the major mechanism for improving oxygen delivery is an increase in cardiac output. Both stroke volume and heart rate are raised at rest. The work of the ventricles is reduced by low viscosity of blood and peripheral vasodilation; the circulation time is short. The blood volume is reduced in about 25% of patients.

Patients are breathless even at rest. There is tachycardia, arterial and capillary pulsation, a wide pulse pressure and haemic ejection systolic murmurs. It is common experience that the patients who are farmers, or others who are solely dependent on manual labour, do not seek medical advice, until they reach this stage of anaemia.

3.10 ANAEMIA WITH LIFE THREATENING COMPLICATIONS

1. Hypoxia and acidosis: If anaemia progresses in children with malaria until Hb falls to < 5 g/dl, respiratory distress develops, showing as tachypnea and at least one of the signs of nasal flaring, in drawing of chest wall or diaphragm, grunting or deep breathing. The children are hypovolaemic and acidotic with lactic acidaemia. Without appropriate treatment mortality is high.
2. Cardiac failure: If anaemia progresses (Hb < 3.0 g/dl approximately), the oxygen supply to the myocardium is insufficient, no further increase in cardiac output is possible, and high output cardiac failure develops. The plasma volume expands; patients who are already suffering from hypervolaemia due to pregnancy and splenomegaly, are most liable to develop heart failure.
3. Patients are severely breathless and may complain of angina, night cramps and claudication. There is cardiomegaly, engorgement of jugular veins, pulmonary oedema, hepatomegaly, peripheral oedema and sometimes ascites. Without appropriate treatment there is a high morbidity rate.
4. Maternal deaths rise sharply when the Hct is below 0.20 at the time of delivery; up to 20% of maternal deaths in Africa and India used to be due to heart failure. This may be true where obstetric and blood transfusion services have not developed. [11]

3.11 MANAGEMENT OF ANAEMIA

The first principle of management is the diagnosis and treatment of cause of anaemia.

By simple bed side test type of the anaemia is first identified. The aetiology is then to be searched out by more elaborate laboratory tests, whenever needed. The detailed diagnostic methods are outside the scope of this chapter. Anaemic patients must be treated by blood transfusion to avoid life threatening complications.

The transfusion of concentrated red cells is required by anaemic patients in three circumstances only: (1) a patient is in danger of dying from anaemic heart failure or hypoxia before specific medication can raise the Hb; (2) a patient is about to experience stress, such as emergency major surgery, obstetric delivery or cytotoxic therapy; (3) the basic pathology of anaemia is irreversible, for example thalassaemia or aplastic anaemia. This will be discussed in details in an appropriate chapter later.

Children with malarial anaemia are suffering from hypovolaemia, not hypervolaemia, and should be transfused whole blood, not concentrated red cells, when the Hb is less than 5.0 g/dl with or without respiratory distress or when Hb is less than 4.0 g/dl with or without respiratory distress. The inappropriate use of blood transfusion is to be condemned, especially since the advent of HIV and the acquired immunodeficiency syndrome (AIDS).

3.12 ANAEMIA IN ASSOCIATION WITH PARASITIC DISEASES

Anaemia is commonly found in Tropics, in a good proportion of cases, in association with a number of parasitic diseases, especially protozoal diseases, which are directly or indirectly responsible for production of anaemia. Some of these diseases, commonly encountered in clinical practice, are discussed below.

Anaemia in Malaria

Out of four different species of Malaria, Plasmodium is most commonly associated with haematological consequences. In endemic regions for Malaria, the severity and progress of the disease passes through different stages according to type of immune response. These are: (1) acute malaria in non-immune children after about 6 months of age when maternally derived immunity is lost; (2) recurrent malaria in children less than about 5 years of age; and (3) recurrent mild parasitaemia in partially immune older children and adults. Malaria, in non-immune adults, such as expatriate visitors to endemic areas or inhabitants of countries where malaria is unstable, has got haematological complications of acute or recurrent malaria.

Acute Malaria

Stages of development

In non-immune individuals there is usually no anaemia within 24–48 hours of the onset of fever, but there is often a rapid fall of the Hb and Hct over 4–5 days, with the degree of anaemia corresponding approximately to the intensity of parasitaemia. The anaemia is normochromic and normocytic. The reticulocyte count is low at this stage, although the bone marrow shows erythroid hyperplasia with minimal dyserythropoietic changes. The total plasma bilirubin and unconjugated fraction are raised; increased conjugated bilirubin indicates complicating hepatic dysfunction. Haptoglobins are reduced or absent.

Mechanism of development

A major mechanism of haemolysis is rupture of red cells at the time of release of merozoites, but anaemia is often more severe and more persistent than can be accounted for directly by parasitaemia. The Hb may continue to fall for between 7 and 21 days following clearing of the parasite, due apparently to both continued haemolysis and delayed release of red cells from the marrow. Survival of both autologous non parasitized red cells and donated red cells is shortened. [12] There is phagocytosis of parasitized and non parasitized red cells, seen easily in the bone marrow. The direct Coombs' test is frequently positive, associated with adsorption by red cells of immunoglobulin G (IgG) and C3 component of the complement; however, autoimmune haemolysis is not an important mechanism, although IgG coated red cells are more rapidly removed by Reticuloendothelial (RES) cells than uncoated cells. Haemolysis of non parasitized red cells appears therefore, due to non specific activation of the RES, hypersplenism, and Fc receptor-mediated uptake. [13]

Malaria is immunosuppressive and is frequently complicated by secondary infections, such as bronchopneumonia, urinary tract infections, and Gram negative septicaemia may be the result of concurrent infection by parvovirus B19, which infects early red cell precursors preferentially and causes a transient red cell hypoplasia. [13]

During acute malaria there is immobilization of iron in macrophages, and low serum iron concentration; serum ferritin is massively increased, being an acute reactive protein. Red cell folate levels are raised above normal through mechanisms which are uncertain, but possibly due to synthesis of folate by the parasites themselves.

Following clearance of parasitaemia and during recovery, the peripheral blood shows reticulocytosis and polychromasia.

Anaemia in recurrent malaria— Children living in endemic area often suffer from general ill health, moderate splenomegaly, and intermittent fever. They have chronic normocytic, normochromic anaemia with low reticulocyte count, anaemia may be profound during acute exacerbation but there is only a scanty parasitaemia, although gametocytes and malarial pigments are seen in the monocytes. The anaemia is a result of both hypersplenism and severe dyserythropoietic disturbance in the bone marrow. The mechanism of dyserythropoiesis is uncertain, but it may be due to hypoxia as a result of packing of bone marrow sinusoids with parasitized red cells or be mediated by an imbalance of cytokines. [14]

Serum tumour necrosis factor (TNF) and Interferon γ (IFNγ) are raised in acute malaria: they play an essential role in the control of parasitaemia and in the inflammatory reactions. Interleukin 10 (IL-10) is also raised, and modulates the inflammatory response. Low IL-10 concentration have been found in African children with severe malaria, and it has been suggested that a failure of IL-10 may allow uncontrolled action of TNF in promoting dyserythropoiesis and erythrophagocytosis.[15]

Disturbed marrow function is reversed by successful antimalarial treatment, which is followed by brisk reticulocytosis and rise in Hb level.

In Haemoglobinuria and Blackwater fever, the majority of patients are glucose 6 phosphate dehydrogenase enzyme deficient and have been treated with some oxidant drugs. Typically such patient is non-immune adult who has been taking quinine irregularly as prophylaxis. Typically patient presents with acute loin pain, tender hepatosplenomegaly, massive haemoglobulinuria, later oliguria with dark colored urine and profound anaemia. The mechanism is probably immune mediated haemolysis by quinine or triggered by mefloquin, artesimin or halofentrine.

Anaemia in Partially Immune Patients with Malaria

In endemic regions older children and adults experience recurrent parasitemia with moderate haemolysis associated with compensatory erythroid hyperplasia. The balance between haemolysis is disturbed in pregnancy, after splenectomy, immune anergy (e.g., malignant disease) or reactive splenomegaly, when the patient suffers from profound anaemia. HIV infection is associated with increased parasite densities and incidence of clinical malaria.

Management of Severe Malarial Anaemia

Malarial anaemia usually responds to antimalarial therapy, but is a major cause of morbidity and mortality. In different series, between 10–16% of all deaths in childhood are found to be due to malarial anaemia. With the advent of HIV in developing countries, thousands of patients may be successfully treated for anaemia with blood transfusion but there is increased risk of HIV transmission, even in the places where the screening for HIV is practiced, because the donor may be in the window period. [16] Therefore, for malarial anaemia, certain guidelines are followed, which prevent mortality from anaemia but minimize the transmission of HIV.

1. Hb > 5.0 g/dl with or without respiratory distress: intravenous normal saline in aliquots of 10 ml/kg.
2. Hb 4.0–5.0 g/l without respiratory distress, intravenous saline as above, with careful monitoring over 48 hours.
3. Hb < 5.0 g/dl with respiratory distress or impaired consciousness: transfusion of whole blood 20 ml/kg without a diuretic, with mild distress (nasal flaring) transfusion should be done for 4–6 hours; with severe distress transfusion 10 ml/kg over 1 hour and the remining10 ml/kg over the next 2–4 hours.
4. Hb < 4.0 g/l, with or without respiratory distress, transfusion should be done in the same manner as in (3).

3.13 MALARIA IN PREGNANCY AS A CAUSE OF ANAEMIA

In women who live in hyper-endemic or holoendemic areas for malaria, the immunity level to P falciparum is high and the frequency and the density of parasitaemia reach a plateau early in the second trimester of pregnancy, especially in the primigravidae. Women in their second pregnancies usually have this abnormality to a less extent. The women are usually asymptomatic or mild symptoms only. Compensatory erythroid hyperplasia leads to high demands for folate, demands which are already increased because of pregnancy. The haemolytic process is often complicated by megaloblastic erythropoiesis and profound anaemia. [16]

The frequency of palpable splenomegaly increases during pregnancy and a peak spleen rate is found at about 16 weeks of gestation, in holo- and hyper-endemic areas.

Even higher spleen rates (about 70%) is found in places like Nigeria, where hyperactive malarious splenomegaly and hypersplenism are also found in 25% of cases, and 5% of women experience haemolysis, all aggravating the anaemia. These perpetuating processes do not respond to antimalarials, but to prednisolone, proving thereby an immune process triggered by malaria, as a cause of profound anaemia. [17] The presentation of malaria with anaemia is of intermediate intensity in mesoendemic areas like Thailand and Zambia.

Clinical pattern is further complicated by co-infection with HIV. Seropositivity during pregnancy has been found to be associated with increased prevalence and density of P faciparum parasitaemia, placental infection, increased incidence of clinical malaria and that of anaemia. The condition shows diminished effectiveness to antimalarials.

The peripheral blood picture of malaria with anaemia in pregnancy is characterized by great anisocytosis, macrocytosis and polychromasia with or without nucleated red cells, but no polikilocytosis; there is reticulocytosis; malarial parasites are usually absent or scanty. The white cell count is variable and there may be a myeloid leukaemoid reaction. The hyper-segmentation of folate deficiency is often masked by a shift to the left. The bone marrow shows megaloblastic changes which may be gross; malarial pigment is present in macrophages; iron stores tend to be increased unless there is concurrent iron deficiency. Maternal morbidity and mortality are extremely high in such conditions.

Blood transfusion is usually indicated only if the patient is in incipient or established stage of cardiac failure, or if the patient is approaching delivery with a Hb < 7.0 g/dl. Anaemia responds rapidly in most patients following antimalarials therapy and folic acid; the haematocrit does not rise but responds by remaining steady in hyperactive malarial splenomegaly and few patients with haemolysis respond to prednisolone 60 mg/day for 1 week and 30 mg/ day maintenance in three divided doses, up to about 30 weeks of gestation.

Malaria and Anaemia can be effectively prevented by the administration of prophylactic antimalarials and folic acid supplementation. There are, however great problem in delivery of effective regime to more than few who attend antenatal clinic regularly. Malaria chemoprophylaxis by administration of sulphadoxin /pyrimethamine in two or more intermittent doses from first attendance to the third trimester has the advantages of compliance and cost-effectiveness, and results in higher maternal Hb, decreased placental malaria and decreased low birth weight. This strategy should be applicable to the remote community. The prevention of malaria in pregnancy, in endemic areas has focused on first or second pregnancies as being the worst affected. With advent of HIV, however, more attention has been paid to multigravidae because of the fact that HIV infection decreases the ability to control malaria and malaria infection may also increase vertical transmission of HIV.

3.14 HYPERACTIVE MALARIAL SPLENOMEGALY (HMS) AS A CAUSE OF ANAEMIA

Hyperactive malarial splenomegaly is an immune mediated clinical condition. This is characterized by (1) residence in malarious area (2) chronic splenomegaly, often massive (3) IgM elevated to more than 2 standard deviations above the local reference mean (4) high malarial antibody titre (5) hepatic sinusoidal lymphocytosis and (6) clinical and immunological response to long-term antimalarials prophylaxis.

Pathogenesis— The basic pathology is overproduction of IgM in response to P or P malariae infection. There is familial and ethnic clustering suggesting a genetic basis.

Genetic polymorphism, in persons living in non-endemic area, and have migrated recently to endemic areas, confer partial protection against malaria. This polymorphism might include genetically controlled processing of malarial antigens and antibody production. During acute malaria, there is transient production of IgM lymphocyto-toxic antibodies which are specific for activated suppressor T lymphocytes (CD8+) and which normally down regulate synthesis of IgM by B cells. It has been shown in Indonesian patients with HMS, this lymphocyto-toxic antibody persists with consequent imbalance of helper T cells (CD4+) cells which are normal, and suppressor cells T cells (CD8+) cells which are greatly reduced, so that there is a lack of inhibition of B cell activity. Recurrent antigenic and mitogenic stimuli from the parasite to the B cells cause overproduction of polyclonal IgM of which only a small part has antimalarial specificity. The IgM forms aggregates and immune complexes which are phagocytosed by RES of liver, spleen, bone marrow.

The apparent anaemia is caused by the expansion of plasma volume up to 130 ml/kg and sequestration of up to one-third of total red cells in the spleen. There is haemolysis of cells pooled in the spleen and erythro-phagocytosis mediated by the adsorption of immune complexes; haemolytic crises are associated with pregnancy and infection. Patients are prone to frequent and prolonged infection due to related neutropenia and disturbed immune function.

Clinical Presentation— is usually found in young to middle aged adults, but can occur as early as 8 years of age and in old age. In some series, women outnumbered men, but in others there is an equal sex distribution. There is massive splenomegaly with dragging pain, hepatomegaly, but lymphadenopathy is usually absent.

Haematological picture— The anaemia is usually moderate but may be severe during pregnancy or acute infections. It is usually normocytic, but macrocytosis and polychromasia with reticulocytosis may occur. The total WBC is usually low, with granulocytopenia. However, in West Africa, in about 10% of cases there may be lymphocytosis, mimicking chronic lymphocytic leukaemia (CLL). There is mild thrombocytopenia, usually not of sufficient severity to cause haemorrhage. Malaria pigments are absent as a rule.

Sickle cell trait confers partial but significant protection against the development of HMS.

The bone marrow shows hyperactivity of erythroid, granulocytic, and megakaryocytic series. Megaloblastic change is rare. An excess of normal lymphocytes is found in West African patients. The frequency of depleted iron store is not more than that seen in normal population. Malaria pigment is not seen.

Distinguishing feature of HMS in comparison to CLL (Chronic Lymphatic Leukaemia)

1. Excessively high serum IgM in HMS, whereas level is lower than normal in CLL, except when there is a monoclonal paraprotein.
2. The normal lymphocyte transformation with phytohaemagglutinin (PHA), whereas transformation is reduced in CLL.
3. Polyclonal lymphoproliferation and polyclonal heavy chain gene rearrangement, as compared to monoclonal proliferation in CLL.
4. Absence of lymphadenopathy in HMS is, of course a useful clinical parameter.
5. Prognosis of HMS— The condition usually runs a benign course in most of the cases, though in some parts of the Tropics, the mortality is found to be as high as 46%–90%, without treatment. Death is due to effect of hypersplenism or overwhelming infection. Some patients show haematological and immune status suggestive of clonal lymphoproliferation sometimes called, 'African CLL' or "Tropical Splenic Lymphoma". The suggestion that the condition is due to proliferation of villous lymphocytes does not stand valid, as the cells are of native B cells in origin; surface markers are consistent with B cell prolymphocytic leukaemia.

Management— Treatment of choice is the administration of antimalarials chemoprophylaxis for life. The choice of prophylactic depends on the local pattern of sensitivity. Proguanil is the most effective agent in Tropical Africa. Failure of treatment may be due to non-compliance, ineffectiveness of anti-malarials, malignant transformation or incorrect diagnosis. There is no place for splenectomy, as it causes high operative and later mortality, transfer of disease from splenomegaly to hepatomegaly, and the need of lifelong chemoprophylaxis to prevent acute malaria.

3.15 HAEMATOLOGICAL CONSEQUENCES OF MALARIA

The degree of anaemia and the rate at which it develops vary enormously. The Hb concentration may fall up to 2 g/dl each day. Anaemia is a particular problem in children, where it may lead to high output cardiac failure and sudden death. These complications are particularly likely when Hb concentration falls below 4 g/dl *i.e.*, 12% of the haematocrit. Some patients appear to tolerate severe malarial anaemia relatively well. These patients usually have an underlying chronic anaemia and have adapted to increased oxygen carriage (right shifted oxygen dissociation curve).Thus it is both the absolute Hb concentration and the magnitude of the fall that determine the clinical consequences.

There is progressive normocytic, normochromic anaemia. The white count is usually normal, but may be raised in very severe anaemia or when a proportion of patients suffer from persistent fever, even after clearance of parasitaemia, due to an identifiable chest or urinary tract infection. Occassionally there is leucoerythoblastic reaction. There is slight monocytosis and reactive eosinopenia. The platelet count is reduced in all cases of acute malaria, usually around 100,000/microlitre, but thrombocytopenia is profound in some cases. Fibrinogen level is usually elevated— a reduction indicates significant disseminated intravascular coagulation (DIC). There is evidence of increased coagulation cascade activity through intrinsic pathway activation with antithrombins III depletion. This is proportional to disease severity and there may be prolongation of prothrombin and thromboplastin time. Polymorphonuclear elastase levels are elevated in severe infection, suggesting neutrophil activation.

3.16 VISCERAL LEISHMANIASIS AS A CAUSE OF ANAEMIA

Infection by Leishmania Donovani causes hyperplasia of macrophages and lymphocytes, massive production of IgG and progressive hepatosplenomegaly. The size of the spleen is directly related to the duration of infection, and to the severity of pancytopenia. Anaemia is produced in Kala-azar, through a number of mechanisms as follows:

1. Expansion of plasma volume, haemodilution, splenic sequestration, as a result of hypersplenism. [18]
2. The adsorption of IgG by red cells and the fixation of complement, plasma anti-I cold agglutinins are noted, but there is no convincing evidence of immune mediated haemolysis contributes to severity of anaemia in Kala-azar. [19]
3. There are evidences of haemolysis due to deficiency of protective enzymes in red cell membrane, both in experimental animals and in patients of Kala-azar. This may be a consequence of dyserythropoiesis and ineffective erythropoiesis found in a good proportion of patients. In India, megaloblastosis due to folate deficiency secondary to increased demand of folate from haemolysis often occurs.
4. Pancytopenia, and therefore, anaemia is particularly severe if there is co-infection with HIV. [21]

Haematological Picture

1. Neutropenia becomes extremely severe with advancing disease. Some workers have reported reduced phagocytic and bactericidal activity of neutrophils.[20] Children in particular are prone to secondary bacterial infection and development of cancarum oris.
2. The eosinophil count is reduced. Lymphocyte and Monocyte counts are raised. Occasionally there may be leukaemoid reaction.
3. Platelets are sequestered in the spleen and platelet survival is short. Thrombocytopenia may be sufficiently severe to cause mucosal bleeding but cutaneous purpura is unusual. Autoantibodies have been demonstrated against red cell, white cell and platelets in visceral Leishmaniasis. [22]

4. Hepatic dysfunction may lead to hypoprothrombinaemia and prolonged coagulation time as well as that of prothrombin time.
5. There is increased fibrinolytic activity and reduced fibrinogen concentration in some patients with advanced disease. Immune complex-mediated vasculitis and disseminated intravascular coagulation (DIC) have been reported in some parts of tropics.[23]
6. Bone marrow is usually (a) Hyperplastic and often megaloblastic, with increased erythroid, granulocytic, and megakaryocytic activity; lymphocytes and plasma cells are numerous, as are macrophages, many of which contain Leishman-Donovan bodies. (b) In long standing Kala-azar there may be bone marrow hypoplasia and fibrosis. (c) Gelatinous transformation has been reported in one patient. [24] (d) Pure red cell aplasia has been reported and this may be due to coincidental infection by parvovirus B19. [25]

Successful treatment of Leishmaniasis is followed by regression of spleen and a return to haematological normality over 9 months following cure. The anaemia response may be delayed due to persistence of dyserythropoiesis as a part of anaemia of chronic disorder.

Anaemia due to Trypanosomiasis

African Trypanosomiasis is accompanied by a haemolytic anaemia, which is usually moderate but may be severe. Haemolysis has several mechanisms:

1. Trypanosomes release haemolysin, which enables parasites to utilize and other nutrients from red cells.
2. There is adsorption of IgM immune complexes on to red cells with fixation of complement, and the sensitized red cells phagocytosed throughout the RES.
3. There is hypersplenism.

Other haematological changes

There is moderate leukocytosis, with raised lymphocyte and monocyte counts, but a neutropenia from hypersplenism. Thrombocytopenia is usual during acute infections, and may be profound due to hypersplenism. With Trypanosoma cruzi rhodesinsae infections, there is, in addition, platelet aggregation and destruction, and in some patients, DIC.

In infections with Trypanosoma cruzi (American Trypanosomiasis, Chagas' disease) there may be a normocytic anaemia, leukocytosis, lymphocytosis and hypoprothrombinaemia.

Anaemia due to Toxoplasmosis

There is high rate of transmission of Toxoplama gondii in childhood in the developing countries, causing only mild disease generally. Some patients may have persistence of lymphocytosis with atypical mononuclear cells like glandular fever cells and thrombocytopenia. Congenital toxoplasmosis is rare as women are most invariably immune. Severe and congenital toxoplasmosis may be seen more commonly as a result of AIDS pandemic.

Anaemia due to Amoebiasis

Patients with chronic disease have a hypochromic microcytic anaemia as a result of either chronic blood loss with consequent iron deficiency and/ or anaemia of chronic disorders. Neutrophil leukocytosis, sometimes amounting to leukaemoid reaction, is associated with perforation of bowel, peritonitis, secondary bacterial infections and amoebic liver abscess, Hepatic disease results in prolonged PT and excessively high B12 levels.

Anaemia due to Giardiasis

Acute diarrhoea due to Giardia lamblia causes malabsorption of folate, whereas about half of the patients with chronic infections have impaired absorption of vitamin B12, which is multifactorial, including damage to ileal receptors, utilization of vitamin by the parasite, and bacterial overgrowth of the bowel.

Anaemia due to Hookworm infestation

One fourth of world population suffers from hookworm disease, anaemia being the commonest clinical presentation. Anaemia is microcytic, hypochromic in nature, often associated with eosinophilia and hypoalbuminaemia. Hookworm anaemia develops from a combination of factors, like prolonged duration of infection, heavy infection, and an inadequate iron intake or poor bioavailability of iron in the diet.

Subjects with poor quality of diet or with depleted iron store may develop anaemia even on light infection. Women have lower threshold than men. Children usually develop heavy infection, in relation to their body weight, due to whole body exposure, while playing on the ground.

The anaemia is essentially a type of haemorrhagic anaemia, as the adult worm by buccal teeth attach to small bowel mucosa and suck blood amounting to 0.2 ml/day. The daily loss of iron has been calculated as 1.2 mg and 0.8 mg per 1000 ova per gram of faeces for A. duodenale and N. Americananus respectively, but as both species are now found more or less worldwide and mixed infections are common, the daily loss of iron of 1 mg per1000 ova regardless of species is a good working figure.

In rural parts of tropical countries, the infection is common in agricultural workers, many of them being barefooted during work. This is more so when the land is fertilized with night soil. The adult worm produces about 1000 eggs/day in the soil and eggs hatch into first rhabitidiform and then filariform or infectious larvae. They gain access into the circulation by penetrating the skin of the foot and ascend up the alveoli into the upper air passages and reaching the pharynx, these are swallowed and gain access into the small intestine. Patients may be asymptomatic if diet contains adequate iron or may develop only abdominal or respiratory symptoms and develop symptoms of anaemia, only when diet is deficient in iron. Adult hookworms may survive over a decade, A. Duodenale live over 6–8 years and N. Americana over 2–5 years. The two species may overlap in certain tropical regions, particularly Southern Asia. A. Duodenale can cross the placenta and infect the infant in utero. Anaemia is from acute blood loss, shows a normochromic picture, and may be life threatening. [26]

Anaemia due to Schistosomiasis

About 200 million people are infected by Schistosoma and transmission is increasing with spread of irrigation. The haematuria from S. Haematobium is short lived but can give rise to a loss of 30–40 mg of iron per day and contribute significantly to iron deficiency especially in adolescent boys, for example in Somalia and coastal South Africa.[27]

The mechanisms of anaemia in S. Mansoni and S. Japonicum infections are complex. Ulcers and polyps in the colon bleed and can result in chronic loss of iron of 7–8 mg / day. Infection of the liver is followed by hepatic fibrosis and the anaemia of chronic disorders; portal hypertension leads to splenomegaly and the pancytopenia of hypersplenism, oesophageal varices may bleed acutely or intermittently, leading to iron loss.

Anaemia due to Trichuris

Trichuris trichuria is one of the most prevalent helminths in the world, infecting about 1000 million people. Blood is lost from the inflamed colonic mucosa. Heavy infection in excess of 800 worms (16,000 ova per gram of faeces) result in a blood loss of 4 ml or iron loss of 1.5 mg per day. Trichuris can contribute to iron deficiency, or be a major cause in children, as has been reported from Central America and Malaysia.

Anaemia due to Diphyllobothrium latum

These tapeworms freely swim in clear water of the pool and embryos are swallowed by freshwater fish like Crustacaea and Cyclops or Diaptons. After development into larvae, they infect the flesh of the fish and grows into plerocercoid Sparganum larva. Human acquires infection by ingesting infected raw fish. Within 3–5 weeks the tapeworm matures into adult worm in the human intestine. The adult worm attaches to ileal and occasionally to jejunal mucosa by its suckers, which are located on elongated scolex. The adult tapeworm absorbs large quantities of vitamin B_{12} and interferes with ileal absorption of this vitamin. Up to 2% of infected individuals develop megaloblastic anaemia, resembling pernicious anaemia and may exhibit neurological sequelae.

Chapter 3

CONCLUSION

Anaemia in Tropics is of diverse aetiology, has got clinical pattern of wide dimension. As parasitic disease covers a broad spectrum of its aetiology, some important parasitic diseases are discussed in this chapter. Other diseases, such as haemolytic diseases and malignant diseases producing anaemia, have got also unique pattern in tropics. These will be dealt in respective chapters.

REFERENCES

1. World Health Organization, Global Program on AIDS. *Global Blood safety initiative. Guidelines for appropriate use of blood*. WHO /GPA/Inf 89; 18, Geneva; WHO; 1989.
2. Lewis SM, Bain B, Bates J, Dacie & Lewis's Practical Haematology, 9th Edition Edinburgh: Churchill, Livingstone, 2001.
3. Lubin BH. *Reference values in infancy and childhood*. In Nathan D.G.7 Oskj F.A. (eds) Haematology of Infancy and Childhood. 4th Edition, Philadelphia; W.B. Saunders, 1993; 1993: Appendix, 1-xx.
4. Gilles HM. *Normal Haematological values in Tropical areas*. Clin Haematol 1981; 10: 897–706.
5. DeMaeyer EAdiels—Tegman M. *The prevalence of anaemia in the world*. World Health Stat Q 1985; 38:302–316.
6. Fleming AF. *Haematological changes in pregnancy*. Clin Obstet Gynaecol 1975; 2: 269–283.
7. Bellingaham AJ. *The red cell in adaption to anaemic hypoxia*. Clin Haematol 1974; 3:577–594.
8. Viteri FE & Toran B. *Anaemia and physical work capacity*. Clin Haematol 1974; 3: 609–626.
9. Baker SJ & D Maeyer EM. *Nutritional anaemia its understanding and control with special reference to the work of the World Health Organization*. Amer J Clin Nutr 1979; 32: 368–417.

10. Harrison KA, Lister UG, Rossiter DE & Chang H. *Perinatal mortality*. Brit J Obstet Gynaecol (1985); 92 (suppl); 51: 86–99.

11. Harrison KA & Rossiter CE. *Maternal mortality*. Brit J Obstet Gynaecol (1985); 62 (suppl 5): 100–115.

12. Fleminf AF.*Haematological manifestations of malaria and other parasitic diseases*. Clin Haematol (1981); 10: 983–1011.

13. Mendeandez C., Fleming AF, Alonso P. *Malaria related anaemia*. Parasitol today (2000); 2000; 16: 469–476.

14. Bryceson A, Fakunle YM, Fleming AF et al. *Malaria and splenomegaly*. Trans B Soc Trop Med Hy (1983); 77: 879.

15. Fakunle YM Tropical Splenomegaly, Part I: Tropical Africa. Clin Haematol (1981); 10: 963–973.

16. Menendez C. *Malaria during pregnancy: a priority area for malaria research and control*. Parasitol Today (1995), 11; 178–183.

17. Fleming AF. Tropical obstetrics and Gynaecology. 1. *Anaemia in pregnancy in tropical Africa*. Trans B Soc Trop Med Hyg (1989); 83: 441–448

18. Kager PA & Rees PH. *Haematological Investigations in Visceral Leishmaniasis*. Trop Georger Med (1986);38:371–379.

19. Pippard MJ, Moir D, & Westherall DJ. *Mechanism of anaemia in resistant visceral Leishmaniasis*. Ann Trop Med Parasitol (1986); 80: 317–323.

20. Lazzarin A, Eposito R & Almaviva. *Modifications of leucocyte function in visceral leishmaniasis*. Bull 1st Seirote Milan (1981); 60: 222–224.

21. Cartwright G.E., Chung HL & Chang A. *Studies on Pancytopenia of Kala-Azar*. Blood (1948); 3:249–275.

22. Kager PA, van der plus-van Dalen C, Rees PH et al. *Red cell, white cell and platelet autoantibodies in visceral leishmaniasis*. Trop Georgr Med (1984); 36:143–150.

23. El Hassan AM, Ahmed MAM, Rahim AA et al. *Visceral Leishmaniasis in the Sudan Clinical and haematological features*. Ann Saudi Med (1990); 10: 51–56.

24. Varma N, Bhoria U, Bambery P, & Dash. *Gelatinous transformation of the bone marrow and Leismania donovani infection*. J Trop Med Hyg (1991); 94: 310–312.

25. Solano C, Gomez-Reino F, & Fernandez-Ranada JM. *Pure red cell aplasia in Kala-azar*. Acta Haematol (1984); 72: 205–207.

26. Report of the WHO informal Consultation on *Hookworm Infection and Anaemia in Girls and Women*. WHO/ CTD / SIP/ 96.I. Geneva World Health Organization, (1996).

27. Ross AG et al. Schistosomiasis. N Engl J Med (2002); 346: 1212.

CHAPTER 4

Iron Deficiency Anaemia

4.1 DEFINITION

Iron deficiency is defined as a decreased total iron content of the body, which when severe enough to suppress haemopoiesis, causes microcytic, hypochromic, anaemia. Usually it results from decreased dietary source or decreased absorption of iron from the diet. But sometimes it results from slow, small persistent blood loss especially from gastrointestinal tract. [1]

4.2 CLINICAL STAGES OF IRON DEFICIENCY

Iron deficiency passes through three stages. In the first stage, there is iron depletion of body's iron store but haemopoiesis is not affected. Plasma ferritin is below normal and staining for iron in bone marrow aspirate shows scanty (1+) or zero iron in macrophages of a cellular fragment. Plasma iron is low or normal, plasma transferrin is raised and its percentage saturation is reduced within normal range. In the second stage iron deficient erythropoiesis occurs, iron stores have been exhausted. Plasma ferritin is reduced further, iron is absent in the bone marrow and there are no sideroblasts, plasma iron and transferrin saturation are below normal. Haemoglobin is likely to be within normal range or there may be slight normochromic anaemia. With further depletion iron is not available for haemoglobin synthesis and iron deficiency anaemia develops. [2]

4.3 IMPACT OF IRON DEFICIENCY ON THE SOCIETY

Iron is essential for many metabolic processes, so its deficiency even without anaemia produces adverse effects on infants, children and adolescents and on outcome of pregnancy. In infants and children it produces motor coordination and language development defects, hampers school performance, psychological and behavioral disorders like lethargy, fatigue, sense of insecurity as well as decreased physical activity.

In pregnant women placental hypertrophy and premature delivery, low birth weight and increased maternal mortality and morbidity are seen to occur. In adults of both sexes, decreased capacity of physical and mental work and easy fatigue affect the earning capacity and capacity of domestic work.

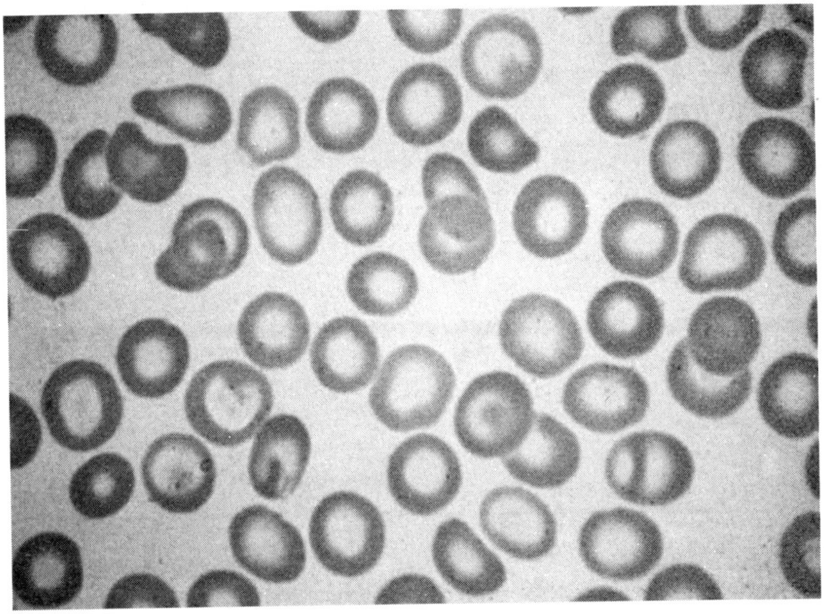

Fig. PBS in case of iron deficency

4.4 IRON BALANCE OF THE BODY

The total body iron is about 4 gm in a 70 kg man. This is to be maintained by a balance between absorption and body losses. Although the body only absorbs 1 mg of iron daily from the diet, to maintain equilibrium, the internal requirement of iron is greater, about 20 to 25 mg daily. An erythrocyte has a lifespan of 120 days so that 0.8% of RBC is destroyed and replaced each day. A man with 5 L of blood volume has 2.5 gm of iron incorporated into haemoglobin, with a daily turnover of 20 mg of iron for haemoglobin synthesis and another 5 mg for other requirements. Iron is required for formation of haem moiety of haemoglobin as well as myoglobin and cytochrome enzymes. Adults loose 1 to 1.5 µg in faeces, desquamated mucosal and skin cells as well as intestinal cells. The haem from destroyed or senescent red cells is recycled into new red cells. Iron is transported by transferrin in the plasma and stored as ferritin and haemosiderin forms in the bone marrow and liver. If more iron is lost or needed than that can be absorbed, iron stores are depleted and becomes gradually deficient. This impairs haemoglobin synthesis and resulting anaemia produces decreased oxygen carrying capacity, low energy level and increased work- load on heart.

4.5 REQUIREMENTS OF IRON AT DIFFERENT AGES

Infants have low requirements, while the red cell mass is diminishing. Requirements in older infants and children increases, relative to body size during growth and in adolescent during growth spurt. Mensturation doubles the demand. Requirement is low in first trimester of pregnancy, but rises rapidly to second and third trimester to 6-7 mg/day amounting to approximately 1000mg in whole pregnancy. Premature infants require more as transplacental passage occurs in last 4 weeks of gestation. In adults average daily requirement is 1 mg.

4.6 IRON METABOLISM

Iron compartments in the body

Haemoglobin is normally the largest iron compartment of the body. It is 34% of total body weight. Thus in an adult, the total iron content of the haemoglobin of iron is about 2 gm, depending on sex and body size.

Storage iron exists in two forms, either as ferritin or as haemosiderin.

Ferritin is a water soluble iron storage protein called apoferritin with a crystalline core that occupies the hollow apoferritin. The crystal is a lettice of hundreds or thousands of ferrihydrite. Within the cytosol ferritin acts as iron buffer.

Haemosiderin is a water insoluble derivative of ferritin. It is aggregated ferritin partially stripped in apoferritin component. Haemosiderin iron turnover is presumed to be rapid than apoferritin. [3]

Transport of iron

Transferrin is a protein of approximately 80000 Dalton, which is found in plasma. Being bound to trivalent iron, each molecule of transferring is attached to two atoms of iron. Approximately one third of iron binding sites on cell membrane of erythrocytes are occupied. A small amount of soluble transferrin receptor is in blood plasma. Iron is taken into cells by interlization of Fe-transferrin complex. Normally the transport iron compartment contains approximately 3 mg of iron.

Myoglobin iron- Skeletal and cardiac muscle cells contain myoglobin and this compartment contains approximately 150 mg of iron.

Other tissue iron- Normally a few grams of iron are bound to various ***enzymes and cytochromes.*** Ribonucleotide reductase required for synthesis of DNA, approximately one-half of enzymes of Krebs cycle, iron responsive protein that interacts with iron responsive elements of messanger RNA are some of the important components of iron.

Labile iron pool- may represent iron in the extravascular compartment i.e. lymph and iron between plasma and cytosol. Normally the labile iron pool contains approximately 80 mg of iron.

Absorption

Limited absorption of iron occurs throughout the whole intestinal tract but in the duodenum it is most efficient. Inorganic iron is absorbed in ferrous state but haem is absorbed in ferric state. The amount of iron absorption increases with the increasing amount of iron ingested. In healthy persons, about 10% of dietary iron is absorbed, and this amount is about 1 mg daily. Ascorbic acid gastric hydrochloric acid and mucin facilitate absorption. The amount of iron absorbed increases when there is iron deficiency or accelerated erythropoiesis and is decreased when there is bone marrow hypoplasia. The effect of ingested alcohol is controversial. [4]

4.7 PATHOPHYSIOLOGY OF IRON DEFICIENCY ANAEMIA

Iron equilibrium in health

Iron is vital for all living organisms because it is essential for multiple metabolic processes, including oxygen transport, DNA synthesis, and electron transport. Iron equilibrium in the body is regulated carefully to ensure that sufficient iron is absorbed in order to compensate for body losses of iron. Whereas body loss of iron quantitatively is as important as absorption in terms of maintaining iron equilibrium, it is a more passive process than absorption.

4.8 IRON DEFICIENCY IN THE BODY

Either diminished absorbable dietary iron or excessive loss of body iron can cause iron deficiency. Diminished absorption usually is due to an insufficient intake of dietary iron in an absorbable form. Hemorrhage is the most common cause of excessive loss of body iron, but it can occur with hemoglobinuria from intravascular hemolysis. Malabsorption of iron is relatively uncommon in the absence of small bowel disease (sprue, celiac disease, regional enteritis) or previous GI surgery. [5, 6]

4.9 IRON ABSORPTION

Most nonheme dietary iron is ferric iron. Iron absorption in mice and rats may involve more ferrous iron because they excrete moderate quantities of ascorbate in intestinal secretions. Humans, however, are a scorbutic species and are unable to synthesize ascorbate to reduce ferric iron.

The iron concentration within enterocytes varies directly with the body's requirement for iron. Absorptive cells of iron-deficient humans and animals contain little stainable iron, whereas those of subjects who are replete in iron contain significantly higher amounts. Untreated phenotypic hemochromatosis creates little stainable iron in the enterocyte, similar to iron deficiency. Iron within the enterocyte may operate by up-regulation of a receptor, saturation of an iron-binding protein, or both.

In contrast to findings in iron deficiency, enhanced erythropoiesis, or hypoxia, endotoxin rapidly diminishes iron absorption without altering enterocyte iron concentration. This suggests that endotoxin and, perhaps, cytokines alter iron absorption by a different mechanism. [7]

In the classical transferrin pathway, the transferrin iron complex enters the cell within an endosome. Acidification of the endosome releases the iron from transferrin so that it can enter the cell. The apotransferrin is delivered by the endosome to the plasma for reutilization.

Iron uptake in the proximal small bowel occurs by 3 separate pathways.. These are the heme pathway and 2 distinct pathways for ferric and ferrous iron. [8]

Haeme iron is not chelated and precipitated by other dietary costituents e.g. tannate, phytatate, oxalate, carbonate, like inorganic iron. Two-third of dietary iron comes from dietary myoglobin and haemoglobin and one-third comes from haem. Haem is maitained soluble and available for absorption by globin degradation products produced by pancreatic enzymes. Heme is digested enzymatically free of globin and enters the enterocyte as an intact metalloporphyrin, presumably by vesicular mechanism.Within the cell iron is released from heme by heme oxygenase to pass into the body as inorganic iron. Haem absorption pathway is distinct and different from inorganic iron pathway but these are non-competitive. [9,10]

Most dietary inorganic iron is absorbed as ferric iron. This can enter the absorptive cell via the integrin-mobilferrin pathway (IMP).Some dietary iron is reduced in the gut lumen and enters the absorptive cell via the DCT-1 pathway (divalent cation transporter). The proteins of both pathways interact within the enterocyte with paraferritin, a large protein complex capable of ferrireduction.

Other proteins related to iron absorption are stimulators of iron transport (SFT) and hepashaestin which are important to transfer iron from enterocytes to plasma. Iron concentration within the enterocytes varies directly with body's requirements. Iron within the enterocyte may operate by upregulation of a receptor, saturation of iron-binding protein or both. [11,12]

Absorptive cells of iron-deficient humans and animals contain little stainable iron, whereas those of subjects who are replete in iron contain significantly higher amounts. Untreated phenotypic hemochromatosis creates little stainable iron in the enterocyte, similar to iron deficiency.

4.10 IRON IN NON-INTESTINAL CELLS

Most iron delivered to nonintestinal cells is bound to transferrin. In the classical transferrin pathway, the transferrin iron complex enters the cell within an endosome. Acidification of the endosome releases the iron from transferrin so that it can enter the cell. The apotransferrin is delivered by the endosome to the plasma for reutilization. The method by which the transferrin receptor–independent pathway delivers iron to the cell is not known.

Nonintestinal cells also possess the mobilferrin integrin and DMT-1 pathways. Their function in the absence of an iron-saturated transferrin is uncertain; however, their presence in nonintestinal cells suggests that they may participate in intracellular functions in addition to their capability to facilitate cellular uptake of iron.

4.11 SOURCES OF IRON IN THE DIET

Although our environment exposes us all to vast quantities of iron, our food contains generally poor quantity of bioavailable iron. This is due to complicated mechanism of iron absorption and variable amount of absorbale iron in different types of food in different countries of world.

Beef, lamb, pork, poultry and fish cotain fair amount of iron. Cereals and flour, even though iron-fortified, provide little absorbable iron,due to presence of phytate. Most fruits and dairy products contain negligible amount of iron. Spinachs and raisins are poor sources of iron. Similarly very little bioavailabe iron is released from cooking utensils, contrary to general belief. Rich sources of iron are liver, oyesters and legumes.

Ascorbic acid increases absorption of ferric and ferrous iron and has little effect on absorption of haem iron. Ascorbic acid chelates non-haem iron to enhance its absorption.

Globin degradation products diminish polymerization of haem into macromolecules to facilitate its absorption. They also increase absorption of non-haem iron because they prevent their precipitation and polymerization by binding with iron, thus absorption of iron in the spinach is increased when it is eaten with meat. Chelation of iron with mucin helps to keep it in soluble form, available in alkaline duodenum.

4.12 PREVALENCE OF IRON DEFICIENCY IN THE COMMUNITY

About one-third of world's population is believed to suffer from iron deficiency.Children, women at all ages, people of lower socio-economic status and elderly people are more vulnerable to iron deficiency. Children, fed only on milk, after first few months of life, develop iron deficiency. Women loose iron due to loss during mensturation and increased need of iron during pregnancy and delivery. Elderly women develop iron deficiency, when they are not compensated adequately in earlier life, or suffer from postmenopausal loss, for example for bleeding fibroid. Poor people get little iron from diet, which is rich in carbohydrate (which hampers absorption of iron) and poor in protein (hence deficient in myoglobin and haeme part of iron). [13]

Iron deficiency anaemia can occur from loss in urine, as in haemoglobinuria or intravascular haemolysis. If urine contains no red cells but is bloody haemoglobinuria is suspected. It should be confirmed that the substance is haemoglobin, but not the myoglobin. This can be accomplished by adding 60% ammonium sulphate which can precipitate haemoglobin but not the myoglobin. Iron deficiency anaemia now becomes rare after heart surgery using artificial valves producing intravascular haemolysis, due to improved valve prosthesis.

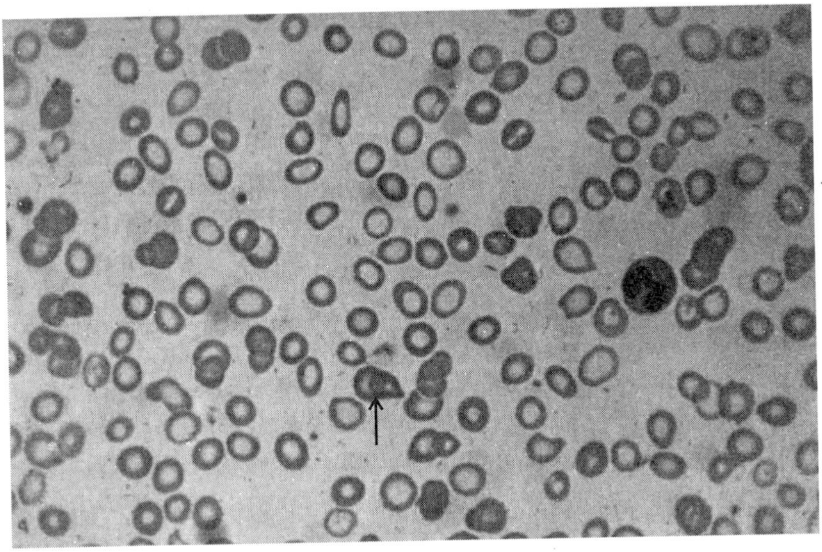

Fig. PBS in case of thalassaeme trait
PBS = Peripheral blood smear
Arrow marked cells are polivilоeyfcs

Regular blood donors are iron depleted until they take iron supplements. Elderly people are often iron deficient due to chronic blood loss from gastrointestinal tract or occult kidney failure. They may also suffer from nutritional deficiency due to failure in procuring balanced food, while living alone.

Iron deficiency seems to be more prevalent in African-American in USA, as seen in Public Health Survey. Microcytosis may be also due to the fact that about 28% of the population has mild form of α thalassaemia (not associated with microcytosis) and 1% have β thalassaemia trait (associated with microcytosis). If microcytic anaemia only indicates prevalence of thalassaemia, its incidence should be about 25% in the population survey. Thus only microcytosis may not be a reliable index of presence of iron deficiency in this ethnic group in subclinical level. [14]

4.13 ADVERSE EFFECTS OF IRON DEFICIENCY AT CELLULAR LEVEL

Many of adverse effects of iron deficiency on cells of different tissues are not due to reduced oxygen transport only.

Immunologic Cellular Mechanisms- These are impaired, specially phagocytosis and killing of bacteria, but it may be offset of reduced bacterial proliferation, as bacteria require iron for their growth and proliferation.

Brain and motor function-Iron depleted animals show reduced activity of α -glycerophosphate dehydrogenase in skeletal musles and reduced exercise tolerance. Brain monoamineoxidase activity is reduced in iron depleted animals.

In human, reduced enzyme activity is not substantiated, but disturbance of motor function and reduction of attention span are found in iron-depleted human infants. [14]

Epithelial changes- The oral and buccal epithelium exhibits thinning and dyskeratotic changes in iron deficient humans, and these changes may occur in iron deficiency alone, even if not associated with sufficient anaemia. The epithelial changes may cause fissuring at the corner of the mouth, glossitis and web formation at the cricoid level of hypopharynx. There is atrophy of papillae of the tongue. There is controversy regarding development of postcricoid carcinoma in chronic iron deficiency.

Kolionychia or spoon nail is a rare complication of iron deficiency. It also indicates reduced tissue iron store, rather than the effect of anaemia.

Chapter 4

4.14 CLINICAL FEATURES OF IRON DEFICIENCY ANAEMIA

Symptoms are vague and nonspecific e.g. weakness, lethergy, tinnitus, vertigo, sore tongue, glossitis, palpitation, reduced exercise tolerance. Pica is symptom, which is unique, and may be present before anaemia develops. It is manifested as compulsive swallowing of clay, laundry starch, or ice. Tachycardia, high volume pulse, innocent systolic murmurs, palpable spleen tip (in 10% of cases) are found in different stages. Kolinychia is commonly seen in United Kingdom but it is rare in United States. The patient with iron deficiency may be asymptomatic, as development of iron deficiency state may be very slow and the ability of body to compensate low iron reserve is enormous. [15]

4.15 LABORATORY FEATURES

Of the common laboratory tests, the serum ferritin (SF) is the first to reflect iron deficiency, often when the blood haemoglobin, erythrocyte count and indices, serum iron,TIBC, and erythrocyte morphology are still normal. Examination of Prussian blue stained film of bone marrow shows iron depletion. As iron deficiency becomes more severe and progressive, further abnormalities develop in sequence, like, anisocytosis, microcytosis,elliptocytosis, hypochromia, of red cells in peripheral blood smear, declining level of haemoglobin concentration,low serum iron concentration.

Maximum changes in RBC cellular indices occur when maximum number of erythrocytes are replaced by microcytes. Before this RBC shows a dimorphic picture, as after a bout of bleeding, This is reflected in Red Cell Distribution Width (RDW) which is a measure of anisocytosis seen in the peripheral blood.

If the serum iron is < 20 mg and microcytosis is present, iron deficiency anaemia is confirmed. If serum ferritin is > 20 μg, it may be also due to anaemia of chronic disease or thalassaemia.

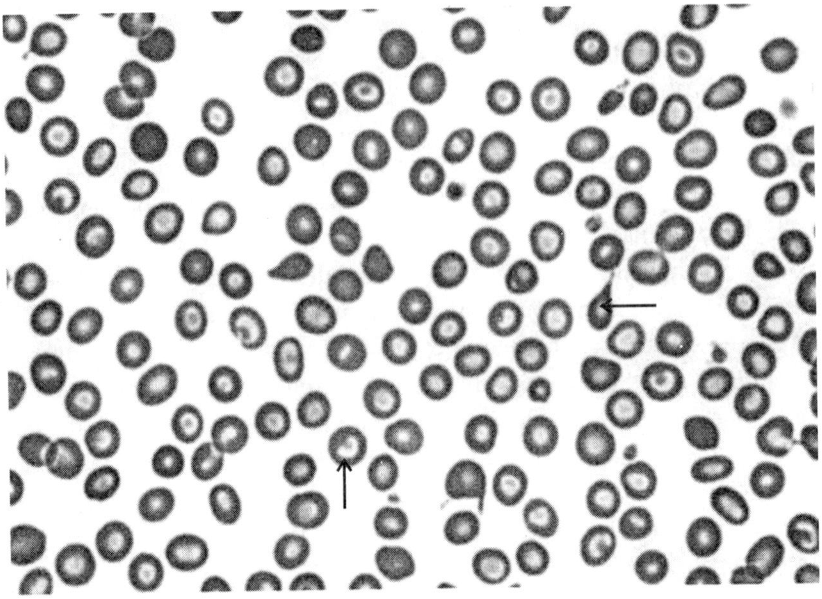

Fig. PBS in case of thalassaemia major
PBS = Peripheral blood smear
Arrow marked cells are fear drop cell (left down)
and poliviloeyfcs (Right up)

Serum ferritin may be 15 to 80 μg in anaemia of chronic disease. Ferritin may be also elevated in hepatitis, Gaucher's disease, chronic lymphocytic leukaemia and Hodgkin disease. Spuriously elevated ferritin level may also occur after oral or parenteral iron therapy for few days to few weeks.

Ferritin is an acute reactive protein and plasma ferritin levels are generally raised in rural population in the tropics. Higher cut off points are to be applied for malaria, recurrent intestinal infections and chronic hepatic disease (prevalent in the tropics). This makes diagnostic value of this measurement of limited value, especially in children.

Erythocyte protoporphyrin is less sensitive than serum ferritin , but it is increased in anaemia of chronic disease, while it is decreased in iron deficiency anaemia.

Serum soluble transferrin receptors are increased in iron deficiency anaemia and myeloprliferatve disorder or haemolytic diseases i.e. the conditions in which haemopoiesis is increased. It is decreased in anaemia of chronic disease, and aplastic anaemia, when haemopoiesis is depressed. The test is non-specific and less sensitive. [16]

4.16 DIFFICULTIES IN DIAGNOSIS OF IRON DEFICIENCY ANAEMIA

There are some important difficulties in diagnosis of iron deficiency anaemia

(1) Limited laboratory facilities in most of the places of rural area where anaemia is commonly prevalent.

(2) Biochemical measurements sometimes give misleading results in patients with occult infection or malignancy.

(3) Differentiation of iron deficiency from β thalassaemia and anaemia of chronic disorder is sometimes difficult

(4) Iron deficiency anaemia is quite common even in the affluent society due to wrong choice of combinations of foodstuff in a particular feed or use of some of the food preferentially.

4.17 FEW IMPORTANT DIFFERENTIAL DIAGNOSIS

Anaemia of chronic disease often accompanies chronic inflammatory disorders like rheumatoid disease or malignancy. Underlying clinical condition is ususally evident. Differentiation is important in chronic inflammatory bowel disease or renal carcinoma, in both these conditions iron deficiency may coexist due to chronic blood loss. In both cases, serum iron concentration is low, but usually the TIBC is also reduced in patients with chronic disease, while it is increased in iron deficiency. On the contrary, percent transferrin saturation is typically normal in the former and low in iron deficiency anaemia. Chronic disease usually causes elevation of serum ferritin. When chronic disease and iron deficiency coexist, serum ferritin concentration may be normal. An increase in erythrocyte sedimentation and CRP that is disproportionate to anaemia helps in distinguishing anaemia of chronic disease and iron deficiency. Differentiation of these two disorders may require bone marrow examination for iron content of the specimen, as it is low in iron deficiency. [17]

Thalassaemia share some morphological abnormalities with iron deficiency anaemia, like micocytosis, target cells (though more common in thalassaemia), anisocytosis, polikilocytosis. Coarse basophilic stippling and polychromasia favour the diagnosis of thalassaemia. An important clue to the diagnosis of thalassaemic trait is that the blood smear may show macrocytosis with normal or increased count, whereas in iron deficiency there is always microcytosis with reduced count. Measurement of haemogobin A_2 by electrophoresis gives the correct diagnosis of β thalassaemia. [18]

Chronic hepatic disease usually is characterised by the presence of round macrocytes, target cells in the peripheral blood film. Hypochromic microcytes may sometimes give erroneous diagnosis of iron deficiency. Usually serum ferritin is normal or increased in liver disease, this test helps to distiguish between uncomplicated liver disease from iron deficiency. Unfotunately iron deficiency often coexists in liver disease due to bleeding oesophageal varices or chronic gastritis. The bleeding may be occult, but clinical evidences of chronic liver disease are usually evident.

Chronic kidney disease is accompanied by burr cells or acanthocytes. (erythrocytes with spiny projections on cell membrane), and the presence numerous schistocytes or fragmented erythrocytes in the peripheral blood smear. This implies abnormalities of small blood vessels as a result of intracellular fibrin deposition. Hypochromic microcytosis is often present because of chronic inflammatory disease or iron deficiency. Deficiency is due to chronic blood loss from urinary tract or repeated haemodialysis. Serum iron concentration are rarely helpful to distinguish and serum ferritin is spuriously normal. Confirmation of iron deficiency can be only done by bone marrow examination which is rarely done in these cases.

Myxoedema is often associated with a mild normocytic normochromic anaemia. The serum iron concentration is reduced, which may lead to erroneous diagnosis of iron deficiency.Further women with myxoedema may suffer from menorrhagia, which may produce iron deficiency.

4.18 GUIDELINE FOR DIFFERENTIAL DIAGNOSIS

1. Mild anaemia, no particular clinical feature, and normal indices- No further investigation may be required other than wait and watch and improvement of nutritional status.
2. Low MCV but normal haemoglobin concentration and normal or increased RBC- Serum ferritin should be measured. If it is < 20 mg/l, the patient has iron deficiency. If serum ferritin is normal or increased, the patient may have thalassaemia or chronic disease. Haemoglobin electrophoresis should be done and HbA_2 and HbF should be measured. Even if these results are normal, patient may have α thalassaemia or chronoc disease. In African-American there may be homozygous α thalassaemia or a thalassaemia-1 trait if the patient is Asian.
3. If in a set up of microcytosis and hypochrmia, serum ferritin is <20 μg/l, diagnosis of iron deficiency is confirmed.
4. If anaemia, microcytosis and serum ferritin >20 μg/l are present together, anaemia of chronic disease should be considered if serum ferritin is >80 μg/l. If the patient has any evidence of chronic disease like rheumatoid arthritis, only bone marrow examination and staining for iron can confirm presence of iron deficincy anaemia. If the patient belongs to a particular ethnic group which shows preponderance of thalassaemia, Hb electrophoresis should be done to exclude thalassaemia. These considerations should be done if the patient has evidence of chronic disease and serum ferritin is between 15 to 80 μg/l and iron stain of bone marrow is required to confirm concomittant iron deficiency anaemia.
5. Peripheral blood smear examination is mandatory in every case of anaemia which gives important clue to the diagnosis of underlying condition like acanthocytosis in microangiopathy or more serious disorder, like leukaemia or myelodysplatic syndrome.
6. Serum iron, TIBC, Ferritin receptor examinations require sophisticated laboratory, are of high cost and less sensitive.

4.19 THERAPY OF IRON DEFICIENCY ANAEMIA

Principle of Therapy

It is obligatory to determine the cause of iron deficiency anaemia before therapy. It is essential to eliminate the cause e.g. Change of milk diet of infant to mixed diet or to remove a bleeding neoplasm e.g. fibroid or treament of oesophageal varices or peptic ulcer.

Iron Therapy

Iron can be administered orally or parenterally. Plain ferrous salt administration is less costly, safe and effective. Enteric coated or sustained release preparation should be avoided because iron is released in places of intestine where it is not efficiently absorbed. The optimal dose is 65 mg of elemental iron i.e.

0.2 g of ferrous salt three times daily between the meals. Such treatment should be continued for 6 months following correction of anaemia to replete the storage iron compartment.

Thus total duration of such treatment is usually 8 months. If bleeding continues, treatment may be continued indefinitely. A small proportion of patients experience nausea, vomiting, constipation, heartburn. In such cases, it may be required to reduce the dose to one tablet once daily and then to increase the dose gradually.

Some patients complain of difficulty in swallowing, this complaint is often of psychological origin , may be treated with Ferrous Sulphate syrup 2 tsf thrice daily. Such preparation contains 32 mg of iron in 4 ml, but it may produce black staining of the teeth, a problem that can be avoided by rinsing the mouth after each dose. "Combination Haematinics" (Iron with vitamins) are unjustified, unless specific deficiency exits. Most of the studies show that use of ferrous fumarate or ascorbate does not increase bioavailability or diminish side effects. Patients on oral iron therapy should be alarmed about black staining of stool.

In infants, dose of iron is 6mg/kg in divided dosage and 12.5mg daily for prophylaxis.

Parenteral Iron Therapy

Iron can be administered parenterally in the form of Iron-dextran. The following are indications of parenteral iron therapy.

1. The patient is unable to take oral preparation due to nausea, vomitting or acidity
2. The patient does not comply due to unwillingness
3. Intestinal malabsorption as in Tropical Sprue, or excessive intestinal resection
4. Continued bleeding from a lesion which can not be surgically treated at such a rate that ingested iron in optimal dosage is insufficient.

Iron-dextran contains 50 mg of iron per millilitre in the ferric form. It is usually administered by intramuscular injection into the buttocks, using a Ztrack technology, in which the skin is pulled sideways before injection to reduce brown staining of the skin. It is generally recommended in a dosage of 2ml (100mg) daily till the full dose is administered. The total dose of iron required is calculated as follows:

Total dose of iron needed= Hb deficit (g/dl) × lean body weight + 1000, Hb deficit is calculated taking normal average for men as 14g/dl and normal average for women as 12 g/dl. The addition of 1000mg is to replenish the iron store in addition to make up the Hb deficit.

Before parenteral therapy, following considerations are to be done.

A test for hypersensitivity should be done,using 0.5 ml of the injection. There should be medical supervision and preparation for treatment of anaphylactic shock. The most common adverse side effect of parenteral therapy is anaphylactic shock, which may occur with both intramucular and intravenous injection. Total dose intravenous infusion of iron-dextran is not approved by US FDA.

The most common adverse effects are pain and swelling at the injection site, arthalgia, fever, which may appear few hours to several days after injection.

These effects are associated with neutrophilia. Rheumatoid arthitis may be excerbated following administration of iron-dextran. There may be generalized lymphadenopathy, splenomegaly or aseptic meningitis. Examination of CSF may show pleocytosis. These benign but unpleasant side effects usually diappear after a few days to few weeks.

A few cases have been reported with sarcomas at the site of injection.

Injudicious administration of parenteral iron therapy in a case of microcytic anaemia, which has got different type of pathology e.g. thalassaemia, or sideroblastic anaemia, may lead to haematochromatosis.

Response to therapy

The rate of response to iron therapy does not depend upon route of therapy, but adequacy of the dose and responsiveness of the bone marrow. The blood haemoglobin deficit should be half corrected within 3 weeks and fully corrected in 8 weeks. Young patients respond more promptly and elderly people respond more slowly.

Failure to respond

The following enquiries must be made:

1. Is there any source of occult bleeding?
2. Does the pharmacist comply with the prescription or the patient comply with the instruction?
3. Is there any sort of malabsorption?
5. Is there any underlying chronic inflammatory or malignant disease?

Some patients respond poorly to iron-dextran either because of mobilizing iron very slowly from the injection site or because of inability of bone marrow macrophages to catabolize iron promptly, so providing iron at insufficent rate to developing normoblasts. Often such patients have ample bone marrow iron, but have low ferritin concentration and microcytic erythocytes. These patients will respond promptly to oral iron therapy.

Transfusion may be needed in severely anaemic patients who may be in danger of ischaemic injury to brain, heart, kidney or other vital organ. Transfusion of packed erythrocytes is better to avoid cardiac decompensation. Erythrocytes prepared from stored whole blood may not promptly improve the oxygen carrying capacity of blood, as low concentration of 2,3 DPG in them produce high oxygen affinity and thus poor uxygen delivery. Modern blood banking anticoagulant solutions alleviate adverse effect of stored blood erythrcytes on oxygen transport.

Tranfusion is the most expensive form of treatment. It also carries the risk of several types of reactions and carries the hazards of different types of infections, including HIV disease and cytomegalovirus infection. Some of these may be lethal also but are largely preventable by modern methods of blood banking.

4.20 PREVENTION OF ANAEMIA

Dietary Modifications

1. On average diet in the tropics, iron content is sufficient to maintain nutrition, but iron absorption is less than adequate due to improper methods of cooking (overboiling and overcooking) and improper use of foodstuff in combinations. This can be ameliorated by proper education.
2. Improved iron status can be achieved by increasing enhancers of iron absorption like ascorbic acid (citrus fruits) and animal protein, decreasing inhibitors of iron absorption (tannin and phytate present in vegetables) or by increasing total food intake, which increases the calorie content as well as total iron content is increased by 30%.

3. Germination, malting and fermentation of grains increase ascorbic acid content and decrease phytate and tannic acid. Folate is present in sufficient amount in leafy vegetables, tubers, liver, red meat, rice, maize, millet, cassava.
4. Though animal protein is difficult to be procured for high cost and social prejudice, vegetables and corn containing folate are often present in daily food of even the poor community. Folate is essential for DNA synthesis in rapidly proliferating cells e.g. bone marrow and G.I. tract. So it is essential for maintaining health of gut mucosa and absorption of iron. Ascorbic acid and folate, are heat labile and water soluble, so can be destroyed by overheating, prolonged boiling or reheating, just like iron.
5. Inhibitors of absorption like tea, coffee, (tannin), rice, maize, wheat (phytate), should be minimized. Polyphenols in nuts and legumes, egg phosphoprotein and fibre contaning food should be properly spaced to avoid impairment of iron absorption.
6. Enhancers of iron absorption like fresh fruits (guava, citrus fruits, pine apple), vegetables like cauliflower, potato, sweet potato, turnip, amino acid containing food like meat, poultry, fish, seafood should be adequate in the diet.
7. Food fortification in the form of acidification of milk and biscuits with added bovine haemoglobin is practiced in some developing countries. Riboflavin deficiency produces erythroid hypoplasia and immobilization of iron in the store and vitamin C deficient diet is deficient in bio-available iron. So supplements of these two essential elements are also recommended in prevention of anaemia.

Chapter 4

4.21 UNICEF RECOMMENDATION DURING PREGNANCY

Elemental Iron 60 μg as ferrous sulphate and folic acid 400 mg taken twice daily without food during second half of pregnancy, and where malaria is prevalent, along with anti-malarial prophylaxis, has been recommended from first antenatal attendance. In the area of heavy hookworm infestation or in remote villages, albendazole 400 mg orally on fist attendance after first trimester, is also standard protocol.

Vitamin A (2-4mg of retinol/day) supplement dramatically enhances affinity of iron when used for prevention of anaemia. Vitamin A deficiency produces distinct haematological effect like immobolization of iron in reticulo-endothelial cells, and infection in anaemic children produces further immobilization. Therefore, Vitamin A dosage should be increased from 10,000 I.U. to 25,000 I.U in children at risk of infection and pregnant women should receive.200000 I.U. after delivery.

REFERENCES

1. Stolzfas R (2001): *Defining iron deficiency anaemia in public health terms*.A iime for rectification J Nutr 131:5655.
2. Fairbanks VF, Beutler E (2001): *Iron Metabolism.* In Beutler E, Lichtman MA, Coller BS et al, eds, Williams' Haematology, 6th ed. :447:470.
3. Charache S, Gittlesohn AM, Allen H, et al., (1987): *Noninvasive assessment of tissue iron stores.* AmJ Clin Pathol:88:333-337.

4. Charlton EW, Jacobs P, Seftel H Bothwell TH (1964): *Effect of alcohol on iron absorption.* Br Med J:1427.
5. Hines JD, Hoffbrand AV, Molin DL (1967): *The haematological complications following partial gastrectomy: a study of 292 patients.* Am J Med 43:555–569.
6. Annibale B, Marignani M, Monarca B, et al., (1999): *Reversal of iron deficiency anaemia after Helicobacter pylori eradication in patients with asymptomatic gastritis.* Ann Intern Med 131:668–678.
7. Wereth E, Tuttle MS, Poulson J et al. (2004): *Hepcidin regulates iron efflux by binding to ferroportion and inducing its internalization.* Science:305: 2090.
8. Conrad ME, Umbriet JN (2002): *Pathways of iron absorption.* Blood Cells Mol Dis 29:336.
9. Tayla PG, Martinnea- Torres C, Romano EL, Layrise M (1986): *The effect of cysteine-compounds containing peptides released during meat digestion on iron absorption in humans.* Am J clin Nutr J 43: 68.
10. Shyaechi M, Sukairs A et al (2005). *Identification of intestinal haem transporter.* Cell 122:789.
11. Cairo G, Pietranglelo A (2000): *Iron regulatory proteins in pathophysiology.* Biochem J 352 Pt. 2241.
12. Meryon Holtz EG, Ghosh MC, Roulat TA (2004): *Mammalian tissue oxygen levels modulate iron regulatory protein activities in vivo.* Science 306:2087.
13. Weintraub LR, Weinstein MB, Husir H, Rafal S. (1968). *Absorption of haemoglobin iron: the role of a haem-splitting substance in the intestinal mucosa.* J Clin Invest 47:531.
14. Grantham Mc Gregor S, Ani C (2001): *A review of studies of the effect of iron deficiency on cognitive development of children.* J Nutr 131:6495
15. Dallman PR (1982): *Manifestations of iron deficiency.* Semin Haematol 19:19-30.
16. Punnonen K et al., (1997): *Serum transferrin receptors and its ratio to on deficiency.* anaemia 89: 1052-1057.
17. Vreugdenhil G, Baltus CA,van Ejik HG et al., (1990): *Anaemia of chronic disease: diagnostic significance of erythrocyte and serological parameters in iron-deficient rheumatoid arthritis patients.* Brit J Rheumatol 29:105-110.
18. van Zeben D, et al., (1990): *Evaluation of microcytosis using serum ferritin and red cell distribution width.* Eur J Haemaol 44:106–108

CHAPTER

5

Megaloblastic Anaemia

5.1 INTRODUCTION

Megaloblastic anaemia is a disorder caused by impaired DNA synthesis. The presence of megaloblastic cells is the morphologic hallmark of this group of anaemia. Megaloblastic cells are larger than normal and have more cytoplasm relative to the size of the nucleus. Promegaloblasts show a blue granule free cytoplasm, a granular chromatin that contrasts with the ground glass texture of the normal counterpart. As the cell differentiates, the chromatin condenses more slowly than normal into dark aggregates that coalesce, giving the nucleus, a characteristic fenestrated appearance. Condensation of chromatin to homogenous mass either fails or delays. The growing maturity of the cytoplasm as it acquires haemoglobin, contrasts with immature looking nucleus, a feature termed nuclar-cytoplasmic asynchrony. Megaloblastic granulocytic precursors are larger than normal. They show nuclear-cytoplasmic asynchrony with cytoplasm that looks less mature than the cytoplasm of normal counterparts. A characteristic cell is giant metamyelocyte, which is a large horse- shoe shaped, containing ragged chromatin. Megaloblastic megakaryocytes may be abnormally large with deficient granulation. In severe megaloblastosis, the nucleus may show unattached lobe.

5.2 AETIOLOGICAL BASIS

Slowing of DNA replication in the megaloblastic anaemia, due to folate and cobalamin deficiency appears to arise from failure of folate dependent conversion of deoxyuridine monophosphate (dUMP) to deoxythymidine triphosphate (dTMP). Because of this failure and the fact that DNA polymerase has difficulty in distinguishing deoxyuridine triphosphate (dTTP) from deoxythymidine triphosphate (dTTP), dTTP is incorporated into DNA of folate deficient cells. Recognizing the mistake, the cells try to repair DNA but the attempt fails. [1]

The frustrated effort at DNA repair ultimately leads to fragmentation followed by cell death. Megaloblastic cells have much more cytoplasm as RNA and protein are synthesized at a faster rate than nucleus and DNA. Not only synthesis of DNA is impaired, joining of DNA fragment lags, migration of DNA fragments fail, and S phase is prolonged. [2]

A curious group of findings suggests megaloblastic cell line appears from a more primitive precursor than from normoblasts. Megaloblasts contain high concentration of foetal haemoglobin, and foetal isoenzyme.

Cytological abnormalities resembling megaloblastosis may appear in other proliferating cells. Epithelial cells of mouth, stomach, small intestine, cervix uteri may look megaloblastic.

5.3 FOLATE COBALAMINE RELATIONSHIP IN PRODUCTION OF MEGALOBLASTIC ANAEMIA

The megaloblastic anaemia of cobalamin deficiency is largely corrected by folic acid supplementation even if no cobalamin is given. Conversely, the anaemia of folate deficiency is not helped at all by cobalamin. These clinical observations indicate that megaloblastic anaemia in cobalamin deficiency actually results from an abnormality in folate metabolism. [3]

The methylfolate trap hypothesis is based on the fact that the folate requiring enzyme N^5 methyl FH_4 homocysteine methyltransferase is dependent on cobalamin, which acts as methyl group transferring agent, methionine being the donor. The hypothesis states that in cobalamin deficiency, tissue folates are gradually diverted into 5-methyl-FH_4 pool, because of slowing of methyl transferase reaction. As a result, in the first instance, N^5 methyl transferase level increases and other folates are decreased. An expanded pool of tissue folate may account for some of the blockade of methyl transferase activity, which is already deficient due to deficiency of cobalamin. Freshly acquired folate can't be converted into a form that can be retained by the cell. The result is development of tissue folate deficiency as the non-conjugated folate leaks out of the cell. [4]

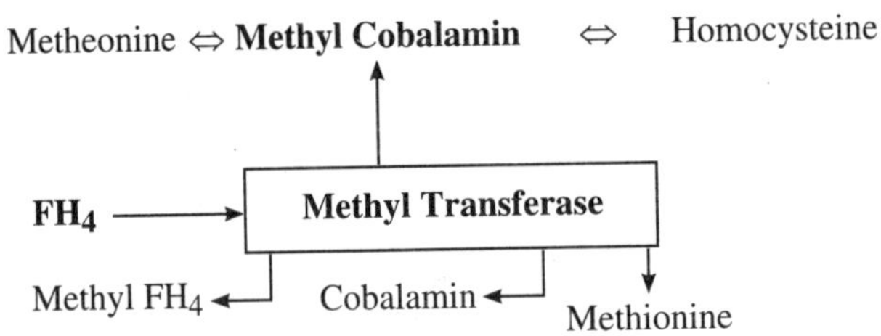

Most evidences point out that deficiency of cobalamin leads to intracellular methionine deficiency, which block availability of reduced folate within the cell, which perturb DNA synthesis by reducing the quantity of thymidylate precursor. This causes pile up of tetrahydrofolate (Folate Trap hypothesis). [5]

Prolonged deficiency of cobalamin deficiency results in defective myelin synthesis within central nervous system. There is defective conversion of propionate to succinyl-CoA which leads to defective myelin synthesis. Elevated levels of methylmalonic acid (MMA) and total homocysteine are positively correlated with cobalamin deficient neurological dysfunction. [6]

Absorption of Cobalamin

Cobalamin in food is absorbed from the terminal part of ileum. Before that it forms complex with intrinsic factor secreted by parietal cells of the body of the stomach. The intrinsic factor-cobalamin complex, which is very resistant to digestion, journeys down the intestine from the stomach until it reaches the microvilli of the ileum, where there is intrinsic factor receptor protein (R protein) found in the brush border epithelium of the microvilli. Following the attachment of the complex to the receptor, the cobalamin is taken up by the ileal mucosal cells by endocytosis. Then it passes into portal blood over many hours, while the receptor recycles to microvilli for another load of complex.

Cobalamin from a small oral dose (10–20 μ gm) starts to appear in the blood after 3–4 hours and reaches peak level in 8–12 hours. Cobalamin, bound by receptor protein (R protein), enters the lumen of the intestine, to be digested by pancreatic lipase. Then it is again taken up by intrinsic factor and gets reabsorbed. Cobalamin then enters enterohepatic circulation, 65–75% of biliary cobalamin, which is estimated to be 0.5–0.9 μ gm/day, is reabsorbed from the intestine. Because of the size of the storage pool, approximately 60 years is required to develop deficiency from a deficient diet. Patients who fail to reabsorb may develop deficiency in 3–6 years.

Cobalamin in the Cell

Transcobalamin II is the plasma protein that mediates the transport of cobalamin in the tissues. Unlike intrinsic factor it is not specific for cobalamin, it can also bind to some chemically related molecules, which have no function in mammalian tissue, and are known as cobalamin analogues. TC II is synthesized by many types of cells *e.g.*, enterocytes, hepatocytes, fibroblasts, haemopoietic precursors in the marrow. Although circulating TC II carries only a minor fraction to which newly acquired cobalamin is first bound, while cobalamin given parenterally immediately associates with this protein which that absorbed from the intestine is carried as preformed cobalamin TC II complexes in the portal blood, these are transported into the tissues within minutes of appearing in the blood. The transport process begins with binding of cobalamin TC II complex to a membrane receptor that is present on a wide variety of cells. The receptor bound complex is internalized by pinocytosis and delivered to a lysoozyme, where the TC II is digested and cobalamin is freed.

R proteins are a group of immunologically related proteins. They are found in milk, plasma, and saliva, gastric juice and numerous other body fluids. They lack the specificity of intrinsic factor. TC I promotes excretion of analogues into the bile as complexes as it binds to these analogues poorly. These complexes are poorly absorbed from the ileum and excreted in the faeces. TC I may serve as storage protein for cobalamin as TC I excretion from plasma is extremely slow. TC I and TC II are detected in plasma in trace quantities *i.e.*, 7–20 μ g/l.

TABLE 5.1: Cobalamin Binding Proteins

Protein	Source	Function
Intrinsic factor	Gastric parietal cells	Promotes absoroption uptake by ileum
Transcobalamin II	Probably all cells	Promotes uptake of cobalamin by cells
R proteins	Exocrine glands, phagocytes	Helps disposal of analogues

5.4 PATHOPHYSIOLOGY OF FOLATE DEFICIENCY

Folate has got multiple dietary sources. Leafy vegetables like spinach, lettuce, lima beans, fruits like banana, melon as well as liver, kidney, yeast and mushroom. In spite of this, folate deficiency occurs because of the fact that folate is easily depleted from the food by excessive cooking and boiling and use of large amount of water during cooking.

Daily requirement is approximately 50 μ g and recommended allowance is 0.4 mg. The body is depleted of folate when intake is reduced to 5 μ g per day and megaloblastic anaemia develops in approximately 4 months.

Effect of Folate Deficiency

Folate deficiency diminishes purine biosynthesis by slowing formylation reaction in the cells. Effect of folate deficiency produces changes in different organs.

1. Folate deficiency produces abnormalities in neural tube closure and poorly developed neuro-psychiatric system. A portion appears to be associated with folate receptor antibodies that may be overcome by higher folate intake.
2. Heart, limb and urinary tract may anomalies also develop when folate deficiency occurs in utero.
3. Polymorphism in gene of glutamate carboxypeptidase increases serum folate level and reduces homocysteine level. Thus folate deficiency diminishes protective value against atherosclerosis and increases risk of athersclerosis. [7]
4. A number of congenital anomalies like fragile site syndromes are associated with folate deficiency.

Folate Deficiency

1. Dietary deficiency: Inadequate folic acid is found in diet deficient in fresh leafy vegetables and citrus fruits. It causes deficiency rapidly as body reserve is small.
2. Hyperalimentation or haemodialysis may cause deficiency.
3. Subtotal gastrectomy may produce subclinical deficiency.
4. Infants or children maintained on synthetic diet or fed on goat's milk may develop deficiency. [8]
5. Premature infants with haemolysis, infection or diarrhoea are prone to develop deficiency.
6. Destruction of folate in over cooked or over-boiled food is another cause of deficiency in the tropics.
7. In alcoholic cirrhosis, there are several reasons of production of folate deficiency Alcoholism causes acute marrow suppression, decreases reticulocyte levels, increases sideroblsts, vacuolisation of erythroid and myeloid precursors, and dysfunction of granulocytes. These changes are observed even if large dose of folate is given with alcohol. [9]
8. In addition to these changes in haemopoietic cells, there are other pathological changes in folate metabolism. [10] These are
   - Dietary malabsorption.
   - Insufficient diet in alcoholics due to high calori intake in alcohol.
   - Decreased hepatic storage.
   - Decreased intracellular folate utilization.
   - Depression of serum folate level by alcoholic.

Intestinal Disorders Causing Folate Deficiency

1. **Non-tropical sprue:** Mucosal atrophy and chronic inflammation of the microvilli of jejunum, more severe proximally along with gluten sensitivity are two characteristic features. Glossitis, dirrhoea, weight loss, osteomalacia and megalblastic anaemia are characteristic features.

2. **Tropical sprue:** It is endemic in West Indies, Southern India, Southern America, South-east Asia. It can be acquired by travellers and can be retained for many years after return. The aetiology is unknown but can be corrected by folate therapy, though folate deficiency is not the cause, response to antibiotics suggests infection. Unlike non-tropical sprue it affects distal small intestine, so leads to cobalamin deficiency as well. Folate deficiency is due to failure of conjugation of polyglutamate. [11]
3. **Other intestinal diseases:** Malabsorption of folate commonly occurs in regional enteritis, after excessive resection of small intestine and conditions such as lymphomatosis, leukemic infiltration, Whipples disease, scleroderma, amyloidosis.

Increased folate Requirement

1. **Pregnancy:** Folate requirement increases 5 to 10 fold because of transfer of folate, which draws down maternal folate store even in the face of maternal severe folate deficiency. It is difficult to diagnose as normal haematological changes obscure it. Absence of hypersegmented neutrophil in peripheral blood smear and MCV 104 fl distinguish it from true megaloblastic anaemia. [12]
2. Conditions producing increased cell turn over, such as exfoliative dermatitis and psoriasis, produces loss of folate up to 5 to 20 μg/day. Methotrexate therapy aggravates the condition which may necessitate pretreatment with folic acid.
3. Conditions producing increased cell turnover are also found in myeloproliferative like CML, lymphoproliferative disorder like lymphoma, metastatic carcinoma, as chronic inflammatory disorders.

5.5 DRUGS CAUSING MEGALOBLASTIC ANAEMIA

Antifolate drugs may cause megaloblastosis by being structurally similar to folic acid thereby inhibiting the enzyme DHFR(dihydrofolate reductase). These are chemotherapeutic agents like **methotrexate, aminopterene, immunosuppessive agents like Imuran, antimalarials like pyrimethamine, trimethoprim and sulfasalazine**. [13, 14]. After they enter cells via the folate carrier and acquire a polyglutamate chain they act as very powerful DHFR (dihydroxy folate reductase inhibitor} inhibitor. By blocking the reaction dihydrofolate to tetrahydrofolate, and perharps by inhibiting other enzymes of folate metabolism,causing a fall in nucleotide (thymidine) biosynthesis that lead to major derangement in DNA application.

Folate itself is ineffective in anaemia caused by folate antagonists unless folinic acid is used. Folinic acid is always in tetrahydro form, so it is effective in spite of DHFR blockage. It is used in a dose of 3–6 μg/day. Larger dose is required in chemotherapy protocol.

Purine analogues like immunosuppressive, azathioprine, retroviral agents like acylovir, pyrimidine analogues like zidovudine act by competitive inhibition and drugs like hydroxyurea, cytarabine act by inhibiting ribonucleotide reductase inhibitor. Zidovudine used to treat HIV infection produces severe megaloblastic anaemia. In HIV infection there is already bone marrow suppression. Azathioprine or trimethoprim used to treat complications of HIV disease may further aggravate the condition.

Hydroxyurea used to treat CML produces megaloblastosis 1 to 2 days after initiation of the therapy. Long term use of **omeprazole or other Na^+/K^+ inhibitors** is associated with reduced cobalamine level, though this is not found in short term use.

Antimalarials and antibacterials (pyrimethamine, trimethoprim) are analogues of purine and competitors of DHFR. Their affinities for bacterial and protozoal enzymes are high and for mammalian enzymes are low, but use in high dosage can lead to megaloblastic anaemia. Antibodies against folate receptors may be overcome by higher dose of folate (1–5 μg/day), as also seen in megaloblatosis produced by **anticonvulsants, like phenytoin.** [15]

Megaloblastic anaemia has been reported in association with long- term **metformin** treatment. [16]

Conditions Causing Megaloblastic Blood Picture

HbC disease is found in 16–20% of all populations of the tropics. Mild macrocytosis is a common feature of this disease and megaloblastic anaemia may complicate the course of pregnancy. Other conditions, which produce macrocytosis, are alcoholic liver disease, hypothyroidism, aplastic anaemia, myelodysplastic syndrome and autoimmune haemolytic anaemia. MCV rarely exceeds 110 fl.in these conditions. In alcoholism macrocytes are oval, whereas in nutritional megaloblastic anaemia macrcytes are round in shape.

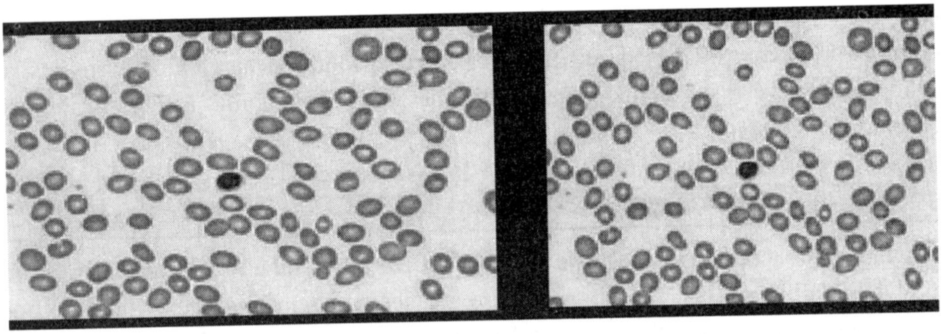

Fig. PBS showing round macrocytes (Left) (a) in $V_1 + B_{12}$ deficency, (b) Oval macrocytes (Right) seen in folic acid deficiency

Non-haematolgical Defects Associated with Megaloblastic Anaemia

In folate deficiency

Folate deficiency is related to a number of serious disorders not involving haemopoietic system. These are congenital anomalies, most important of which is neural tube closure defect, rare disorder like fragile site syndrome, and homocysteinaemia as well as atherosclerosis. A proportion of neural tube closure defects is associated with folate receptor antibodies that may be overcome by higher folate intake. Another proportion is due to mutation involving metabolizing enzyme of folate. Deficiency of cobalamin may be responsible in another group, as level of TC II in normal pregnant women correlates with the likelihood of developing neural tube defect. [17]

In cobalamine deficiency

Neurological defects develop due to deranged methyl group methylation. The development can be prevented by methionine, which is produced in cobalamine dependent reaction, and which is the precursor of the biologic methylating agent SAM. A finding is that the brain of catecholamine deficient pigs contain increased levels of SAH, a powerful inhibitor of methylation. Catecholamine does not produce any effect on methylation of phospholipids or myelin basic protein of in the brains of fruit bats.

Effect of Folate and Requirements During Pregnancy, Lactation and Infancy

Folate prevents congenital defects in neural tube, heart, limb and urinary tract. In three-fourth cases of anemia in pregnancy, folate deficiency is the cause. High demands for folate occurs in normal pregnancy, especially multiple pregnancy, primigravidae and pregnancy with pyrexia and haemoglobinopathies.

In infancy, prematurity of enzyme system, feeding boiled cow or goat milk in which folate is unavailable, poor weaning food, diarrhoea, repeated systemic infections and haemoglobinopathies put extra demand of folate. Folate deficiency anaemia usually occurs over 6 months of postpartum period, this is more so in women mainly on maize based diet not meeting the demand of prolonged lactation.

High demand in pregnancy, especially multiple pregnancy, malarial haemolysis particularly in primigravidae, pyrexia and haemoglobinopathies are common aetiologies in these groups of populations.In three fourths of anaemia in pregnancy, women present with megaloblastosis about 6 months post patrum, due to low intake of maize in the poor community, not meeting the demand of pregnancy and prolonged lactation.

5.6 COBALAMIN DEFICIENCY

In adults, deficiency may result from following diseased conditions:

1. Nutritional deficiency is quite common in tropical developing countries with comparatively poor economic status or social prejudices for avoidance or restriction of animal protein in the diet. In such people, only microorganism in the intestine is the source of cobalamin. Gastric peptic digestion at low pH is a prerequisite for cobalamin release from methyl cobalamin complex. Therefore hypo- or achlorhydria in elderly people over 70, may account for 20–25% cases of megaloblastic anaemia.
2. Pernicious anaemia: This arises as a consequence of long standing gastritis leading to eventual atrophy of all secretory cellular components of stomach due to deficiency of intrinsic factor (IF), there is almost complete malabsorption of ingested cobalamin and development of megaloblastic anaemia. Some indirect evidences point to an immunological abnormality in the form of autoantibodies directed towards IF, which is found in two-third of cases of pernicious anaemia. All patients have low serum cobalamin level, usually less than 100 μg/ml. Serum folate levels are either decreased or normal. Gastric IF as measured by radioimmunoassay is almost undetectable. Radiolabelled B_{12} absorption or schiling test establishes the correct diagnosis. Clinical manifestations usually appear after the age of 40. In prolonged deficiency neurological manifestations due to demyelination of dorsal column appear.
3. Gastrectomy syndromes: It is inevitable after subtotal or total gastrectomy, if the patient survives 4 years without supplementation. The delay is due to slow exhaustion of storage in the liver. All patients need monthly or bimonthly parenteral supplementation of vitamin B_{12}.

4. Small intestinal syndromes: The following intestinal diseases cause cobalamin deficiency.
   - Surgical resection of the distal ileum
   - Regional ileitis
   - Tropical Sprue
   - Chronic pancreatic insufficiency
   - Chronic ingestion of *p*-aminosalicylic acid and colchicines
   - Associated with hypothyroidism
   - These conditions are not usually associated with clinical symptoms.

Small intestinal parasitic disease: There are two well known parasitic disease giving rise to cobalamin deficiency, infection with cestode, diphyllobothrium latum, fish tapeworm, prevalent in Baltic sea and Great Lake as well as Escheria coli infection and gram negative infection superimposed on blind loop due to stricture or surgery. In the first one, quinacrine or nicolosamide is needed for eradication, In the second one, therapeutic trial of tetracycline for 2 weeks, normalizes the absorption. In severe deficiency, parenteral therapy is needed.

5.7 DIAGNOSIS OF MEGALOBLASTIC ANAEMIA

Clinical Presentation

It is emphasized that initial clinical presentations in either folate or cobalamin deficiency may be indistinguishable from each other. Depending on severity of the deficiency, patients may present with minimal symptoms or with anorexia, glossitis,fatigue, and other symptoms of anaemia. The only clinical feature that occurs in some patients with cobalamin deficiency, but not with folate deficiency, is neurological deficit, either peripheral neuropathy or dorsal spinal column disease. This is seen exclusively in cobalamin deficient patients with megaloblastic anaemia. With more severe degree of anaemia, the liver may become readily, but clinically detectable splenomegaly is uncommon. Physical signs may include pallor, 'a lemon yellow colour' in fair colored individual due to mild icterus, a smooth tongue, a cardiac 'haemic' systolic murmur. Neurological picture in cobalamin deficient patients ranges from subtle changes mental inattentiveness to mental confusion, with or without dorsal column tract signs. Fortunately, in most patients, cobalamin therapy results in significant objective reversal of these neurological abnormalities.

Blood Picture

All cell lines of blood are affected. Erythrocytes markedly vary in shape or size and in severe cases may show basophilic stippling and nuclear remnants (Cabot ring, Howel Jolly bodies). The anaemia is macrocytic, MCV being 110–150 fl or more. Neutrophils often have 3–5 lobes. Typically more than 5% neutrophils contain more than 5 lobes. In nutritional megaloblastic anaemia, hypersegmented neutrophils may be the earliest sign and may persist for many days after treatment.

In cobalamin deficiency, platelet production is only 10 p.c. of that expected from the megakaryocytic mass, perhaps reflecting ineffective thrombopoiesis.

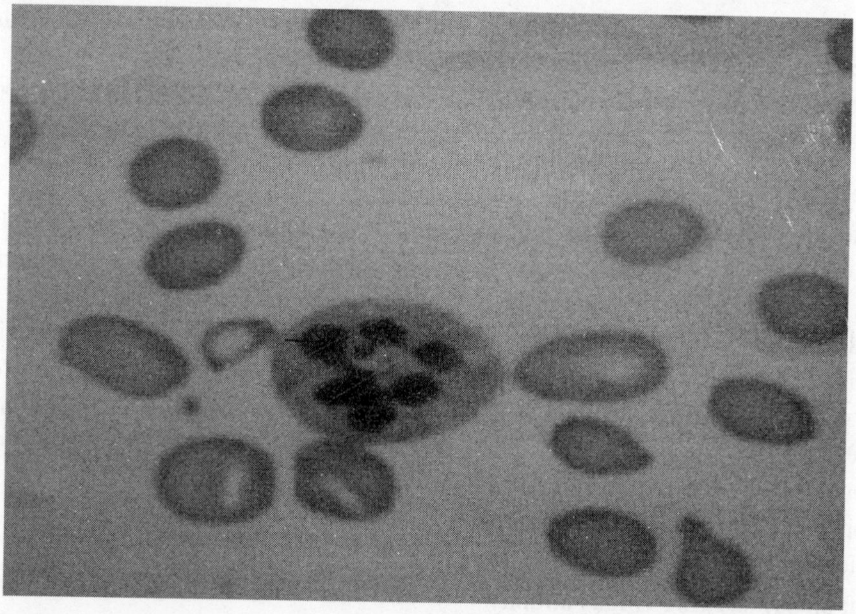

Fig. PBS showing hypersegmented neutrophils with oral macrocytes anaemia (magnifried)

Biochemical Changes

Two abnormalities in erythrocytes are ineffective erythropoiesis and haemolysis. Red cell life span is decreased by 30 to 50 p.c.

The first one increases red cell precursor reticulocyte ratio as well as iron turnover and LDH 1 and LDH 2 levels, LDH 1 being greater than LDH 2, unlike other haemolytic anaemia, in which LDH 2 is greater. Increased serum muramidase may be caused by increased granulocyte turn over, while serum glutamic transaminase level is normal. Plasma bilirubin, ferritin, iron levels are increased.

Erythropoietin level is high but rise is less than other types of anemia. The level falls sharply within days of beginning of treatment.

Bone Marrow

Aspirated marrow is cellular and shows striking megaloblastic changes, especially in erythroid series. Ratio of myeloid erythroid precursors falls to 1:1 or lower. Granulocytic reserve may be decreased. In severe cases promegaloblasts containing an unusual number of mitotic figure, are plentiful. Macrophage iron content is often increased.

5.8 ACUTE MEGALOBLASTIC ANAEMIA

May develop in acute toxic deficiency of folate or cobalamine. The condition arises acutely with rapidly developing thrombocytopenia and/or leukopenia but with little change in red cell parameters. The most common cause is nitrous oxide anaesthesia, approximately 6 hours after exposure. Gross anaemia develops in 12 to 24 hours. Hypersegmented neutrophils do not appear until 5 days. The condition can be prevented by folinic acid (30 mg at surgery and 12 hours later). Effects spontaneously disappear after several days, but the recovery can be hastened by folic acid or cobalamine.

Chapter 5

Nitrous oxide destroys methylcobalamin. Phenomenon may occur without previous deficiency but more frequent and severe in preexistent deficit. [18]

Case report is found in a patient of femoral fracture in Portugal. (Acta oled Port 2000 Sep-Dec, 13(5–6): 309–12).

Aetiological Diagnosis

The serum folate level is not a precise indicator of depleted body store of the vitamin, though it is a single most useful test for the diagnosis of folate deficiency. In most laboratories, the normal range is 5–15 ng/ml. Values of 3–5 ng/ml are considered indeterminate in interpretation. Red cell folate is not usually used as diagnostic test, as it lacks the precision.When red cell folate concentration becomes subnormal, it is always associated with cellular folate deficiency. A subnormal red cell folate always accompanies cobalamin deficiency, though serum folate is increased and it does not fall until all body stores are depleted.

Diagnosis of non-tropical sprue rests upon

1. Demonstration of malabsorption by urinary excretion of less than 1.5 g of D-xylose 5 hours after a 5 g loading dose
2. Jejunal biopsy showing villous atrophy
3. Response to gluten free diet

The use of so-called FIGlu (Formiminoglutamic acid) excretion after oral histidine is no longer used in the diagnosis of folate deficiency. Occasionally the so-called deoxyuridine test suppression test is used when inborn errors of cobalamin metabolism are suspected.

Adequate treatment of folate deficiency is achieved by administration of folic acid in 1–5 mg daily dose, while cobalamin-deficient patients may exhibit a haematological response to physiological dose of 200 μg of folic acid. However, this test is not used for distinguishing folate and cobalamin deficiency, as use of only folic acid in cobalamin deficient aggravates neurological symptoms.

5.9 REFRACTORY MEGALOBLASTIC ANAEMIA

Response to therapy is indicated by

1. Rise of haemoglobin level at the rate of 1g/wk
2. Reticulocytosis becoming evident within 3-5 days
3. Level of LDH and indirect bilirubin falling rapidly within few days
4. Leucocyte and platelet counts usually restored to normal within few days
5. Anaemia proves to be refractory if response does not occur after adequate therapy for 2–4 weeks.

Three categories of patients show megaloblastic bone marrow morphology and yet do not respond haematologically to cobalamin or folate therapy. The first and most commonly observed category is that associated with anti-neoplastic therapy. The second category is the megaloblastic haematopoiesis that results from myelodysplastic syndrome or later on develop AML M6. The third category is the megaloblastic anaemia resulting from inborn errors of metabolism or chromosomal disorder of cobalamin or folate metabolism.

1. Megaloblastic anaemia due to anti-neoplastic agents:
   (a) Purine inhibitors-most commonly used drugs are 6-mercaptopurine, 6-thioguanine, and azathioprine. The megaloblastic bone marrow develops prior to aplasia. The condition resolves on cessation of therapy.
   (b) Pyrimidine inhibitors- include 5-uracil. 5-fluro-2-deoxyuridine, 5-azauracil.
   (c) Deoxyribonucleotide inhibitors-include cystosine arabinoside, used in acute leukaemia, and hydroxyurea, used to treat chronic myeloid leukaemia. These agents produce pronounced megaloblastic changes in bone marrow soon after administration.
   (d) Intercalating agents include doxorubicin, daunorubicin, amascrine,and mitoxantrone. All these are used to treat leukaemia and lymphoma and can produce megaloblastic haematopoiesis and other dysplastic changes before producing profound myelosuppression.
2. Inborn errors of metabolism and folate malabsorption
   (a) Orotic aciduria is a rare disorder of pyrimidine metabolism which gives rise to megaloblastic anaemia.
   (b) Dihydrofolate reductase deficiency— such anaemia responds to folinic acid.
   (c) Homocysteine methyl transferase deficiency— this condition responds to folate, cobalamin or pyridoxal phosphate.
   (d) Congenital folate malabsorption— associated with mental retardation.
3. Cobalamin deficiency
   (a) Selective malabsorption of normal IF, associated with albuminuria.
   (b) Congenital abnormality of IF.
   (c) Congenital R binder protein deficiency.
   (d) True Pernicious anaemia of childhood.
   (e) Transcobalamin II deficiency— it is autosomal recessive condition,associated with irreversible nerve damage in early infancy.

5.10 THIAMINE RESPONSIVE MEGALOBLASTIC ANAEMIA

Characterised by megaloblastic anaemia, sensorineuronal hearing loss, diabetes mellitus onset is between infancy and adolescence anaemia is corrected by 25–75 mg of thiamine in contrast to pharmacological dose of 1–5 mg. Macrocytosis and hearing loss persist, though anaemia may recur on withdrawal.

This is a rare hereditary disorder. Defective gene is found on chromosome 1. The nature of biochemical defect is unknown. This is an autosomal recessive disorder, 25% of offspring being affected, 1/3 of unaffected ones are carriers, 50% of affected children are asymptomatic. Erythroid cells in the bone marrow contain iron filled mitochondria. SLC 19A2 which encodes for high affinity thiamine transporter, is the gene associated. All with this phenotype can be identified by sequence analysis. Cancer testing for at risk individuals and prenatal testing are essential. [19]

Recently some cases of such type of anaemia have been studied in the department of Genetics and Genomics, Mount Sinai School of Medicine, and published on Oct. 24, 2003.

Chapter 5

5.11 MEGALOBLASTIC ANAEMIA IN THE TROPICS

Recognition of megaloblastic anaemia is difficult in the developing countries of the tropics due to following reasons:

1. insidious onset and general unawareness of the public about health.
2. tendency to be masked by use of multivitamin preparations, containing folic acid.
3. typical presentations.
4. diverse aetiology.
5. complex laboratory procedure for diagnosis.

Macrocytosis in peripheral blood may occur in a number of conditions prevalent in the tropics. These are alcoholic liver disease, hypothyroidism, any case of reticulocytosis *e.g.*, thalassaemia, autoimmune haemolytic anaemia, myelodysplastic syndrome. The common causes of megaloblastic anaemia are folate and/or vitamin B_{12} deficiency.

Low serum folate (3 ng/day) only indicates a drop in intake in past few days. Red cell folate is a better indicator of folate deficiency.

In tropical countries, most common causes are intestinal diseases affecting the ileum like tropical sprue, or colonization of intestine by bacteria (as in blind loop syndrome), which take up cobalamine before its absorption. It occurs also in parasitic infection like diphyllobothrium latum (fish tapeworm). Infection comes from under cooked or raw fish. The anaemia develops in 5–6 weeks. Only 3 p.c. of persons, such infected, are affected by anaemia. [20]

Among the diagnostic procedures, measurement of red cell folate and serum B_{12} are not available in remote parts of developing countries and antibody measurements are more difficult and require more sophisticated laboratories.

5.12 MANAGEMENT OF MEGALOBLASTIC ANAEMIA

Folate deficiency induced megaloblastic anaemia: Irrespective of the etiology of folate deficiency, adequate therapy is provided with the administration of folic acid tablet in 1–5 mg doses between 1–7 days in a week depending on the degree of deficiency. It should be reemphasized that initial therapy of any patient presenting with megaloblastic anaemia should consist of parenteral B_{12} therapy until the serum vitamin concentrations are known with certainty. The rationale of this treatment strategy is that cobalamin deficient patients can exhibit a haematological response to 100 μg of folic acid. Once the serum assay results are available, the clinician's responsibility is to direct investigations into the specific cause of the deficiency.

Treatment of Cobalamin Deficiency Induced Megaloblastic Anaemia

Transfusion therapy: There exists a significant mortality among severely anaemic elderly patients with Hb level below 5 g/dl . These patients often have incipient cardiac failure with a greatly expanded plasma volume. Generally patients older than 50 years of age should receive 1 unit of packed red cells given over 10 to 12 hours with appropriate diuretic therapy. In subjects with Hb level below 8 g/dl, it may be prudent to remove judiciously 250–300 ml of anaemic blood while administering packed red cells.

Treatment of Concurrent Infections

Urinary and pulmonary tract infections are common in elderly people. Close culture surveillance is required and appropriate antimicrobial therapy should be given at the earliest sign of infection.

Specific replacement therapy: As soon as blood is obtained for serum B_{12} and folate assay, treatment with parenteral B_{12} should be instituted. The daily requirement of cobalamin is 1 μg and an initial loading of 1000 μg is customary. Oral folic acid is administered as 1mg each day until serum assay results are available to establish specific deficiency. Pernicious anaemia patients are subsequently administered monthly dose of 1000 μg of cobalamin for life. Many pernicious anaemia patients present with subnormal K^+ level. On institution of parenteral therapy, most patients require careful monitoring, and supplemental K^+ therapy is often necessary.

Follow –up of Cases Presenting with Megaloblastic Anaemia

Haematologist should be consulted if there are neurological symptoms, or pregnancy, or there is suspicion of haematological malignancy.

Gastroenterologist should be consulted if evidences of gastric malignancy or coeliac disease are detected.

Dietician should be consulted if folate deficiency is due to strict vegetarian habit, or coeliac disease.

Follow-up should consist- Annual peripheral blood smear examination, and repeated endoscopy to exclude gastric malignancy.

REFERENCES

1. Hunneckens FM (1968): *Folic acid coenzyme in the biosynthesis of purines and pyrimidines.* Vitam Haem 26 : 378.
2. Blount BC, Mack MM, Mehr CM, et al., (1997): *Folate deficiency causes uracil misincorporation into human DNA and chromosome breakage: Implications of cancer and neuronal damage.* Proc Natl Acad Sci USA 94 : 3290.
3. Herbert J, Zalnsky R (1962): *Interrelations of vitamin B_{12} and folic acid metabolism:Folic acid clearance studies.* J clin Invest 4 : 1263.
4. Shane B, Stockstad EL((1985): *Vitamin B_{12} interrelationships.* Annu Rev. Nutr. 5 : 115.
5. Chararin I, Perry J, Lumb M (1974): *The biochemical lesion in vitamin B_{12} deficiency in man.* Lancet 1 : 1251.
6. Alfman LA, Van den Put MM, et al., (2001): *Reduced vitamin B_{12} metabolism: Folic acid binding by transcobalamin II increases the risk of neural tube defect.* J Med 94 : 159.
7. Klujijtmas LA, Young RS, Boheran CA et al., (2003): *Genetic and nutritional factors contributing to hyper-homocysteinaemia in young adults.* Blood 101 : 2483.
8. Ford JD, Scott KJ ((1968): *The folic acid activity in some milk foods for babies.* J Diary Res. 35 : 85.
9. Savage D, Lindenbann J. (1985): *Anaemia in Alcoholics.* Medicine (Baltimore) 65: 322.
10. Eichen ER, Hillman RS (1973): *Effect of alcohol on serum folate level.* J clin Invest 52:584.
11. Klipstein FA (1972): *Folate in tropical sprue.* Brit J Haematol 23 : 119.

12. Chanari I, Mc Feyden IR, Kyle R ((1977): *The physiological macrocytosis in pregnancy.* Brit J Obst Gynaecol 84 : 504.
13. Magee J, O'Sullivan H, Mac Cann SR (1981): *Megaloblastosis and low dose trimethoprim sulfamethoxazole (letter).* Ann Intern Med 95:657.
14. Bertino JR (1990): *Folate antagonists: toward improving the therapeutic index and development of new analogs.* J clin Pharmacol 30 : 291–295.
15. Carl GF, Smith ML, Furman GM, et al., (1991): *Phenytoin treatment and folate supplementation affect folate concentration and methylation capacity in rats.* J Nutr. 121 : 1214.
16. Callaghan TS, Hadden DR, Tomkin GH (1980): *Megaloblastic anaemia due to vitamin B_{12} malabsorption associated with long term metformin treatment.* Brit J 280 : 1214.
17. Alfman LA, Van der Put MM, Thomas CM et al., (2001): *Reduced vitamin B_{12} binding by transcobalamin II increases the risk of neural tube closure.* J Med 94 : 59.
18 (a) Koblin DD, Tomerson BW, Waldman FM, et al., (1990): *effect of nitrous oxide on folate and vitamin B_{12} metabolism in patients.* Anaesth Analog 71 : 610-70.

(b) Nunn JF, Chanarin I, Tanner AG et al., *Megaloblastic bone marrow changes after repeated nitrous oxide anaesthesia.* Brit J Anaesth 58:1469–1470.

19. Bazarbachi A, Mukkit S, Ayas M, et al., (1998): *Thiamine responsive myelodysplasia.* Brit J haematol 102 : 1098.
20. Giannela RA, Broitman SA, Zamechk N (1971): *Vitamin B_{12} uptake by intestinal microorganisms: mechanisms and relevance to syndromes of bacterial overgrowth.* J clin Invest 50 : 1100.

CHAPTER

6 Anaemia of Chronic Disease

6.1 INTRODUCTION

Most patients of the tropic suffer from chronic infection or inflammation like tuberculosis or inflammatory bowel disease Anaemia of chronic disease (ACD) is probably the second most common cause of anaemia in the tropics. The inflammatory process produces suppression of bone marrow through inflammatory cytokines. This type of anaemia is characterized by low serum iron and iron binding capacity, low to normal transferrin level and increased macrophage store of iron in the bone marrow. Anaemia is normocytic, normochromic but may be also microcytic, hypochromic. Even when underlying disease can not be alleviated, anaemia often responds to erythropoietin in pharmacologic dosage. Anaemia of critical illness is an alike condition, which rapidly develops within few days and develops in some elderly persons without identifiable chronic disease. This type of anaemia is often exaggerated by suppressive effects of infection on bone marrow, disease-related or iatrogenic blood loss, or red cell destruction, which themselves are not severe enough to cause anaemia. Elderly patients in this defined subset have an elevated ESR and/or elevated C-reactive protein, a high plasma IL-6 concentration.

6.2 HISTORY

Physicians have known the pale appearance of patients with chronic infections for hundreds of years. In the 19th century Europe, tuberculosis was the major killer and the pallor associated with the disease was romanticized in the art literature of the time. The measurement of red cell mass revealed the association between inflammation and anaemia. Discussing "the alterations in the condition of the blood in inflammation" in section 372 of the 1859, William B Carpenter described the connection between the inflammation and anaemia. In 1961, 100 years later, Maxwell Wintrobe, in the 5th edition of Clinical Haematology, used the term "Simple Chronic Anaemia". Thereafter Wintrobe proposed "profound alteration in iron and porphyrin metablism," as the likely cause.

Incidence of anaemia of chronic disease is expected to increase all over the world as there is proportionate increase of elderly population and upsurge of HIV disease, which also sets up an inflammatory process.

6.3 PATHOGENESIS

The key questions about pathogenesis of anaemia of chronic disease still remain unanswered: (1) what accounts for the inability of the marrow to increase erythropoiesis (2) how is the deficit connected to the characistic hypoferraemia and sequestration of iron in macrophages and hepatocytes.

The diseases, which are often associated with chronic infection or inflammation, seem to be unrelated to ACD. Renal, hepatic and endocrinal disorders are not consistently associated with the characteristic abnormalities of iron metabolism. Hypoferremia does not usually accompany the anaemia of hypothyroidism or Addison disease. Renal insufficiency and cirrhosis are also not associated with the characteristic disturbances in iron metabolism unless inflammation or infection is present.

Disturbance in iron kinetics is the hallmark of ACD. Hypoferremia with normal to increased body iron store is the common presenting feature. Impaired flow of iron from the tissues to plasma appears to be the major explanation for the decreased serum iron. Multiple factors seem to be responsible.[1]

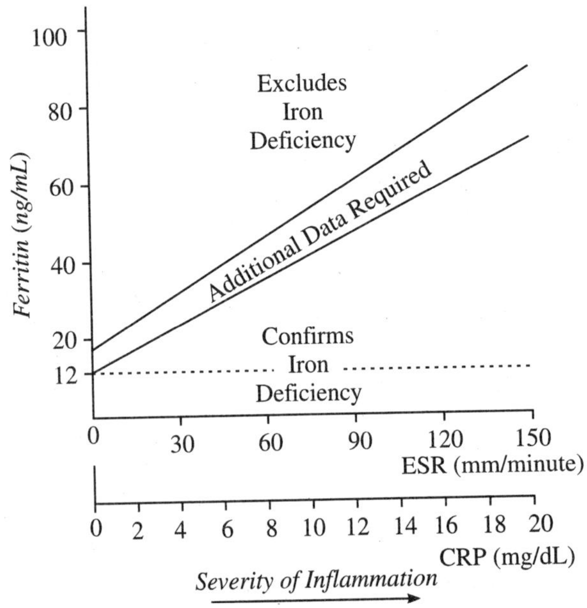

Fig. Diffrential diagnosis of ACD and IDA by graph of ferritin level plotted against ESR & CRP

It appears that iron is not released from intracellular sites when infection or inflammation is present. Macrophages, normally responsible for break down of senescent RBC in RE system, seem to sequester iron and produces hypoferremia. Hepatocytes and epithelial cells of GI mucosa also sequester iron and fail to release it to the plasma at a normal rate and to other storage compartments such as bone marrow.[2]

The macrophages of bone marrow of RE system are the major cells controlling the iron dynamics. The iron extracted from senescent red cells, is not released into plasma promptly, as in iron deficiency anaemia. Thus these macrophages contain an increased amount of iron. The factors leading to this restricted iron release in ACD is poorly understood. There are some possible mechanisms like:

(1) Interleukin-1 is a low molecular weight inflammatory mediator substance. Its effect on hepatocytes and macrophages may induce acute phase response seen with infections and inflammation. Erythropoietin (EpO) level is increased but less so as in iron deficiency anaemia. Production of erythropoietin is inhibited by inflammatory cytokines, IL-1 and TNFa and this inhibition is mediated through effects of transcription factor GATA-1 on EpO promoter. The patients who had renal disease with inflammation, as measured by increased serum CRP(>20mg/l) require on an average 80% higher dose of EpO than the patients with simple EpO deficiency due to renal disease.

(2) Another inflammatory cytokine, is IL-6, which induces Hepcidin, which, in turn, inhibits iron release from macrophages, and probably from hepatocytes, leading to hypoferremia.

(3) Inhibition of intestinal iron absorption is also probably due to inhibition by IL-6 and hepcidin-induced mechanism.

(4) Lactoferrin is an iron-binding protein found in milk and virtually in all body secretions, in fairly high concentration. Its concentration in plasma, is, however, very low. It is synthesized and stored in granulocytes and its release is stimulated during phagocytosis, by IL-1.Lactoferrin is almost similar to transferrin, the major transport protein of iron. Though structurally and immunologically it is different from transferrin, it can compete with and remove iron from transferrin, but it does not cause decrease iron absorption from GI tract. As a result of diversion of iron from the dynamic pool to the intracellular storage pool and an insufficient supply of iron for erythropoiesis in the bone marrow.[3]

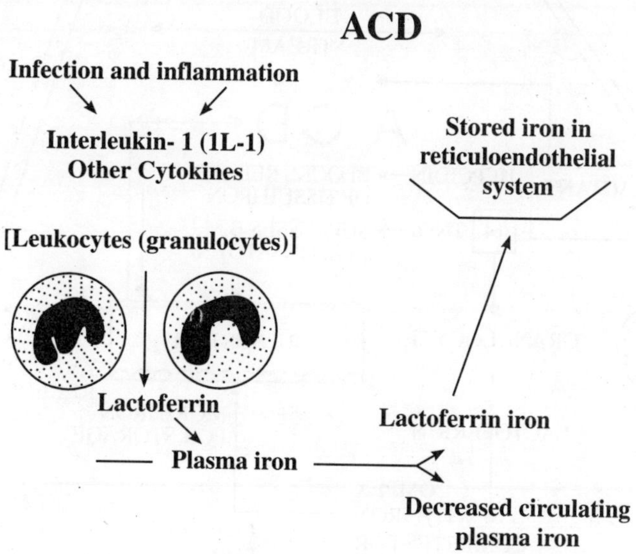

Fig. Pathogeneses of ACD in infection (Role of Lactoferrin)

(5) There is a haemolytic component that contributes to the development of anaemia in ACD. The RBC survival is mildly decreased (80-90 days). Cross-transfusion studies show that

haemolytic factor is outside the RBC. Hyperactivity of the RE system with increased phagocytic activity of the macrophage is believed to be responsible for increased RBC uptake and their shortened survival. Activated macrophages have an increased number of membrane receptor sites. This phenomenon is also related to inflammatory cytokines. [4]

6.4 CONSEQUENCES OF HYPOFERREMIA

Hypoferremia stimulates ferritin synthesis. This surplus binds to a larger (than normal) proportion of iron entering the cell and prevents its rapid release. Apoferritin behaves like an acute phase reactant and increases before there is increase of intracellular iron. Serum ferritin level reflects the amount of storage ferritin (intracellular). The serum ferritin level increases within 24 hours of infection or inflammation and remains so for several weeks and persists in chronic inflammation. The fundamental process of ACD seems to divert intracellular iron in to storage iron rather than its release in plasma, making the storage iron unavailable for erythropoiesis.[5]

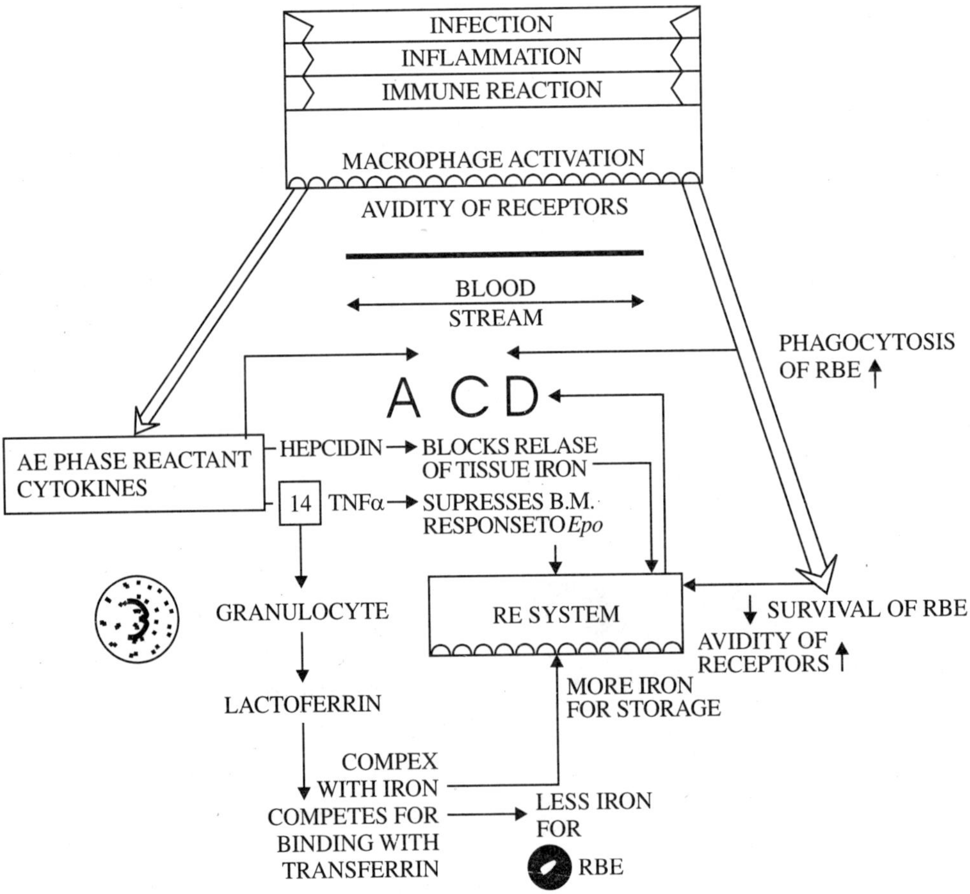

Fig. Pathogeneris of Anaemia in ACD

6.5 RELATION OF IRON METABOLISM TO INFECTION/INFLAMMATION

It is well known that most microorganisms require a specific iron concentration for optimal growth. When infection occurs, there is competition for iron between iron binding protein in the plasma and microorganisms. Thus transferrin and lactoferrin have an indirect effect to intracellular compartments, by binding to available iron and transporting it to intracellular compartments, where it is unavailable for utilization by microorganisms. The high concentration of lactoferrin in human breast milk is thought to have antibacterial effect through this mechanism.

It has been shown that induced by endotoxin or IL-1 administration increases resistance to infection. Thus it appears that mechanism to sequester iron have evolved as part of host response to infection, and, if chronic, could lead to anaemia [6]

Generally ACD is regarded as refractory to iron therapy, but when iron is given in parenteral saccharated form, a reticulocytosis can be elicited with mild increase in haemoglobin level. However, such therapy is never practiced as it may be dangerous to the patient.

6.6 RELATION OF CYTOKINES AND ACD

It is possible that IL-1 inhibits EpO synthesis or a precursor of EpO. IL-1 can cause a decrease in the synthesis of a number of proteins by the liver and other tissues while stimulating or increasing the synthesis of a variety of mediators of inflammation. It suppresses activity of bone marrow when inflammation is active.

Other elegant studies have shown direct inhibitory effect of IL-1, tumour necrosis factor, interferon^{g} and interferon^{b}. Other studies have shown that a number of cytokines play an adjuvant role in inhibiting erythropoiesis in ACD. [7]

6.7 ERYTHROPOIETIN LEVEL AND ACD.

Unique features of ACD are that the EpO level is not increased proportionate to the degree of anaemia. RBC 2,3-DPG levels are increased producing reduced affinity of haemoglobin, corresponding to degree of anaemia and hypoxaemia.

Erythropoiesis is also increased if erythropoietin is administered but a greater degree of hypoxaemia is necessary to stimulate erythropoiesis.[8]

6.8 MALIGNANCY AND ACD

The anaemia associated with malignancy is far less clear than that associated with inflammation and infectious disease. It is well established that suppression of erythropoietin by certain malignancies may occur In other studies, there are evidences that there may be a defect in bone marrow's ability to respond to erythropoietin. Thus factors operating in malignancy in producing anaemia may be somewhat different from those producing ACD.[9]

6.9 THERAPY OF ACD

To be brief, therapy of ACD is entirely dependent on underlying pathological condition, The anaemia usually resolves after amelioration of infection or inflammation or effective chemotherapy of malignant disease. However, associated aggravating factors like blood loss or iron deficiency needs proper attention. Here it is worthy to mention that any existing iron deficiency must be evaluated and this has been discussed in chapter of "Diagnostic Approaches"

REFERENCES

1. Biergard G (1980): *The source of serum ferritin during infection: studies with concavalin A-sepharose absorption*. Clin Sci 59:385-387
2. Brock Jh, Esparaza I (1979): *Failure of reticulocytes to take up iron from lactoferrin saturated by various methods*. Brit J Haematol 42:481-483
3. Catwright GE (1966): *The anaemia of chronic disorders*. Brit J Haematol 21:147-152.
4. EastagateJA, Symons JA, Wood NC, et al (1988): *Correlation of plasma Interleukin I levels with disease activity in rheumatoid arthritis*. Lancet2: 706-709.
5. Fillet J, Cook JD, Finch CA, . (1974): *Storage iron kinetics: VII. A biologic model for reticulo-endothelial iron transport*. J clin Invest 53:1527-1533.
6. Konijn AM, Hershko C. (1977): *Ferritin synthesis in inflammation:1. Pathogenesis of impaired iron release*. Br J Haematol 37: 7-16.
7. Means RT, KrantzSB (1992); *Progress in understanding of the anaemia in chronic disease*, 80: 1630-1647.
8. Zaroulis CG, Kourides IA, Valeri CR.(1977): *Red cell 2,3 –diphosphoglycerate and oxygen affinity of haemoglobin in patients with thyroid disorders*. Blood52: 181-186.
9. Zucker S, Lysik RM, Distefano M. (1980): *Cancer cell inhibition of erythropoiesis*. Lab clin Med. 96:770-782.

CHAPTER

7 Enzymopathy and Membrane Defects of Red Cells

7.1 GLUCOSE 6 PHOSPHATE DEHYDROGENASE DEFICIENCY

Introduction

Erythrocytes are non-nucleated but living cells, which are dependent on several enzymatic pathways for their metabolism. They obtain energy from breakdown of glucose, 95% of which is metabolized by anaerobic glycolysis to lactate and in the process ATP is produced. 5% of glucose is metabolized via HMP shunt pathway, during which reduced NADP is produced. Red cell membrane is also not an inert cellular membrane, but contains several enzymes, which give protection against breakdown of red cells. There are many inherited enzymopathies, which are governed by defective genes, controlling the expression of these enzymes. Among these Glucose 6 phosphate dehydrogenase (G6PD) deficiency needs special mention in the tropics, not only for the fact that this enzyme is the first and foremost rate limiting enzyme of HMP shunt pathway, but also due to the fact that this condition produces diagnostic dilemmas along with a number of important drug reactions in the tropical countries. [1]

Pathogenesis of the clinical condition

In red cells reduced glutathione is synthesized at high concentration and has the function of restoring oxidized sulfhydryl group. NADPH is essential for the regeneration of glutathione sulfhydryl group. Glucose 6 phosphate dehydrogenase deficiency and a reduction of synthesis of NADPH exposes red cells to oxidation of haemoglobin with intracellular precipitation of Heinz bodies, as well as of several enzymes and of several lipids and proteins in the membrane, with consequent haemolysis. [2]

About 400 million of world population, carry one or two gene for G6PD deficiency. Highest frequency is found in sub Saharan African countries, where 32% of males are affected. In Saridinans and Kurdish Jews, prevalence in male exceeds 50%.

TABLE 7.1 : Genetic variants of G6PD deficiency

Class	p.c. of G6DP activity	Manifestations	Genetic polymorphism	Zone
Class I	Nearly absent	Cong non-spherocytic anaemia	—	—

Class II	<10% (severe deficiency)	Severe Intermittent haemolysis	Medeterranen, Mali, Union	Zone I Mediterranean area, North Africa, Western Asia, Indian subcontinent
Class III	10-60% (moderate deficiency)	Less severe Intermittent haemolysis	Canton, Mahidal	Zone II SE Asia, China, Korea
Class IV	60-100% (normal)	None	B, A, Gambia	Zone III Subsaharan Africa
Class V	>150% (Increased)	None	--	--

In zone II two severely deficient classII variants $Gd^{Medeterranean}$ and Gd^{Union}as well as two moderately deficient $Gd^{Mahidol}$ and Gd^{Canton} are commonly prevalent..

Asia is remarkable for frequency of number of variants e.g. in population of Tawii, at least nine variants are prevalent, of which $Gd^{Tawian\ Hakka}$ is most prevalent. Zone II population achieves high polymorphic frequency, and in zone III up to 40% carry the GdA variant with normal enzyme activity [3]

In Australia or America, deficient variants usually occur in descendants of Africa, Mediterranean area and Asian immigrants, but not in indigenous population.

7.2 CLINICAL PICTURE

Episodes of haemolysis and jaundice occur in four situations: (1) In neonates (2) Severe infections (3) Ingestion of certain food (4) Exposure to certain drugs and chemicals. These intermittent episodes are more severe with class II variants..

Usual presentations are:

(1) Anaemia is generally moderate with microcytosis, spherocytosis, anisocytosis and polychromasia. On the fourth day of life, serum bilirubin is often elevated, and this is found in all parts of world

(2) Neonatal jaundice is recognized as major health problem in Greece, Saudi Arabia, tropical Africa, South-East Asia, China, Hong Kong (12%) and Singapore (10%)

Clinical picture depends upon severity of enzyme deficiency and prematurity of infant and the liver enzyme system thereby. [4]

Haemolysis may take place under following conditions:

(1) Infections: umbilical sepsis, pneumonia, septicaemia, may precipitate episodes of haemolysis in infants. Infection induced haemolysis is found in adults, in viral infections like hepatitis or viral enteritis or respiratory tract infection. In bacterial infections like pneumonia, typhoid, paratyphoid, also haemolysis is triggered.

Possible mechanism of haemolysis in infection is generation of H_2O_2 by activated neutrophils and macrophages triggering haemolysis and consequent liver dysfunction leads to hepatocellular jaundice.

Infection also produces suppression of bone marrow, which makes the anaemia more severe. The course is further complicated in cases of concomittant UTI, renal ischaemia, tubular obstruction by released haemoglobin. Life threatening renal failure may also occur. Treatment is mainly supportive

(2) Exposure of mother or infant to oxidant drugs like primaquin, pamaquin, chloroquin, sulphonamide, dapsone, sulfasalazine, chloramphenicol, vitamin k analogues, may precipitate haemolysis. Use of mentholated powder around umbilicus in neonates, (as practiced in many parts of developing countries) may predispose to haemolysis. Drugs that produce haemolysis in G6DP dehyrgenase deficient red cells are of two groups (1) drugs which cause oxidative damage to red cells e.g. phenylhydrazine, phenylbutazone, acetanilide, (2) drugs that cause haemolysis only in deficient subjects but not in subjects with normal enzyme activity e.g. primaquin, pamaquin. Drug induced haemolysis may occur in adults due to nephrotoxic drugs

7.3 THERAPY FOR DEFICIENT INFANTS

When bilirubin is > 250mmol/dl or 15mg/dl, in the serum, in mature or otherwise healthy infant, phototherapy is indicated, which is effected by fluorescent tubes of 20 watt placed 40 cm above the naked infant, eyes being shielded. Alternatively exposure to morning sunlight with shielding of eyes and cooling of body is also effective. Exchange transfusion from donors with normal level of Glucose-6-phosphae-dehydrogenase and with compatible blood for mother and infant, is a form of therapy. This is indicated when uncojugated bilirubin is > 300mmol/l and brain damage is inevitable. Transfusion is given in a dose twice that of infant's blood volume i.e. 2x 85 ml/kg BW, in 20 ml aliquots over a period of two hour, This usually combats haemolytic episode, when it is severe. Phototherapy and exchange transfusion are indicated at lower bilirubin level in low BW and ill infants [5]

Malaria and G6DP deficiency- This enzyme deficiency confers advantage in case of P falciparum infection. Global deficiency reaches highest where P falcilarum infection is endemic. Here limitation of malaria is seen in heterozygotes only. In severe malaria, in west and east Africa, significant protection is seen in both male and female heterozygotes, whereas in mild malaria, it is found in females only. Parasitic growth is impaired in parasitized cells and due to hemolysis, there is early engulfment of parasites by macrophages. Sometimes oxidative stress is required for this process, oxidant radicals cause growth impairment and early phagocytosis of red cells with damaged membrane.

Prophylactic therapy for vivax malaria should be guided by G6DP dehydrogenase measurement, if the deficiency is prevalent in the community [6].

(5) Ingestion of fava beans (vicia faba) or inhalation of its pollen may produce haemolysis inGlucose-6-phosphate deficient subjects. It may occur after ingestion of fresh, dried, or frozen beans, in breast fed infants may follow ingestion of beans by mother. [7]

In Nigeria, haemolysis may occur after ingestion of roasted meat (kabab) cooked with an orange colouring agent. This is a napthol derivative. Starting from a few hours to 3 days there is rapidly progressive anaemia reaching a nadir in 7-8 days. Continued exposure to the offending agent may produce severe anaemia or renal failure. [8]

7.4 CONTROL PROGRAMME

(1) Glucose-6-phosphate dehydrogenase deficiency is screened in cord blood of all infants in vulnerable areas.
(2) All these infants are observed in the hospital for 2 weeks and treated promptly if jaundice appears.
(3) Both the general public and health professionals are educated in this respect.
(4) Information is carried during delivery of the next baby.
(5) Card is issued to the deficient babies warning against haemolyzing drugs.
(6) Non-traumatic delivery should be always attempted to avoid haematoma on the infant with G6PD deficiency.
(7) Strict hygienic measures are maintained in the puerperium to avoid infection.

7.5 MEMBRANE DEFECTS

Red cell membrane is supported by protein skeleton, sides of which are spectrin tetramers, these are linked at corners of hexagons by actin, tropomyosin and protein 4.1 and is attached to lipid bilayer by anykrin and band 3 (the major transmembrane protein and anion transporter).

Red cell membrane defects are inherited diseases due to mutations in various membrane skeletal proteins, resulting in decreased red cell deformability, reduced red cell life span and premature removal of erythrocytes from the circulation. There are four main types: (1) Hereditary Spherocytosis (2) Hereditary Elliptocytosis (3) Hereditary Ovalocytosis and (4) Hereditary Stomatocytosis.

Hereditary Spherocytosis- this condition displays autosomal dominant inheritance in 75% of cases, the remaining cases show recessive forms and de novo mutations. The chief clinical features comprise of haemolytic anaemia, which can range from compensated to severe forms, sometimes require exchange transfusion at birth or need repeated transfusion. Patients may have variable jaundice, splenomegaly, and cholelithiasis. Abnormal protein may be detected by SDS-PAGE (sodium dodecyl sulphate-polyacramide gel) analysis of red cell membrane. Deficiency of band 3 and anykrin has been found in 54% and 31% of cases and the rest of the cases are found to be unclassified by this method. Splenomegaly and gall- stones are more frequent in band 3 deficiencies, and anaemia, neonatal jaundice and need for transfusion is commonly found in spectrin than in band 3 deficiencies. Spectrin deficiency is usually detected in childhood and band 3 deficiency is detected in adult. Splenectomy corrects anaemia usually in all cases but spectrin-deficient patients show a slightly lower median rise in haemoglobin level. Red cell osmotic fragility, when tested show sensitivity in 48% to 95% of cases, independent of the cytoskeletal abnormality and the amount of protein band deficiency.

Clinically there are three varieties: mild, moderate and severe. The classification is based on haemoglobin level (mild 11-15, mod 8-12, severe 6-8mg/dl); haemolytic parameters (reticulocyte count: 3-6% mild, >6% mod, >10% severe); Serum bilirubin (17-34mg/l mild, >34 mg/l mod, >51mg/l severe).

Hereditary Elliptocytosis- this condition is an autosomal dominant disorder, more common in malarial endemic regions of West Africa. Usually patients are asymptomatic, 10% of cases have moderate to severe anaemia, including a few reported cases of hydrops foetalis. The severe variant form of the condition, known as pyropolikilocytosis, is characterized by reduced elasticity of red cell cytoskeleton and membrane fragmentation. The mutations responsible lie in the SPTA1, SPTB gene and EPB 41 gene encoding for protein band 4.1. Very few cases need surgery.

Hereditary Stomatocytosis- this condition presents in two varieties: (1) Over-hydrated and dehydrated. The first one is characterized by increased cell volume without concomitant increase in membrane surface area due to marked increase of intracellular sodium as a result of cell's inability to regulate its cation homeostasis. Cells are oval and seen to be marked on its periphery by two transverse ridges, (hence its name), in peripheral blood smear. Dehydrated form is characterized by loss of cell water, increased cytoplasmic viscosity and a typical increased MCHC. Clinical features include well-compensated mild to moderate anaemia and enlarged spleen. Splenectomy is strictly contraindicated in dehydrated variety as it may precipitate venous thrombosis.

Ovalocytosis-Molecular basis of South East Asian ovalocytosis is a deletion of 27 nucleotides, resulting in 9 amino acids in band 3, increased membrane rigidity and oval shape. Inheritance is autosomal dominant. Homozygotes have not been found. The condition is lethal. It is prevalent in Malayasia, Indonesia, New Guinea. Reduced parasitic invasion into rigid membrane causes lower rate of P. vivax and falciparum infection. Malarial anaemia is aggravated by ovalocytosis. The mechanism of protection against cerebral malaria is likely to be related to differences of adherence of parasitized red cells to endothelium [9].

Treatment of haemolytic anaemia due to red cell membrane defect depends on the clinical variety. Supportive therapy is done in mild cases; surgery is indicated in moderate type before puberty and necessary in severe forms. Supportive therapy consists of folate therapy in first few years of life. In moderate and severe forms, in which surgery is usually delayed up to six years, supportive therapy is indicated. It is also indicated during pregnancy, during aplastic crisis and infection. Usual prophylactic therapy with vaccination and antibiotic therapy along with proper counseling should be done. Re-immunization of the child is not usually recommended. Iron overload and gall stone should be monitored and treated [10].

In the tropics, particularly in ethnic areas, awareness of G6DP dehydrogenase deficiency and of various membrane defects of red cells is essential for evaluation of unexplained anaemia, neonatal jaundice and haemolytic episode after drug ingestion or particular type of food intake.

REFERENCES

1. WHO Working Group.(1989): *Glucose-6-phosphate dehydrogenase deficiency*. Bull World Health Organ 67:601-11.
2. Luzzato L (1993): *G6PD deficiency and haemolytic anaemia*. In Nathan DG and Oski RA (eds) Haematology of Infancy and childhood, 4th ed. Philadelphia WB Saunders: 674-695.
3. Huang C-S, Hung K-L, Huang M-J et al (996): *Neonatal jaundice and molecular mutation in glucose 6 phosphate dehydrogenase deficient new born infants*. Am J Haematol 51:19-25.
4. HO NK (1992). *Neonatal jaundice in Asia*. Beullerias Clin Haematol 5: 131-142.
5. Chan MCK (1992): *Glucose-6-phosphate dehydrogenase deficiency*. Postgrad Doct Middle East 5:10-15.
6. Rawande C, Hill A. (1998): *Glucose06-phosphate dehydrogenase deficiency and Malaria*. J Mol Med 76: 581-586:

7. Galiano S, Gatani GE, Barbino A et al,(1990): *Favism in the African type of glucose-6-phosphate deficiency*. (A). BMJ300:236.

8. William CKO, Osotimethim BO, Ogunmola GB and Awotedin AA. (1988): *Haemolytic anaemia associated with Nigerian barbecued meat (red Suya)*. Afr J Med Sci 17:71-75.

9. Coppadora M, Girbaldi G, O'Brian E,et al (1998): *Early phagocytosis of erythrocytes parasitized by P falciparum may explain malaria protection in G6PD deficiency*. Blood 92:2527-2534.

10. W Barcellini, P Bianchi, E Ferns, FG Imperiale, Anna P Marcello, C Varcellati, A Zanininoic, A Zanella (2011): *Hereditary red cell membrane defect: diagnostic and clinical aspects*. Blood Transfusion July, (3): 874-77.

Part III

Malignant Disorder

CHAPTER

8 Acute Myeloid Leukaemia

8.1 INTRODUCTION

Acute Myeloid Leukaemia represents a group of clonal haemopoietic stem cell disorder in which both failure to differentiate and over proliferation in the stem cell compartment results in accumulation of non-functional cells termed myeloblasts. While the specific cause of this biological abnormality is unknown in any individual patient, the genetic background has been well established by modern researches and this helps to a great extent to a rational approach to the therapy, which is, now-a-days, designated as targeted therapy. The targeted therapy means the therapy which is directed towards the molecular defect of the cells which undergo malignant proliferation. Molecular pathogenesis of leukaemia has been studied in great detail recently and a vast amount of knowledge and information has been accumulated in this area in recent times. We first elaborate this for better understanding of its different aspects.

8.2 MOLECULAR PATHOGENESIS AND CLASSIFICATION OF LEUKAEMIA

Molecular pathogenesis has greatly changed the classification of acute myeloid leukaemia, which is essentially required for planning therapy. The traditional classification of AML was based on morphological and histochemical characteristics of peripheral blood and bone marrow cells. This is now superseded by new WHO classification. This is because of the fact that all the subtypes of AML may have overlapping clinical syndrome, (described later), but they may belong to the same variety and may respond to identical therapy. For example, increased incidence of Disseminated Intravascular Coagulation (DIC) in promyelocytic variety and increased incidence of extramedullary leukaemia in monocytic variety are frequently seen, but they fundamentally represent the same disease. The most important prognostic factor determining the outcome of therapy are the acquired genetic changes in the leukemic cells, determined by cytogenetics technique, fluorescence hybridization analysis (FISH) or polymerase chain reaction (PCR).

Acute myeloid leukaemia is a consequence of acquired somatic mutation of haemopoietic progenitor cells that confers a proliferation growth advantage to the affected cells. The mutation involves a balanced reciprocal chromosomal translocation, which results in creation of a new fusion gene. These translocations involve the genes that normally have a major role in the maturation and differentiation of hemopoietic progenitor cells. By transferring these genes and fusing them with other genes, their function is distorted and a block in maturation and differentiation can occur. The progression to acute leukaemia may require multiple genetic events until the transformed genotype is able to be expressed.

8.3 CLASSIFICATION OF AML

I. FAB Classification

Classification within this category is based on cell features of morphology, cytochemistry, and maturation.

The different categories are:

M0: Acute myeloblastic leukaemia, minimally differentiated (no visible myeloid feature)

M1: Acute myeloblastic leukaemia without maturation (undifferentiated myeloblastic)

M2: Acute myeloblastic leukaemia with maturation (undifferentiated myeloblastic with classic myeloblasts and Auer rods)

M3: Acute promyelocytic leukaemia (AML with t(15; 17)(q22; q12); (PML/RARÎ±) and variants)

M4: Acute myelomonocytic leukaemia

M5: Acute monoblastic leukaemia and acute monocytic leukaemia (classic monocytic)

M6: Acute erythroid leukaemia

M7: Acute megakaryoblastic leukaemia

II. Histochemical Classification

Two types of histochemical stains are used to delineate the immature malignant cells: These are enzymatic (peroxidase and esterase), and non-enzymatic (Sudan Black and periodic Acid Schiff) stains. Peroxidase and esterase stains are particularly useful for accurate morphological classification of AML. Unequivocal peroxidase positive staining of the cells is usually diagnostic of AML. The esterases are often helpful when peroxidase is negative. It must be emphasized that a negative peroxidase or esterase stain may still be found in AML, when we have to depend on other characteristics of the cells, for identification.

III. WHO Classification

The World Health Organization (WHO) Classification System incorporates clinical, morphologic (i.e., FAB Classification information), immunophenotypic, cytogenetic, and molecular data. [1] There are also some differences for defining the criteria of diagnosis.

The threshold of blast cells, for the diagnosis, of AML is reduced from 30% to 20% blasts in the blood or marrow. In addition, patients with the clonal, recurring cytogenetic abnormalities t(8; 21)(q22; q22), inv(16)(p13q22) or t(16; 16)(p13; q22), and t(15; 17)(q22; q12) should be considered to have AML regardless of the blast percentage.

8.4 CLASSIFICATION PROPER

1. AML with recurrent genetic abnormalities:

1. AML with t(8; 21)(q22; q22); (AML1(CBF alpha)/ETO.
2. AML with abnormal marrow eosinophils.
   (*i*) inv(16)(p13q22).
   (*ii*) t(16;16)(p13;q22) (CBFb/MYH11).

3. Acute promyelocytic leukaemia (AML with t(15; 17)(q22; q12) (PML/RARa) and variants (included as M3 in the FAB classification).
4. AML with 11q23 (MLL) abnormalities.

2. AML with multilineage dysplasia (de novo or following a myelodysplastic syndrome):
Most cases of refractory anemia with excess of blasts in transformation fall in the latter category.

3. AML, therapy-related:
1. Alkylating agent-related AML.
2. Topoisomerase II inhibitor-related AML.

4. Acute leukaemia of ambiguous lineagae:
1. Undifferentiated acute leukaemia (leukaemic blasts show no or minimal signs of morphologic and/or protein expression signs of maturation).
2. Bilineal acute leukaemia (more than one cell lineage that demonstrates leukemic transformation).
3. Biphenotypic acute leukaemia (a single population of leukaemic blasts have simultaneous expression of protein expression markers of different hemopoetic cell lineages).

5. AML not otherwise categorized (including the FAB morphology-based M0 to M2, and M4 to M7 categories):
1. AML minimally differentiated (FAB M0).
2. AML without maturation (FAB M1).
3. AML with maturation (FAB M2).
4. AML (FAB M4).
5. Acute monoblastic and monocytic leukaemia (FAB M5a and M5b respectively).
6. Acute erythroid leukaemia (FAB M6).
   (*i*) Erythroleukemia (FAB M6a).
   (*ii*) Pure erythroid leukaemia (FAB M6b).
7. Acute megakaryoblastic leukaemia (FAB M7).
8. Acute basophilic leukaemia.
9. Acute panmyelosis with myelofibrosis.
10. Myeloid (granulocytic) sarcoma.

8.5 IMMUNOPHENOTYPIC ANALYSIS

This is especially useful to detect minimal residual disease. Myeloid blasts are characterized by the presence of CD13 and CD33 antigens. AML M0 and M5 types may present with undifferentiated peroxidase negative cells. Immuno-haemotyping, in such cases, may help to determine the diagnosis of blast cells. AML blasts may simultaneously express both myeloid and lymphoid antigens. These may include CD2, CD5, CD7, CD10 and CD19. [2]

It is not surprising, however, that many patients with so-called AML, present with ALL, especially when analyzed for leukaemia-specific immunophenotype. In the past, these leukaemias were often termed biphenotypic leukaemias. It is now recognized that these are AML with lymphoid markers and should be treated as typical AML. True biphenotypic leukaemia is rare.

Terminal deoxynucleotidyl Transferase (TdT), typically a marker commonly associated with lymphoblastsis has been reported in increasing number of patients of AML. Though its prognostic significance is still being debated, it is often used as a marker of acute leukaemia.

8.6 HIERARCHICAL CYTOGENETIC PROGNOSTIC CLASSIFICATION

Favorable

t(8;21), t(15;17), inv(16), either alone or in conjunction with other changes

Intermediate

1. Normal, +8, +21, +22, del(7q), abnormal 11q23, or other structural/numerical abnormalities
2. Lack of additional favorable or adverse abnormalities

Adverse

–5, del(5q), –7, abnormal 3q, complex (> 4 unrelated changes) alone or in conjunction with intermediate-risk or other adverse-risk abnormalities. [3]

8.7 CYTOGENETIC ABNORMALITIES AND ITS RELATION WITH THERAPY AND PROGNOSIS

The most common targets of AML-associated chromosomal translocations are genes that encode DNA-binding transcription factors or regulatory components of transcriptional complexes. Cloning of AML-associated (8, 21) translocation led to the identification of AML1-CBF beta, a transcription factor that regulates a number of haemopoiesis-specific genes and is essential for normal development of hemopoietic system. Therapeutic approach with differentiation-inducing agent, all-trans-retinoic acid (ATRA) which targets the chimeric protein encoded by t (15, 17) translocation is the most successful attempt.

Abnormalities of chromosome 5& 7 (del 5q, del 7q) are commonly associated with alkylating agent related AML or in elderly patients with de novo AML. These variants often have a more resistant form of disease with a somewhat less likelihood of attaining complete remission with therapy. [4] Most of these types are preceded by a more indolent form of leukaemia that is often referred to as myelodysplastic syndrome. Topoisomerase inhibitor related AML tends to develop without a pre leukaemic phase and involve mainly the 11q23 chromosome.

In general, patients with a normal karyotype have a better prognosis. Patients with a single karyotype abnormality, have a better prognosis than patients with multiple or complex cytogenetics abnormalities. Exceptions are those with inversion16, t (8; 21), (15; 17). These patients have a better prognosis than patients with a normal karyotype. [4]

8.8 PROGNOSTIC INDICATORS

Different clinical studies show that, the following factors are the prognostic indicators.

1. Unfavourable karyotype
2. Age > 60 years with de novo AML

3. Poor performance status of the patient
4. Secondary AML
5. Multi-drug resistance
6. High WBC count at diagnosis

In multivariate analysis, however, only the karyotype is found to be true predictive of outcome.

8.9 INCIDENCE AND EPIDEMIOLOGY

The incidence is approximately 2.4 per 1000,000. It increases progressively with age. Acute leukaemia accounts for 10% of all human malignancy and is the leading cause of cancer deaths in young adults, the incidence of AML being much higher than that of acute lymphoid type, which is reverse of the incidence pattern in childhood.

8.10 PREDISPOSING FACTORS

Although exact cause of chromosomal aberration is unknown, several risk factors have been found to be related with increased incidence. Leukaemia following radiation exposure has been documented after atomic explosion in Hiroshima and Nagasaki. Leukomogenesis has been also observed after therapeutic irradiation for such diseases as ankylosing spondylitis. Benzene exposure has been closely associated with subsequent development of leukaemia. Exposure to phenylbutazone, arsenic, thorotrast and chloramphenicol may lead to the future development of leukaemia. Cytotoxic therapy, especially with alkylating agents, like mephalan, chlorambucil etc. increases the risk of leukaemia 4–7 years later. The risk seems to be related to the total dose of the agent than to the duration of therapy.

The combination of radiation with alkylating agent, which are frequently used for treatment of Hodgkin lymphoma, is found to carry the highest risk of leukaemia, especially, AML. Therapy-related or secondary leukaemia has a poorer prognosis than de novo leukaemia, not associated with prior cytotoxic therapy.

There is evidence implicating RNA viruses in the aetiology of animal leukaemia. A similar etiologic agent has been implicated in adult T-cell leukaemia, which is human T-cell leukaemia type I (HTLV-I). Congenital factors and immunologic deficiency may be also important in the pathogenesis particularly in acute leukaemia of childhood.

8.11 CLINICAL AND LABORATORY FEATURES OF AML

Most patients with AML present with progressive fatigue and commonly have evidence of infection or bleeding diathesis. The white blood cell (WBC) count is usually elevated but may be low or normal. It is not necessary for leukaemic blasts to be present in the peripheral blood for the diagnosis of AML to be made. In fact the term leukaemia is a misnomer in this instance because the diagnosis can be made in the presence of leukaemic cells in the bone marrow. Anaemia is present and often profound. thrombocytopenia is also common.

Patients may present with petechiae, ecchymoses, haematuria, or gastrointestinal bleeding. Haemorrhage in the CNS is often a fatal complication. It occurs most commonly in patients who present with very high leucocyte count. Disseminated intravascular coagulation presents with petechae, gingival bleeding or even life threatening bleeding. It is most often seen in patients with promyelocytic leukaemia, but can also occur in myelomonocytic and monocytic leukaemia. In the last two varities, signs of extramedullary involvement, including gingival hypertrophy, skin infiltration (leukaemia cutis) or meningeal leukaemia, may be seen. Rarely, a solid tumor mass, known as chloroma or granulocytic sarcoma, may be seen and is the only presenting feature of AML.

Examination of peripheral blood smear may reveal dysplastic changes in the red cells, granulocytes and platelets. Diagnosis is based on the presence of typical blast cell in the peripheral blood. Blast cytoplasm frequently contains Auer rods (azurophilic granules in the lysosomes). The rapid turnover of leukaemic blasts produces a hypermetabolic state with increased levels of lactate dehydrogenase (LDH) and uric acid. The bone marrow is usually hypercellular and often is replaced by leukaemic blast cells.

Uncommonly the bone marrow is hypocellular. In this csase, the diagnosis is somewhat more difficult to establish and depends on very precise delineation of the cells that are present. Ideally the cytogenetics and immunohaemotypic analysis is used for confirmation.

Electrolyte imbalances, such as hypokalaemia or hypophosphataemia are common features at presentation. However, these abnormalities depend upon the ongoing metabolism or lysis of blast cells before collection.

Pseudo-hyperkalaemia may be present, usually in patients with high WBC count, and may be confirmed by checking an anti-coagulated specimen of plasma. Pseudo-hypoglycaemia may be present as a result of glucose utilization by blast cells. The rapid oxygen consumption by large number of leukocytes, also known as leukocyte larceny, leads to pseudohypoxaemia, which may make it impossible to determine the arterial blood oxygen accurately.

8.12 TREATMENT OF ACUTE PROMYELOCYTIC LEUKAEMIA (APL)

Induction Therapy

Several studies confirm that APL is sensitive to Anthracycline, due to significantly lower Pgp expression and other resistance marker in leukaemic cells. Both daunorubicin and idarubicin, used as single agent, or with anthracycline, induce a complete remission (CR) in 60–80% of patients. Study of Southwest Oncology group showed an improved survival time when dose of anthracycline is increased without a change in cytarabine dose. However, induction mortality remains 10% and acquired resistance contributes to 20–30% of patients. [5]

The incidence of coagulopathy and bleeding diminished significantly with ATRA therapy but the retinoic acid syndrome remains the major toxicity. Incidence of toxicity is approximately 15%. The mortality has been reduced significantly with institution of Dexamethasone which also reduces incidence of RAS. Consolidation Chemotherapy is mandatory and lower dose of cytarabine appears to be efficacious.

Maintenance Therapy

It appears that patients with APL may benefit from maintenance ATRA, with or without cytarabine.

8.13 TREATMENT OF AML OTHER THAN APL

Induction Therapy

For patients less than 55–60 years old standard regimen of daunorubicin 45 mg IV for three days plus cytarabine 100 mg IV by continuous infusion for 7 days usually produce remission completely. Anasarmine, Mitoxantrone, aclacinomycin have been shown to produce an improvement in overall result, when compared with daunorubicin 45 mg/m^2 dose. Intensifying induction therapy through higher dose of cytarabine or etoposide, clearly have an effect on disease free survival, although not affecting initial CR. [6]

8.14 POST REMISSION THERAPY

AML with favourable cytogenetics

Only two of large prospective studies of post-remission therapy have rigorously analyzed post remission data by cytogenetics prognostic group. The initial response rate in favourable group was approximately 85%. With intensive post-remission therapy the overall survival at 5 years exceeds 50%. Recently based on CALBG data it has been postulated that it may be appropriate not to administer high dose cytarabine to patients with t (8; 21) abnormality, in which the disease free survival was 60% without using high dose cytarabine.

Whether autologous stem cell transplantation should be offered as post remission therapy to patients with favourable cytogenetics remains controversial. US Inter-group study suggested that autologous stem cell transplant after four cycles of therapy may be particularly useful. Except for young patients in whom fertility remains a consideration, it is reasonable to use autologous stem cell transplantation. Experienced centers show a data of low morbidity and therapy related mortality of 3–5%.

Patients who do not have HLA-matched sibling should receive high dose cytarabine of 1.5 mg/m^2 to 3 mg/m^2, the optimal duration and number of total dose vary with the patients. Cycles are better than single dose of chemotherapy. For patients up to 55–65 years of age and those having intermediate risk, allogenic transplant show 3 year survival rate of 65% and relapse risk at 3 years at 18%, therefore this is the recommended therapy in this group. Patients with unfavourable prognosis show poorest outcome, though initial response rate is 50%. The overall long time survival is poor, whatever may be the mode of post-remission therapy. The MRC AML 10 study reported that among the group with unfavourable cytogenetics, allogenic graft did not offer any advantage. Because of extremely high rate of relapse and poor long term outcome either matched unrelated donor or matched family donor is selected.

8.15 BONE MARROW TRANSPLANT

The preponderance of data demonstrates that autologous transplant i.e., reintroduction of patient's own bone marrow provides better anti-leukaemic activity, than allogeneic bone marrow transplant. Bone marrow transplant is effective in younger age group. The anti-leukaemic benefit is negated by high procedural mortality (14% in US Inter-group and 18% in MRC AML group).When bone marrow is used as source of stem cells, by this procedure morbidity is considerable with a median time of neutrophil recovery of 25 days and over 7 weeks for platelet recovery. Bone marrow transplant (BMT) in AML will be discussed in detail in "guidelines of management".

8.16 AML IN OLDER PATIENTS

Older patients, who do not have significant co-morbidities, should be treated with standard induction therapy. 50% can have complete remission. The major difficulty is in selection of post-remission therapy. Though patients can tolerate one cycle of cytarabine at somewhat lower dose than that in younger adults, it has never been shown to improve the long term outcome. Current strategy to treat these patients is by non-myeloblastic immunomodulation following induction and limited post-remission therapy. Phase III studies evaluating role of IL-2/histamine, IL-2 and Fit-3 ligand are conducted in these patients. [7]

8.17 TARGETED THERAPY OF AML IN SIGNAL TRANSDUCTION PATHWAY

Receptor tyrosine kinase (RTK) has an immunoglobulin like domain on membrane and an intracellular domain with tyrosine kinase activity. Grb2 and SOS are two adaptor proteins that bridge the association of RTK with ras (a family of guanosine nucleotidase). Receptor gets dimerization and RTK gets phosphorylated when attracted by extracellular ligand. RTK in turn activates the ras through adaptor protein. This causes a conformational change in ras by GTP binding and products interact with effector protein. As a result signal transduction occurs, which promotes normal cellular proliferation and maturation. Abnormal signal transduction occurs in AML due to Tyrosine kinase receptor mutation and ras mutation.

8.18 INHIBITORS OF ABNORMAL SIGNAL TRANSDUCTION

Farnesyl-transferase inhibitors target the post-translational modification of ras to prevent sub-cellular localization necessary for participation in signal transduction. FT inhibitor R 11 5777 is given in doses from 100 mg to 1200 mg twice daily for 21 days. Dose-limiting neurotoxicity was encountered at 1200 mg twice daily.

1. SU 5416 blocks the activity of both vascular and endothelial growth factor receptor 2 (VEGFR2) and stem cell factor (SCF) receptor. Treatment with SU 5416 has been recently been described in AML patients on refractory relapse.
2. Blocking ligand binding or RTK activation is in preclinical stage of development. [8]

8.19 IMMUNOTHERAPY

Monoclonal antibodies may halt the malignant process in three ways:

1. Immunologic injury to cells, which may be either complement-mediated or cell dependent
2. React with cell receptors resulting in modulation of signal transduction
3. Directly leads to apoptosis.

Three types of monoclonal antibodies are studied in AML:

1. **Unconjugated Monoclonal Antibody:** This targets CD33 antigen, a glycoprotein present in blasts in 90% of cases of AML. It is also expressed on normal early myeloid or erythroid progenitors but not in haemopoietic stem cells or non-haemopoietic tissue. Current trials are examining HuM 195 in combination with retinoic acid or arsenic trioxide in first relapse. [9]

2. **Drug Conjugates or Immunoconjugates:** The drug conjugate, Mylotarg has been developed, which joins a humanized anti-CD33 IgG antibody to the potent calicheamicin. Phase I trial has been conducted with escalation dose of 0.25–9 mg/m^2 for 14 days up to 3 weeks. It is stopped at 9 mg/m^2 dose as antigenic sites are saturated [10]. The common side effects are fever, chill, elevated liver enzyme and expected myelosuppression. Peripheral blood counts dropped at 6 mg/m^2 dose. It has been tried in older patients in combination with cytarabine and anthracycline in de novo treatment and in maintenance therapy with cyclosporin in younger patients in remission stage.
3. **Radio–immunoconjugates:** The only hope to irradiate leukaemic cells, sparing the stem cells would be radionucleotide possessing extremely short wave length, such as alpha emitter ^{213}Bi. HuM conjugated to 0.28–1.0 m Ci/kg, ^{213}Bi has been tried in AML. Although blasts decreased, no complete remission occurred and pancytopenia was significant at higher level. It has been tried as stand-alone treatment and in the context of stem cell transplantation. [11]

8.20 OTHER TARGETED THERAPY

1. As an alternative to targeting CD33 antigen a fusion protein consisting of GM-CSF combined with Diphtheria toxin has been tried as a specific means targeting myeloid cells. Phase I trial showed 90% reduction of marrow blasts. Fever and chill are common side effects.
2. Like CD33 antigen, CD45 and CD66 antigen are other two targets against which monoclonal antibody has been used. CD45 antigen is present in all haemopoietic cells, save mature red cells and platelets. ^{131}I anti-CD45 has been used for radiation of spleen (13 fold radiation than conventional) and marrow (4 fold radiation than conventional). Re^{88} anti-CD66 antibody has been used as an adjunct standard preparative regime before bone marrow transplant. [12]
3. **Targeted Therapy against MDR1/ Pgp**

   The presence of multi-drug resistant protein with attendant high dose of efflux of drugs that bind it (e.g., daunorubicin, mitoxantrone, and probably Mylotarg) unfavourably affects outcome of AML. This prompted clinical trial of drugs e.g., Cyclosporine (CSA) and PSC 833 (which is a cyclosporine analog and 10 times more effective than it) that inhibit Pgp1. [13]
4. **Proteasome Inhibitor**

   The 20S proteasome is an ATP dependent multicatalytic enzyme. Increased degradation of protein (p53, 21, 27, KkB) leads to apoptosis and/ or cell cycle arrest. PS 341 is a specific inhibitor of 20S proteosome that is in phase-I trial in AML. [14]

8.21 ROLE OF ARSENIC TRIOXIDE IN AML

This unique agent now used in haematological malignancy, produces its antineoplastic effect by:

1. Hyperacetylation of histones and thereby modulation of apoptosis
2. Inhibition of farnesyl group to ras, leading to inhibition of cellular proliferation and differentiation. [15]

8.22 DISCOVERY OF NEW MOLECULAR TARGETS

The study of molecular biology in leukaemia has opened the possibility to identify a set of gene that can distinguish ALL from AML. This adds considerable promise for new biologic classification of leukaemia and lymphoma. As a novel study this technology may reveal uninterrupted and unique pathways in leukaemic cells which are amenable to treatment. The vaccine therapy now seems unlikely to be useful as there is no universal antigen for all subtypes of AML, but such methodologies are more likely to isolate immuno-dominant tumour antigen, which may be useful in the production of vaccine.

8.23 GUIDELINES FOR MANAGEMENT OF AML

Conventional management of AML consists of induction therapy, Post-remission therapy and Consolidation therapy (as described earlier). In each phase of treatment, good supportive care, comprising of adequate blood transfusion, appropriate antibiotics and management of complications is essential.

Induction Therapy mainly consists of an anthracycline, such as doxorubicin, or idarubicin or mitaxantrone, (the last two are used more recently) together with cystosine arabinoside. These are given in a typical regime of doxorubicin 45 to 60 mg/m^2 for 3 days, together with cystosine arabinoside, 100 to 200 mg/m^2 continuous infusion for 5 to 7 days. About 65% of patients under the age of 40 years obtain complete remission.

A bone marrow sample is collected on day 10–14. If bone marrow is not hypocellular in this repeat examination, there is unequivocal residual leukaemia, a second course of therapy with similar dose is administered. Approximately 25% to 40 % of patients require two courses of chemotherapy. The length of hospitalization is usually 4–6 weeks.

Post-remission Period Therapy Clinical trials have confirmed an almost 100% rate of relapse occurs in patients subjected to observation only in the post-remission period. Several treatment modalities have been tried and there is no clear evidence that one form of therapy is superior to the other. The regime usually consists of high dose cystosine arabinoside with or without anthracycline. It may require as high as 106 complete cycles. Another alternative consolidation includes mitoxantrone and etoposide.

Allogeneic Bone Marrow Transplant (BMT) is most effective in the first complete remission in younger patients who have histocompatible sibling. BMT offers a 50% long term disease free survival in 50% of cases in patients younger than 50 years. Relapse rate following transplantation is low, in the order of 15–20%, but the post transplant mortality, primarily from growth-versus-host disease and interstitial pneumonitis may be as high as 25–30%.

Autologous BMT is an alternative venue for post-remission therapy. The advantage of the procedure is that patient's own marrow is transplanted and there is minimal chance of GVHD. The procedure can be offered to patients up to age 65 to 70 years. The procedural mortality is less than that with allogeneic transplant. The overall mortality for AML patients who undergo transplant in first remission is less than 1%.

The disadvantages of autologous BMT are that there is absence of anti-leukaemic properties of GVH reaction and potentiality for transplantation of some of the leukaemic cells. There is evidence, however, that relapse after such transplant is mostly due to presence of residual leukaemia in such patients rather than reintroduction of leukaemic cells.

Many methods of "purging" the bone marrow before autologous transplantation have been practiced. The methods using cytotoxic agent such as 4-hydroperoxycyclophosphamide or use of mafosafamide is more commonly used. At present the role of autologous BMT compared to conventional consolidation therapy in post-remission period is being evaluated. With the use of peripheral blood as source of stem cells, the morbidity and mortality rates have been further lowered and this form of therapy is gaining widespread acceptance.

8.24 SUPPORTIVE THERAPY

Supportive therapy is very much important in patients' care in AML. It includes:

1. Control of infection in neutropenic patients
2. Transfusion therapy
3. Administration of Haemopoietic growth factors
4. Control of DIC
5. Management in hyperleukocytic phase
6. Management of Meningeal Leukaemia

8.25 CONTROL OF INFECTION

Infection becomes the main threat to absolutely neutropenic patients. The management of febrile neutropenia must be empiric because infections in such patients are life threatening, and delaying therapy until results of cultures are available, is not possible. When absolutely neutropenic patients are febrile, even without an obvious source of infection they must be placed on broad spectrum antibiotics that provide effective coverage against gram negative organisms. Traditionally two types of antibiotics are used. One is a semi-synthetic penicillin e.g., pipercillin or methicillin, along with an aminoglycoside. The other is a broad spectrum antibiotic like imipenem, ceftazidine. The empiric addition of anti-staphylococcal antibiotic is recommended in leukaemic patients with central venous catheter.

With advent of newer broad spectrum antibiotics, death from bacterial sepsis is rare. A major cause of death in young patients in AML of young patients is fungal infection like Candidiasis or Aspergillosis, which are so-called "opportunistic infections" in immunocompromised patients. If the patients remain febrile 24–72 hours after institution of broad spectrum antibiotics, antifungal agents like Amphotericin, or fuconazole or voriconazole is recommended according to clinical signs. At present there is no equivocal evidence of role of prophylactic antifungal agent in preventing sepsis. However, it is recommended in high risk individuals e.g., patients with protracted neutropenia, prior therapy with high dose corticosteroid, previous fungal sepsis during the preceding few months. The mainstay of prophylaxis is meticulous handwashing by all healthcare personnel and barrier nursing.

8.26 TRANSFUSION THERAPY

Management of profoundly pancytopenic patients requires repeated red cell and platelet transfusion. With multiple platelet transfusion patients develop alloimmunization and become progressively refractory to further platelet transfusion. Alloimmunization may be reduced by using leucocyte filters, both for red cells and platelets special washing of platelets, and using platelets from ABO compatible donors or HLA-matched donors. The effect of white cell transfusion remains controversial. Variations in leukocyte product are marked, administration is usually fraught with adverse reactions. The inability of blood banks to provide leukocytes within few hours of collection is also responsible for ineffectiveness.

Leukocyte transfusion is usually reserved for life threatening situations like gram negative sepsis with haemodynamics compromise or resistance to antibiotics or invasive canadiasis or aspergillosis. As many patients subsequently undergo BMT, all blood products including fresh frozen plasma should be tested for cytomegalo virus and, if positive, should be irradiated to avoid GVHD.

8.27 THERAPY WITH HAEMOPOIETIC GROWTH FACTORS

The use of haemopoietic growth factors like granulocyte-colony-stimulating factor (G-CSF) or granulocyte-macrophage-colony-stimulating factor (GM-CSF) has been evaluated in several clinical trials, whether they can reduce period of neutropenia as well as morbidity and mortality related to infections. Multiple trials show that these cytokines are safe when administered at the neutropenic nadir after induction therapy, in the sense that they do not induce leukaemic clone proliferation significantly. Growth factors also shorten the period of neutropenia, duration of fever and infections are also shortened in some observations, though there is no reduction of number of documented infections. Data also indicate that growth factors reduce the period of neutropenia following BMT. Another role is to mobilize stem cells from the bone marrow or peripheral blood stem cells collected after growth factor therapy.

8.28 THERAPY FOR HYPERURICAEMIA

Therapy for reducing serum uric acid is essential to prevent renal damage and subsequent failure. Serum uric acid rises due to rapid lysis of large tumor burden. This is prevented by adequate hydration and administration of Allopurinol during therapy.

8.29 THERAPY FOR DIC

This unique complication is more likely to develop in promyelocytic leukaemia and it may also develop during therapy, even if not developed initially. Optimal management is controversial, but certain guidelines are followed.

1. ATRA treatment is helpful in reducing DIC. So it must be given before or concurrent with chemotherapy.
2. Frequent monitoring of coagulation parameters is essential.
3. If there is no evidence of clinical bleeding and only mild abnormality of coagulation factors is present, addition of prophylactic heparin with close observation is needed.
4. If evidence of clinical bleeding or severe DIC is present, platelet cryoprecipitate and fresh frozen plasma should be instituted according to laboratory results.
5. Only in life threatening bleeding, unresponsive to treatment, should low dose of heparin, 300–500 units per hour by continuous infusion, should be considered.

8.30 MANAGEMENT OF MENINGEAL LEUKAEMIA

This type of leukaemia is commonly seen in lymphoblastic type but is also seen in monocytic variety of AML. If the patient's CNS symptoms or signs do not develop, CSF should not be examined till blasts disappear from peripheral blood. If meningeal leukaemia develops, methotrexate 12 to 15 mg or cystosine arabinoside 30 to 50 mg, given by lumbar puncture or via Omaya reservoir. Intrathecal therapy is given every 3 to 4 days until the CSF is clear on at least two or three occasions. The use of cranial irradiation in cases of uncomplicated AML is not considered.

8.31 MANAGEMENT OF HYPERLEUCOCYTIC LEUKAEMIA

These leukaemias require urgent therapy, especially if leukostasis develops. Clinical features include dyspnoea, CNS signs and symptoms as well as fundoscopic findings e.g., distended vessels and blurred disc margin, and haemorrhagic infiltrates. Patients are treated with leukapheresis unless the blast count is less than 50,000 per microlitre at which point standard antileukaemic therapy is instituted.

8.32 REMISSION IN AML

Different Oncology groups laid down different criteria for remission, based on different clinical studies. However, the most common criteria which are followed for evaluation from time to time, after induction therapy, are described below. Complete remission has been defined as:

Patient has no symptom or sign of leukaemia

Hb > 10 g/dl

Neutrophilic granulocytes > 1.5 × 10^9/L

Platelets > 100 × 10^9/L

Bone marrow should show < 5% blast cells

The marrows are rated as M1, M2, and M3.

M1 contains 0–5% blasts, 0–40% of total cells for mature cells and blasts together

M2 contains 6–25% blasts, 41–69% of total cells for mature cells and blasts together

M3 contains > 25% of blasts, > 69% of total cells for mature cells and blasts together

This classification holds good for ALL

Complete remission in AML, should not be considered until all granulocyte precursor cells disappear from peripheral blood. Complete remission is present so long as the

(*i*) patient is well,

(*ii*) there are no abnormal cells in the peripheral blood,

(*iii*) more than 0.5 × 10^9/L neutrophils,

(*iv*) more than 75 × 10^9/L platelets, and

(*v*) persistent M1 marrow.

Onset of persistent M2 or M3 marrow changes, meningeal infiltration, testicular mass, or signs or symptoms definitely attributable to leukaemia indicate the end of remission, and onset of relapse.

8.33 CONCLUSION

Acute myeloid leukaemia is a disease of rather obscure aetiology, but study of its molecular pathology shows many well defined and specific feature some of which are now amenable to therapy. This opened up a vast field of research and better understanding of pathogenesis of hematological malignancy. Probably some day in future we can conquer this type of malignancy with combined weapon of targeted therapy and immunotherapy, avoiding the risk of toxicity of chemotherapy.

REFERENCES

1. Vardeman JW, Harris NL, Bruning RD. *The World Health Organization (WHO) Classification of myeloid neoplasm.* Blood (2002); 160: 2292–2302.
2. Bain BJ, Barnett D, Linch D, Matutes E, Reilley JT. *Revised guideline of immunophenotyping in acute leukaemia and chronic lymphoprpliferative disorder.* Clin Lab Haematol. (2002); 24: 1–13.
3. Arbar DA. *Realistic pathologic classification of acute myeloid leukaemia.* (1996); 10: 1826–31.
4. Byad JC, Dodge RK, Carroll A, et al. *Patients with the t (8; 21) (q22; q22) and acute leukaemia have superior failure free and overall survival when repetitive cycle of high dose cytarabine are administered.* J Clin Oncol (1999); 17: 3767–3775.
5. Tallman MS, Andersen JW, Schiffer CA, et al. *All-trans-retinoic acid in acute promyelocytic leukaemia.* N Engl J Med. (1997); 337: 1021–1028.
6. Greenberg P, Advani R, Tallman M, et al. *Treatment of refractory/relapsed AML with PSC 833 plus mitoxantrone, etoposide, cytarabine (PSC-MEC) vs MEC: randomized phase III trial (E2995).* Blood. (1999); 94 (Suppl 1): 383a. (Abstr)
7. Baer MR, George SC, Jodge RK. *Phase III study of PSC 833 modulation of multi-drug resistance (MDR) in previously untreated acute myeloid leukaemia (AML) patients (PTS) > 60 years (CALBG 9720).* Blood (1999); 94 (Suppl 1): 383a (abstr).
8. Heinrich M, Zigler A. Griffith D, et al. *Selective pharmacological inhibition of mild type and mutant c-kit receptortyrosine kinase activity in haemopoietic cells.* Blood (1999); 94 (Suppl.): 265a (abstr.)
9. Jucie JG, DE Blasio, Durnint L, Yao-T-J, *Scienberg DA Molecular remission induction with retinoic acid and anti-CD33 monoclonal antibody HuM 195 in acute prolymphocytic leukaemia.* Clin Cancer Res (2000); 6; 372–80.
10. Seivers EL, Applebaum FR, Speilberger RT, et al. *Selective ablation of Acute Myeloid Leukaemia using antibody-targeted chemotherapy, a phase I study of anti-CD33 calcheamicin immunoconjugate.* Blood (1999); 93: 3678–84.
11. Jurcic JG, McDevitt MR, Sgouros G, et al. *Phase I trial of targeted alpha-particle therapy for myeloid leukemias with bismuth-213-HuM195 (anti-CD33).* Proc Am Soc Clin Oncol. (1999); 18: 7. (abstr)
12. Mathews DC, Applebaum FR, Eary JF, et al. *Phase I study of ^{131}I-anti CD45 antibody plus cyclophosamide and total body irradiation for advanced acute leukaemia and myelodysplastic syndrome.* Blood (1999); 94: 1237–47.
13. Leth CP, Kopecky KJ, Cher IM, et al. *Frequency and clinical significance of the expression of the multi-drug resistance proteins MDR1/ P-glycoprotein, MRP1 and LRP in acute myeloid leukaemia.* A Southwest Oncology group study. Blood (1999); 94: 1086–99.
14. Perez-Soler R, Ling Y, Mendoz S. et al. *Effect of proteosome inhibitor PS 341 on cell cycle progression and cell dependent agents.* Am Soc Clin Oncol (2000); 19: 190a (abstr.)
15. Perkins C, Kim CN, Fang G, et al. *Arsenic induces apoptosis of multidrug-resistant human myeloid leukaemia cells that express bcr-abl or overexpress MDR, P, Bcl, or Bcl-xL.* Blood (2000); 95: 1014–1022.

CHAPTER

9 Acute Lymphoblastic Leukaemia

9.1 INTRODUCTION

Acute lymphoblastic leukaemia (ALL) is a malignant disorder that originates in a single B or T lymphocyte progenitor. It involves multi-step somatic mutation in a single lymphoid progenitor cell at one or several stages of development. The immuno- haemotyping reflects the level of differentiation achieved by the dominant clone. The clonal origin is established by cytogenetic analysis of polymorphic X-chromosome linked genes. In these patients both alleles are expressed in normal cell, but only with a single active parental allele is expressed in leukaemic lymphoblasts. Analysis of T cell receptor or immunoglobulin gene has documented the monoclonal nature of the disease.

9.2 AETIOLOGY AND PATHOGENESIS

Initiation and progression of ALL is driven by successive mutations that alter cellular function, including enhanced self renewal, a subversion of control of normal proliferation, a block in differentiation and an increased resistance to death signals (apoptosis). Environmental agents e.g. ionizing radiation and chemical mutagens have been implicated in some patients. [1]

A. Genetic Syndromes

Only a minority is associated with inherited genetic syndromes. Children with Down syndrome have 10 to 30 p.c. greater risk of leukaemia. B cell precursors are more likely to be involved. Autosomal recessive disease like ataxia telengectasia and Bloom syndrome are associated with greater predisposition. The causative gene encodes a protein, involved in DNA repair, regulation of cell proliferation, apoptosis.

B. Environmental Factors

Exposure to diagnostic X-Ray confers to slightly increased rate of ALL, which correlates positively to number of exposures. Exposure to natural terrestrial, occupational or cosmic ionizing radiaton or paternal radiation exposures, prior to conception carries increased risk. Exposure to low magnetic fields produced by a residential power supply has been largely excluded. Administration of vitamin K in neonates, maternal alcohol consumption during pregnancy and increased consumption of dietary nitrites, all have been suggested but highly controversial.

C. Host Pharmacokinetics

Low penetrance polymorphism of folate metabolizing enzymes, and various inactivating polymorphism of detoxifying enzymes have been advocated for drug interaction unraveling leukaemic condition.

D. In-utero Development

Development of concordant leukaemia in identical twins with t (4:11)/ MLL-AF4, suggest that fusion of gene increases the frequency of ALL. All childhood cases develop in utero. Some researchers are of opinion that delayed exposures to common infection at a time of increased lymphoid cell proliferation serves as postnatal instigating agents. Mechanisms include aberrant expression of oncoproteins, and chromosomal translocations, that generate fusion genes encoding transcription factors or active kinases. The common genetic abnormalities are translocation, (most common), deletion, inversion, point mutation, amplification. Change in growth regulatory key pathway controlled by p53 gene, which function as a sensor of aberrant cellular changes, and by tumor suppressor gene (RB protein), which control the entry into cell cycle, is responsible for leukaemic proliferation. Components of p53 pathway are frequently mutated in ALL. [2]

9.3 CLINICAL FEATURES

Incidence: ALL constitutes 12% of all leukaemias, 60% of leukaemia in younger than 20 years of age, 20% of adult leukaemia. The disease affects male more than female in all age groups. The incidence is higher in Europeans than in Africans. Improvement in diagnostic facilities increases the incidence from late 70s.

Clinical presentation depends on the degree of marrow failure and the extent of extramedullary spread. The presentations may be as follows:

1. In half of patients fever is the chief presentation. This may be due to pyrogenic cytokines (IL-1, IL-6, TNF) released from leukaemic cells. There may be also associated infection.
2. Fatigue and lethargy are next common presentations, often related to anaemia. In older patients dyspnoea may occur due to anaemia.
3. More than a fourth, especially young children, suffer from bone pain, arthalgia due to leukaemic infiltration or expansion of marrow cavity by excessive haemopoiesis. Young patients with prominent bone pain and normal peripheral blood count are diagnosed late. In a small proportion of patients, marrow necrosis causes severe bone pain, very high lactate dehydrogenase and fever.
4. Less common presentations are headache, vomiting, altered mental function, oliguria, anuria.
5. Occassionally life threatening infection or intracranial haematoma may produce high leukocyte count more than 400×10^9/l.
6. Very rarely no symptom or sign occurs, when routine examination may reveal the condition.

9.4 PHYSICAL FINDINGS

1. Pallor, petechiae, ecchymoses on skin and mucous membrane are common findings. Bone tenderness may occur due to leukaemic infiltration in the marrow or haemorrhage, that stretches the periosteum.

2. Bulky anterior mediastinal masses composed of mediastinal lymph glands may compress great vessels and trachea, producing mediastinal syndrome. Patients may present with cough, dyspnoea, orthopnoea, dysphagia, stridor, cyanosis, facial oedema, sometimes syncope. Such patients tolerate anaesthesia poorly. Thymic mass is seen in 7-10% of children and in 10% of adult cases.
3. Painless enlargement of scrotum, or hydrocoele, resulting from lymphatic obstruction, is another presenting feature in male patients, though overt testicular disease is rare. This presentation is common in infants with T cell leukaemia and hyperleukocytosis. Priapism due to leukostasis of corpus cavernosa, and dorsal veins or scrotal nerve involvement is the other mode of presentation in this group.
4. Rather uncommon presentations are leukaemic infiltration of the orbit, optic nerve, retina, iris or subcutaneous nodules, enlarged salivary glands (Mickuliz syndrome) as well as cranial nerve palsy. Epidural spinal cord compression may result in paraparesis or paraplegia.
5. Infiltration of tonsil, adenoid, appendix or mesenteric lymph node may require surgical intervention.

9.5 LABORATORY FEATURES

1. Blood count

   Anaemia, neutrpenia, thrombocytosis and leukocytosis are usual presenting features. The degree of the first two indicates the degree of replacement of marrow by leukaemic tissue. Brunt of the disease is determined by total leukocyte count, which varies from $0.5\text{-}1.5\times10^9$/l up to $10\text{-}12\times10^9$/l.

   Hyperleucocytosis occurs in 10-16% of cases, when count may go up to 100×10^9/l. [3] Profound neutropenia may occur in 20-40% of cases, where neutrophil count falls to $<0.5\times10^9$/l. Hyper-eosinophilia may occur in male patients and usually precedes several months of onset of the disease. [4]

   In patients with cardiomegaly, congestive cardiac failure and pulmonary infiltration, as well as chromosomal aberrations like t (5:14), q (31:32), circulating lymphoblasts may not be present in the peripheral blood and a relatively small percentage of blasts occur in the marrow.

   Decreased platelet counts are often seen at diagnosis, e.g.52×10^9/l. Leukaemic condition thus differs from immune thrombocytopenia as it is associated with anaemia or leukocyte abnormalities or both. Occassional patients, principally male, present with thrombocytosis, the count may be as high as $>400\times10^9$/l. Pancytopenia with spontaneous recovery may precede. [5]
2. Coagulation

   Coagulopathy, usually mild, may be seen in 3 to 5% of cases, most of them have T-cell leukaemia.
3. Blood Biochemistry

   (i) Increased serum uric acid is common in patients with large leukaemic cell burden.

   (ii) Patients with massive renal infiltrate may have increased levels of urea, creatinine, and blood urea nitrogen.[6]

(iii) Level of LDH is increased in most of the cases and related to the degree of leukaemic infiltrate.

(iv) Rarely patients present with hypocalcaemia, which result from release of PTH-like protein from hypothalamus and there may be leukaemic infiltration of bone.

(v) Serum IgG and IgM are moderately increased in one-third of children with ALL.

(vi) Liver dysfunction due to leukaemic infiltration occurs in 10-30% of cases.

4. Examination of CSF is an essential diagnostic procedure to exclude CNS leukaemia. Leukaemic blasts are present in CSF in one-third of patients at diagnosis. They usually have neurologic symptoms, and are associated with increased risk of CNS relapse. This is an indication of intensified therapy. Many therapists perform the test at diagnosis and a second diagnostic test is needed to verify.

9.6 DIAGNOSTIC TESTS

Morhologic test for lymphoblasts in peripheral blood smear and bone marrow is established by staining the smear with Romanowsky stain. Lymphoblasts appear relatively small twice the size of small lymphocytes with scanty light blue cyto-plasm , a round cleft or slightly indented nucleus, fine to slightly coarse chromatin and inconspicuous nucleoli. The granules are readily distinguishable from deep purple granules. [7]

Among **cytochemical stains** esterase doesn't recognize lymphoblasts. A low level of myeloperoxidase is detected in bone marrow due to presence of low level of normal myeloid precursors.

Immunophenotyping is done by antibodies, that distinguish clusters of differentiation antigens (CD). These antigens are same cellular antigen but of different isotope. The panel used includes lineage for highly sensitive markers CD 19 for B-lineage, CD 7 for T-cell lineage, CD 13 and 33 for myeloid cells are generally used. CD10+ve B cells (common ALL), CD 10 –ve (pre -, pro-B) cells and T-cells are of therapeutic importance. Myeloid associated antigens are found in 5to 30 % of children and 10 to 50% of adults with ALL. [8]

9.7 CYTOMETRIC AND CYTOGENETIC STUDIES

Two ploidy groups are of clinical relevance. More than 50 chromosomes means hyperploidy less than 45 chromosomes indicates hypoploidy. Hyperploidy is seen in 25% of childhood cases and 6-7% of adult cases It is considered to be of favorable prognosis. That may reflect an increased accumulation of methotrexate polyglutamate and indicate an increased sensitivity to therapeutic antimetabolites and marked propensity of cells to undergo apoptosis. Hypoploidy is associated with poor prognosis. [9]

Flow cytometric studies can sometimes identify a small but drug-resistant subpopulation of near haploid cells that may have been missed by standard cytogenetic analysis. Reciprocal translocations can mobilize promoter/enhancer element of immunoglobulin chain on heavy or light chain or T cell antigen receptor. More often genetic rearrangements result from fusion of two genes encoding different transcription factors. Such chimeric transcription factors activate the genes, which regulate differentiation, renewal and proliferation of stem cells. [10]

9.8 MANAGEMENT OF ALL

Management includes supportive care by maintaining metabolic stability, by controlling hyperleukocytosis to avoid thrombotic complications, by effective control of infection, and by haematological supplement like platelet and concentrated RBC, on one hand, as well as treatment of leukaemic condition by judicious chemotherapy. Supportive therapy is indicated in the following conditions.

1. **Metabolic Complications** may be hyperuricaemia, hypocalcaemia or hyperphosphataemia. Hyperuricaemia is treated plenty of oral or intranenous fluid (according to clinical condition) by allopurinol or rasburicase. By inhibiting de novo synthesis allopurinol can reduce peripheral blast cell count. It reduces both anabolism and catabolism of 6-mercaptopurine (used in therapy of ALL), by inhibiting xanthine oxidase and by depleting intracellular phosphoribosyl pyrophosphate. The dosage of both the drugs should therefore be reduced. Rasburicase breaks down uric acid to allantoin, which is ten times more soluble than uric acid, and is readily excreted in urine. This is a potent uricosuric agent that obviates the need of alkalinization of urine. It is contraindicated in glucose-6- phosphate dehydrogenase deficiency, because hydrogen peroxide accumulated as bye product of uric acid metabolism, can cause methaemoglobinaemia or haemolytic anaemia.[11]
   Hyperphosphataemia may be treated by a phosphate binder e.g. aluminium hydroxide. Calcium carbonate may be given if serum calcium is low.
2. **Hyperleukocytosis**- The condition develops when leukocyte count rises up to $400 x 10^9/l$. Leukopharesis or exchange transfusio is indicated. Vincristine or cyclophosphamide used for therapy can reduce the cell burden. Preparatory to induction therapy, low dose steroid with addition of vincristine and cyclophosphamide may help lessen the cell count.
3. **Infection**- About 50% of patients present with infection. Therapy increases susceptibility to infection further. Protective isolation of the patients with infection, air filtration in the ward, avoidance of certain food e.g. raw cheese, uncooked vegetables, unpeeled fruits, use of antiseptic mouth wash for the patients with mucositis are some of the preventive measures. Administration of GM-CSF hastens recovery but increases risk of acute myeloid leukaemia. Use of dexamethasone early in the course of infection may produce disseminated fungal infection. For Pneumocystis carnii infection, prophylactic therapy with sulphamethoxazole-trimethoprim should be instituted for 2-3 days per week, 2 weeks after remission induction. And should be continued 6 weeks after control. For those who can not tolerate this form of therapy, aerosolized pentamidine, dapsone, atovaquone, are indicated. Live virus vaccine should not be used during therapy. Inactivated polio vaccine may be used for sibling and other contacts. Zoster immunoglobulin within 96 hours of exposure should be administered.
4. **Haematological Support** - ALL or its therapy may lead to thrombocytopenia. Bleeding in CNS, lungs or GI tract may be life threatening. Patients under chemotherapy, hepatic dysfunction can have such complication. Patients having L-asparaginase therapy and a glucocorticoid, generally are in hypercoagulable state and may develop DIC with consequent thrombocytopenia. Platelet transfusion is given therapeutically for overt bleeding or when

count is 10×10^9/l at diagnosis. A higher threshold is considered for active toddlers and patients with fever or infection. Packed red cells transfusion may be necessary to treat chronic anaemia to prevent congestive cardiac failure, and transfusion should be given very slowly. Absolute neutropenia may necessitate granulocyte transfusion, in cases of septicaemia or disseminated fungal infection, though it is required rarely, when there is poor response to antibiotics. Blood components should be irradiated before transfusion, to avoid viral infection and to prevent graft-versus-host disease. Gram-negative septicaemia must be treated before any form of transfusion.

5. **Anti-leukaemic Therapy - For B cell ALL-**Success has been achieved with event free survival in 68%-84% of cases, using cyclophosphamide, methotrexate, in higher than usual dose and vincristine and cytarabine, in conventional dose, in different studies.. Others use a small multi-agent regime that incorporates fractionated cyclophosphamide, high dose methotrexate ($5g/M^2$/dose), etoposide and cytabirine ($2g/M^2$/dose). Effective CNS therapy (described later) is essential side by side. A cure rate of 50% has been achieved for adult patients. Some prefer reduced dose of methotrexate and cytarabine for adults older than 60 years to reduce toxicity and to add Rituximab (Anti-CD 20 monoclonal antibody) for its demonstrated efficacy in B cell malignancy. [12]

For B cell precursor and T cell ALL therapy is usually conducted in three phases: (1) Induction of remission (2) Intensification of remission (3) Consolidation or continuation or maintainance therapy

A.Induction Therapy- This usually consists of a glucocorticoid (prednisolone, dexamethasone), an antracycline, (such as daunorubicin or mitoxantrone) for adults and L-asparaginase for children. A typical regime involves two phases

Phase I consists of daunorubicin 45-60mg/M^2 on days 1,8,15,and 22, vincristine 1.4mg/M^2 on days 1,8,15 and 22 and prednisone given at a dose of approximately 60mg/M^2 for a total of 28 days. L-asparginase 5000-10000 units/M^2 is usually added for 7 to 12 days beginning on day 15 to 17 of phase I. **Phase II** which is administered very soon after completion of phase I, usually includes cyclophosphamide, cytarabine and 6-mercaptopurine as well as prophylactic intrathecal methotrexate. Usually the therapy is given at intervals of 2 weeks, for 6-8 doses.

For **maintainance chemotherapy** methotrexate is given in a dose of 2.5 mg/M^2 once or twice weekly may be given orally with other agents, like purinethol (merccaptopurine) or singly by intravenous infusion in high dose. Leucovorin calcium or folinic acid in 75 mg doses by intravenous infusion within next 12 hours, when a large dose of methotrexate is administered, or given intrathecally as a "bone marrow rescue." [13] Induction therapy along with supportive care produces 80-85% complete remission.

The concept of haematologic remission means 0.01 p.c. of involvement of marrow cells. But patients in clinical remission may have as many as 10 billion of leukaemic cells.

Perhaps, because of increased penetration in CSF and longer half life, dexamethasone can produce better control of systemic and CNS leukaemia than other steroids.

Out of other important therapeutic agents, L-asparginase (derived from Eruinca chrysanthami, E coli and a third made of polythelene glycol derived from E coli). The third one Pegasparase has got longest half life and it is used in 2500 IU/M^2 dose every other week. By contrast Eriwina preparations are used at 20,000 IU/M^2 three times per week for twelve doses. E coli preparations are used in 6000-10,000 IU/M^2 doses. It is administered 2-3 times per week for 6 to 12 doses. This is often used for induction of remission on fourth or fifth day of therapy in each cycle.

B. Intensification therapy - The value of this therapy is less certain in adults. Most commonly used regime is high dose methotrexate (5gm/M^2). It is more effective than 1gm/M^2 dose. High dose methotrexate with or without mercaptopurine, high dose L-asparginase and doxorubicin or a combination of dexamethasone, vincristine, L-asparaginase and doxorubicin followed by thioguanine, cytarabine, thioguanine. In randomized trial prolonged four month consolidation therapy with methotrexate, cytarabine, thioguanine, cyclophosphamide, L-asparaginase yield essentially the leukaemia-free survival rate. [14]

C. Consolidation or continuation therapy- A combination of methotrexate weekly and mercaptopurine administered daily constitutes the usual regime for children, Following induction therapy, patients require prolonged therapy for 9 to 24 months. Most such maintenance program can be administered on an outpatient basis.

Considerations to be taken in continuation therapy::

(a) Mercaptopurine should not be administered with milk or milk products containing xanthine oxidase as it may degrade the drug.

(b) Prolonged oral administration of methotrexate in divided doses is inferior to intermittent intravenous administration at higher doses. By contrast mercaptopurine is most effective when administered orally.

(c) Antimetabolite treatment should not be withheld because of isolated increases of liver enzyme, as such liver enzyme abnormalities are tolerable and reversible.

(d) A few patients are deficient in enzyme that inactivates mercaptopurine by methylation. The drug should be used in much lower doses (10-fold reduction) in these subjects.

(e) Patients with enzyme deficiency have higher risk of drug-induced leukaemia. Emphasis has been laid on inherited differences in drug metabolism and disposition resulting from genetic polymorphism. Intermittent pulses of vincristine and glucocorticoid improve the efficacy of antimetabolite based continuation therapy.

9.9 CENTRAL NERVOUS SYSTEM (CNS) PROPHYLAXIS

Even if no meningeal invovement is documented at presentation, CNS treatment is mandatory. Although CNS treatment is not considered during induction therapy, it is used throughout intensification and maintenance therapy. Cranial irradiation, intrathecal prophylaxis or systemic therapy appears to provide satisfactory CNS prophylaxis, thus preventing late CNS relapses, is recommended with high dose cystosine arabinoside or high dose methotrexate. Intrathecal administration consists of slow intrathecal injection of 12.5mg of methotrexate in 1 ml of normal saline, after slow withdrawal of same amount of CSF. [15]

9.10 ALLOGENEIC STEM CELL TRANSPLANTATION

Human Stem cell transplantation during first remission remains controversial. In adults, event free survival rates range from 30 to 40 p.c. with chemotherapy alone and 40 to 60 p.c. with allogenic transplantation along with chemotherapy. The procedure appears to improve outcomes of adults (t 4:11) but not that of children with the same genotype. The general consensus is to arrange allogeneic transplantation for all patients under 50 years of age, after induction and intensification chemotherapy, if they have histocompatible sibling. The patients of 15 to 20 years of age, if they lack in poor prognostic factors, may be treated with standard chemotherapy and transplantation is considered only when relapse occurs. The one group of patients in whom transplantation is considered in first instance, are those with Ph-1 chromosome. This group of patients have uniformly poor prognosis and multiple clinical trial shows that the long term outcome is dismal with modern therapy. Early trials with BMT shows that about one-third of patients have long term survival with this form of therapy.

9.11 RELAPSE OF LEUKAEMIA

Relapse is defined as reappearance of leukaemic cells at any site in the body. Most relapses occur during treatment or within first 2 years of completion of therapy, although initial relapses have been observed 10 years or more after diagnosis. Anaemia, leukocytosis, leukopenia, thrombocytopenia, enlargement of liver and spleen, bone pain, fever or sudden decrease in tolerance to chemotherapy, may signal the onset of marrow relapse. [16]

Leukaemia relapse may occur at sites other than marrow e.g. CNS, testicle, eye, ear, ovary, uterus, bone, muscle, tonsil, mediastinum, pleura, paranasal sinuses. Prolonged second remission >3 years, can be achieved with chemotherapy, in as many as half of the patients with late relapses i.e. 6months after cessation of therapy. In patients who develop relapse while on therapy or shortly thereafter, allogenic HSC transplantation is the treatment of choice.

For patients with ALL, relapses after allogenic transplantation, a second transplant or donor T lymphocyte infusion occasionally results in sustained remission. Adults with isolated CNS relapse fare much more poorly than children. No firm evidence indicates an advantage of either autologous or allogenic transplantation over intensive chemotherapy. One-third of patients with early testicular relapse become long term survivors after salvage chemotherapy and bilateral testicular irradiation. However prognosis for extramedullary relapse is unclear. [17]

9.12 PROGNOSIS OF ALL IN ADULTS

Unlike ALL of childhood, of which most children can be cured, long term survival for adult patients with ALL is rather uncertain. Established poor prognostic factors are high white count at presentation (>25,000-30.000/ml), the presence of Philadelphia chromosome with 9:22 translocation, pure B-cell ALL, long duration to attaininitial complete remission (>4 weeks), adult age. Clinical and laboratory presentations are similar to those of AML. Once patients have had a relapse, irrespective of duration of first relapse the outcome is always fatal without BMT. Patients who have relapsed should be referred for allogenic transplantation after a second subsequent remission has been attained. If no donor is available they should be referred to centers that have trials using autologous BMT or transplant centers offering experimental treatment with matched unrelated or mismatched related donors.

REFERENCES

1. Stock W, Tsai T, Golden C, et al. (2000): *Cell cycle regulatory gene are important determinants of leukomogenesis and disease, biology in adult acute lymphoblastic leukaemia.* Blood 95:2364
2. Westbrook Ca, Hooberman AL, Spino C, et al (1992): *Clinical significance of the BCR-ABL fusion gene in adult acute lymphoblastic leukaemia: a cancer and leukaemia group B study(8762).* Blood 80:2963
3. Lowe EJ, Puri C-H, Hanock ML, et al (2005): *Early complications in children with acute lymphoblastic leukaemia presenting with hyperleucocytosis.* Paeditr Blood Cancer 45:16
4. Hasle H, Heim S, Schroeder H, et al. (1985): *Transient pancytopenia preceding acute lymphoblastic leukaemia (pre ALL).* Leukaemia 9:665.
5. Blatt J, Penchansky L, Hom M (1989): *Thrombocytosis as a presenting feature of acute lymphoblastic leukaemia in childhood.* Am J Haematol 31: 46,1989
6. Jones DP, Stapleton FB, Rabrinsky D et al. (1990): *Renal dysfunction and hyperuricaemia at presentation and relapse of acute lymphoblastic leukaemia.* Blood66:Med Paeditr Oncol 18:283
7. Gassmann W, Loeffler H, Thiel E et al (1997): *Morphological and cytochemical findings in 150 cases of T-lineage of acute lymphoblastic leukaemia in adults.* Br J Haematol 97:372
8. Bene MC, Benier M, Castoldi G, et al ((2002) : *Impact of immunophenotyping on management of acute lymphoblastic leukaemia.* JAMA 288:2001
9. Harrison CJ, Moorman AV, Broadfield ZJ et al (2004): *Three distinct subgroups of hypoploidy in acute lymphoblastic leukaemia.* Brit J Haematol 125:552
10. Yeoh EJ, Ross ME, Sturtleff SA, et al (2002): *Classification, subtype, and prediction of outcome of acute lymphoblastic leukaemia by gene expression profiling.* Cancer Cell:1:133
11. Goldman SC, Holcenberg JS, Finuelstein JZ, et al (2001): *A randomized comparision between rasburicase and allopurinol in children with lymphoma or leukaemia at high risk of tumour lysis.* Blood 97:2998
12. Kei briaei P, Larson RA (2003): *Progress and challenges in therapy of adult acute lymphoblastic leukaemia.* Curr Opin Haematol 10:284
13. Larson LA, Dodge RK, Burns CP et al (1995): *A five drug remission induction regimen with intensive consolidation for adults with acute lymphoblastic leukaemia: Cancer and leukaemia.* Group B study 8811. Blood 85:2025
14. Hussein KK, Dahlberg S, Head D et al. ((1989): *Treatment of acute lymphoblastic leukaemia in adults with intensive induction, consolidation and maintainance chemotherapy.* Blood 73:57
15. Puri C-H (2003): *Toward optimal central nervous system directed treatment in childhood acute lymphoblastic leukaemia.* J clin Oncol 21: 179
16. Mayer RJ (1988): *Allogenic transplantation versus intensive chemotherapy in first remission acute leukaemia: is there a best choice?* Blood 6:1532
17. Puri C-H, Compana D (2000): *New definition of remission in childhood acute lymphoblastic leukaemia.* Leukaemia14: 783

CHAPTER

10 Myelodysplastic Syndrome

10.1 EVOLUTION OF CONCEPT

At the beginning of twentieth century, reports of highly morbid cytopenic disorders that were refractory to therapy, began to appear in medical literature. This was designated as odo-leukaemia. (Odo is a Greek word which means threshold). Chevallier proposed the name leucosis. In 1949 Hamilton-Peterson used the term preleukaemia *i.e.*, refractory anaemia antecedent to acute myeloid leukaemia (AML). In 1953 Block and his co-workers introduced current concept of a clonal myeloid haemopathy prior to AML. In 1975, at a conference on unclassified leukaemias held at Paris, Mercel Bersis, Jean Bernard, and others suggested the term haematopoietic dysplasia, later shortened to myelodysplasia, for the group of disorders having a more indolent course than AML. [1]

10.2 DEFINITION

Myelodysplastic syndrome (MDS) is a term to encompass a spectrum of clonal (neoplastic) myeloid disorders marked by ineffective haematopoiesis, cytopenias, qualitative disorders of blood cells and their precursors, clonal chromosomal abnormalities, and a variable predilection to undergo evolution of florid AML. Spectrum varies from non-progression to slow progression to AML. [2]

10.3 EPIDEMIOLOGY

The overall incidence of MDS is 3.5 to 12.6 per 100,000 per year. The actual incidence may be much higher, however, as the result of difficulties in diagnosis, classification and recording. Approximately 25% to 30% of patients with MDS will transform to acute myelogenous leukaemia (AML) Transformation varies by subtype from 10% to 60% for the low-risk to high-risk groups, respectively. [3]

The disorder may appear in childhood but the incidence increases exponentially after age of 20 years. Most cases occur between the ages of 50 to 90 years [4] Most cases are sporadic, but a proportion result from stem cell injury during treatment of lymphoma or solid tumor with cytotoxic chemotherapy. The disorder may develop in inherited syndrome that predispose to AML *e.g.*, Fanconi's anaemia, Down syndrome. [5(a) (b)] Familial myelodysplasia occur rarely as a result of as yet unidentified germline susceptibility genes. [6]

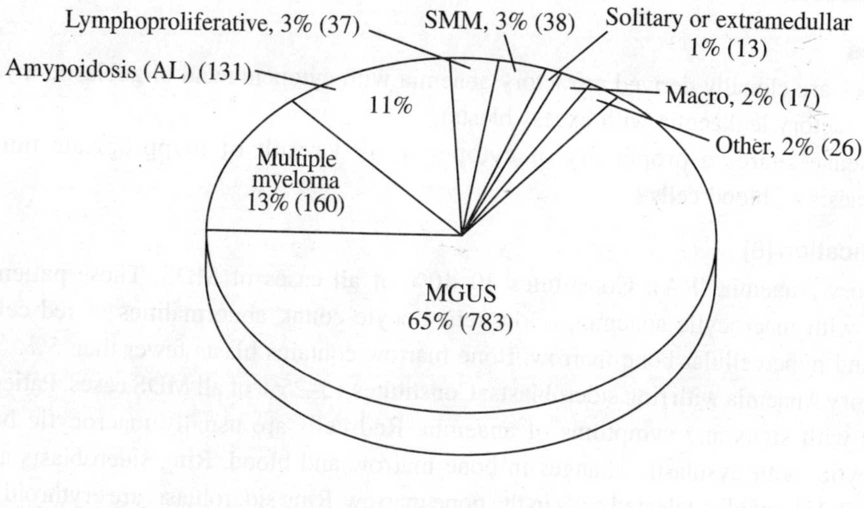

Fig. Incidence of different types of myeloma as descrived in mayo clinic 1999.

10.4 ORIGIN OF THE DISEASE

Clonal origin of the disease is supported by the studies of women who are heterozygous for G6PD isoenzymes A & B. Haematopoietic progenitors and in some cases B lymphocytes of such patients have only one isoenzyme present.

FISH study with probe for chromosome7 or 8 in patients with monosomy 7 or trisomy 8 indicates chromosome abnormalities may not be present in lymphocyte populations. Studies of immunoglobulin heavy chain gene rearrangement and assay of human androgen receptor and other genes on X chromosome also have concluded that lymphocytes are not derived from neoplastic clones. [7]

10.5 AETIOLOGY

The aetiology of the MDS in most patients is unknown; however, several factors are associated with an increased risk for the development of MDS.

1. Cytotoxic chemotherapy: A prior exposure to alkylating agents (cyclophosphamide, chlorambucil, and mephalan) is associated with increased risk of MDS. The risk is in part related to the dose and duration of therapy and generally occurs 3 to 7 years of exposure. MDS occurring after chemotherapy exposure is called secondary or therapy-related MDS and has a poor prognosis.
2. Patients who received the combination of radiation therapy plus chemotherapy have an increased risk of MDS. Patients who have received chemotherapy as part of the preparation regimen for autologous stem cell transplantation are at higher risk of MDS. The incidence of MDS is increased in patients who have been exposed to benzene and related compounds.

10.6 CLASSIFICATION

Clinical Types

Two main types are clonally derived refractory anaemia with cytopenia and oligoblastic myelogenous leukaemia (refractory leukaemia with excess blasts).

The disease shares a propensity of cytopenia, as a result of inappropriate multilineage dysmorphogenesis of blood cells.

WHO Classification [8]

1. Refractory Anaemia (RA): Constitutes 30–40% of all cases of MDS. These patients usually present with macrocytic anaemia, a low reticulocyte count, abnormalities of red cell size and shape and hypercellular bone marrow. Bone marrow contains blasts fewer than 5%.
2. Refractory Anaemia with ring sideroblasts: Constitutes 15–25% of all MDS cases. Patients usually present with signs and symptoms of anaemia. Red cells are usually macrocytic but may be normocytic, with dysplastic changes in bone marrow and blood. Ring sideroblasts account for more than 15% of all nucleated cells in the bone marrow. Ring sideroblasts are erythroid precursors with iron staining in the mitochondria forming a necklace around the nucleus.
3. Refractory Anaemia with multilineage dysplasia.
4. Refractory Anaemia with excess blasts (RAEB) and isolated 5q abnormality.

FAB (French-American- British) Classification further Categorizes the last mentioned type as [9]

1. Refractory anaemia with excess blasts. This constitutes 15–25% of MDS cases. Patients usually present with signs and symptoms of anaemia or bruising. Cytopenias usually involve two or more lineages and dysplastic changes in all three lineages with fewer than 5% circulating blast forms. The bone marrow is hyper cellular with increased blast forms, more than 5% but less than 20%.
2. Refractory anaemia with excess blasts in transformation (RAEB-T). This constitutes 5–10% of MDS cases. This category includes patients with 5–10% blasts in peripheral blood and 21–30% blasts in bone marrow Auer rods, (which are nothing but aggregates of lysozomes appearing as thin rods in the cytoplasm of immature myeloid cells) are seen. More than 50% of these patients will transform to AML. This type is classified as MDS with multilineage dysplasia in WHO classification. World Health Organization (WHO) proposed that 20% blasts should be the dividing line between MDS and AML.

Regarding course and prognosis, RA with < 15% ring sideroblasts is same as RAEB with < 21% blasts, and RA with > 15% ring sideroblasts is same as RAEB with > 21% blasts, the condition being equivalent to AML.

Myelodysplastic syndrome includes entities that have marrow blast p.c. ranging from < 2% in RA to 20% in RAEB. It is myelogenous leukaemia but not refractory anaemia. If the marrow contains blast cells, the question does not arise whether p.c. is 5% or 50%. There is an unclassifiable myelodysplastic syndrome, which does not fit into any of the above mentioned category.

Classification According to Clonal Cytogenetic Abnormality [10]

Classic 5q syndrome
Clonal (refractory) sideroblatic anaemia
Clonal bi- or tri- cytopenia (multilineage)
Oligoblastic leukaemia (RA with excess blasts)
Apparent clonal myeloid disease that does not fit into any category (chronic clonal monocytosis)

TABLE 10.1: International Prognostic Scoring System and its age related survival [11]

	IPPS score value				
Variable	0	0.5	1.0	1.5	2.0
Marrow Blast (%)	<5	5 – 10	5 – 10	11 – 20	21 – 30
Karyotype*	Good	Intermediate	Poor	Poor	Poor
Cell lines**	0 – 1	2 – 3			

*Good, normal, 5q-, 20q-; Poor, >3 Abnormalities –7, multiple; intermediate, all others.
**Neutrophils < 1,800/cmm; Platelets < 100,000/cmm; Haemoglobin < 10 g/dL.

TABLE 10.2: Age related survival

	Median survival	
Score	**Age < 60 yrs**	**Age > 60 yrs**
Low (0)	11.8	4.8
Intermediate 1 (0.5 – 1.0)	5.2	2.7
Intermediate 2 (1.5 – 2.0)	1.8	1.1
High > 2.5	0.4	0.5

Pathogenesis

The specific abnormality in myelodysplasia is **defective maturation and death of marrow precursor cells** due to decreased proportion of cells in DNA synthesis phase of mitotic cycle and a marked increase in the formation of late precursor cells undergoing apoptosis. Stepwise degradation of precursor cells is seen, which is a marker of apoptosis.

Apoptosis, an active process that controls programmed cell death, is increased in MDS progenitor cells. The bone marrow is typically hypercellular with increased haematopoietic activity but with peripheral cytopenia because of abnormal and impaired maturation within bone marrow. [12]

Increased level of apoptotuc mediators *e.g.*, TNF α (tissue necrosis factor), FAS antigen (CD 95), and calcium dependent nuclease activity is seen. Alkylating agents, topoisomerase inhibitors, and radiation cause **DNA damage, impair DNA repair enzymes** and induce loss of chromosome integrity. Most post-treatment MDS occur as a second clonal myeloid disease.

Abnormal oncogene expression in progenitor cells and dysregulation of cell cycle kinetics has been implicated in MDS. Alterations in N-ras oncogenes, p 53 expression, tumor suppression genes, and transcription factors have been described in MDS progenitor cells.

Immunoregulatory abnormalities in MDS manifest as impaired T-cell, natural killer cells and B-cell function. MDS is associated with a number of autoimmune disorders, including immune haemolytic anaemia and immune thrombocytopenia.

Pathology

The marrow usually contains **increased erythroid precursors with dysmorphic features,** including nuclear distortions, and scanty, poorly haemoglobinised cytoplasm. Ring sideroblasts are almost constant feature. **Neutrophils have anomalies including bilobed nuclei and hypergranulated cytoplasm**, in association with increased marrow granulocyte precursors. **Giant and microcytic platelets with abnormal granulation** in the blood are associated with megakaryocytic hyperplasia, and atypical lobulation of the nucleus. In progressive syndrome, anaemia may be accompanied by mild variations, usually in neutrophil and platelet levels, but blast cells are not increased to greater than 2 p.c. in the marrow.

In classic 5q syndrome, anaemia (usually in older women) is accompanied with **hypercellular, dysmorphic erythropoiesis in the marrow with lobulated erythroblast nuclei, hyper-lobulated micromegakaryocytes,** but usually **normal or elevated platelet count.** It is the most indolent type of MDS with lowest propensity of evolution to AML. In the more progressive syndrome, leukaemic blast cells are increased, cytopenias are more severe and the disease has high morbidity and mortality from infection and bleeding. Each of the syndromes has a high propensity to evolve into frank AML ranging from approximately 40 to 50 p.c. of patients with trilineage cytopenias and increased marrow blast cells. Mortality from infection is a high risk to patients with leukopenia.

Cytogenetics

Clonal cytogenetic disorders occur in approximately three-fourths of patients. Chromosomal abnormalities include an extra chromosome 8, loss of long arm of chromosome 5, 7, 9, 20, 21 and monosomy of chromosome 7 & 9. Loss of part or all of chromosomes 5 & 7 and complex chromosome aberrations are particularly common in the oligoblastic myelogenous leukaemias (and overt leukaemias) associated with prior treatment with cytotoxic drugs, radiation or exposure to benzene. In these circumstances, the deletion in 5q is at band 31.1 in distinction to classic 5q syndrome, in which deletions occur at the band q, 32, 33.3. The Ph chromosome t (qqt; 22q) and a variety of other chromosomal abnormalities rarely seen in MDS have been described on occasion.

The more favorable risk category includes a normal karyotype and isolated deletions of 5q 32-33.3, 20q or y. The poor risk category includes 5a 31.1, –7, del (7q), and complex chromosomal abnormalities. The intermediate risk group includes other abnormalities in de novo MDS chromosomal abnormalities occur in 15% of cases and in treatment-induced MDS cytogenetic abnormalities are very common. Chromosome abnormalities are more frequent in patients with oligoblastic myelogenous leukaemia than in patients with clonal (refractory) anaemia.

10.7 SPECIFIC MYELODYSPLASTIC SYNDROME

Classic 5q syndrome: Deletion of chromosome 5 at band 32–33.3 is distinguished from that associated with AML Anaemia, observed most frequently in older women, is accompanied with marked dyserythropoiesis, erythroid multinuclearity as well as hypolobulated and frequently small "dwarf" megakaryocytes. Neutropenia and thrombocytopenia are highly uncommon. The syndrome occurs infrequently in children. The somatic mutation resides in a very primitive multipotential cell, which has been defined as myeloid progenitor in some studies and lymphopoietic progenitors in others. Patients who correspond to WHO criteria of 5q syndrome have a median survival of approximately 7 years. The much less morbid course of the classic 5q syndrome is associated a lower degree of pathological apoptosis.

Deletion of 5q may be a feature of oligoblastic myelogenous leukaemia or other AML. In these situations, two of the classic features of 5q syndrome are often absent, macrocytic red cells and normal or elevated platelet count. Blast cells are evident in oligoblastic leukaemia and basophilia and eosinophilia are evident in over half of patients. 5q cytogenetic abnormalities confer a somewhat better prognosis if marrow blast is less than 10 p.c. [13]

There are several favored candidate genes in the initiation of clonal mutation disease. In the 5q syndrome there is a gene encoding for a member of E-cadherin family and that is homologous for Drosophilia fat tumor suppressor gene and gene encoding RAS guanosine triphosphatase activating protein. An epigenetic change, probably hypermethylation accounts for the loss of tumor suppressor activity of the gene. [14]

The q or long arm of chromosome 5 also contains the genes that encode for a number of growth factors, including interleukin 3, 5 and 9 and granulocyte macrophage-colony-stimulating factor (GM-CSF). How the loss of these factors contributes to the development of this syndrome is unclear. [15]. The syndrome runs an indolent course with least propensity to transform into AML. Most patients present with refractory anaemia, which is transfusion-dependent, so measures to prevent iron load must be undertaken.

Monosomy 7: It is the second most frequent cytogenetic abnormality in MDS. The marrow cells exposed to radiation or chemotherapy is associated with poor prognosis and rapid transformation to AML. A critical region carrying the gene may reside within bands of 7q. The syndrome is not usually associated with special clinical features in adults, but in children they are characterized by an atypical myeloproliferative disorder, abnormal expression of neurofibromatosis and Wilm's tumor gene, unusual susceptibility to infection and Fanconi's anaemia. A variant translocation1:7 is also seen in adults and children and may be preceded by previous exposure. The ERBB gene, which encodes a shortened form of epidermal growth factor receptor, is amplified in this syndrome. Patients with aplastic anaemia have a predisposition to this syndrome. [15]

Paediatric MDS: MDS is uncommon in children, but higher incidence is found in Down syndrome. Abnormalities of chromosome 7, monosomy 7, and 7q are more frequent in paediatric MDS. Unlike in adult patients, however, this cytogenetic abnormality is not associated with an adverse prognosis. The rate of progression to AML is higher in paediatric MDS. Juvenile chronic myelomonocytic leukaemia, one of the most common feature of paediatric MDS has features of both myeloproliferative disorder and MDS. [16]

Hypoplastic MDS: Most patients with present with a hyprcellular or normal cellular bone marrow with ineffective haematopoiesis. A subset of patients will present with hypocellular bone marrow (< 15% cellularity of bone marrow on biopsy) and minimal dysplasia. Hypocellular bone marrow must be differentiated from aplasic anaemia and hypocellular AML. A characteristic MDS cytogenetic abnormality helps to differentiate this disorder (*i.e.*, –5, –7, +8, 20q-). The course and treatment of these patients are similar to those patients with aplastic anaemia.

Myelodysplasia with bone marrow fibrosis: MDS with bone marrow reticulin deposition is generally associated with a poor prognosis. MDS with myelofibrosis must be differentiated from the M7 subtype of AML and myelofibrosis from myeloid metaplasia. In this type of MDS, patients present with trilineage dysplasia, < 30% blast forms in the bone marrow, and an absence of hepatomegaly or prominent splenomegaly.

Therapy related MDS: MDS that occurs following exposure to cytotoxic chemotherapy or ionizing radiation is referred to as secondary or therapy-related MDS. Trilineage dysplasia is common in this type, and the prognosis is generally worse than de novo MDS. For alkylating agent-related MDS the latency period is 3 to7 years. The condition is associated with abnormal cytogenetics involving loss or deletions of chromosome 7 or 5.

Topoisomerase II inhibitors-related MDS have a latency period of 18 months to 3 years after exposure. This condition is associated with a balanced translocation involving chromosome bands 11q 23 and 21q 22. [17]

Myelodysplastic syndrome with myeloproliferative disorder (MDS/MPD): These are clonal stem cell disorders characterized by increased but ineffective haematopoiesis resulting in increased peripheral blood levels of one or more cell lines. Bone marrow is typically hypercellular with dysplasia and defects in maturation. MDS/MPD disorders resemble both a chronic MPD and a syndrome of ineffective and impaired maturation and function. Patients present with hepatosplenomegaly. The disorder has a poor prognosis and an increased incidence of leukaemic transformation.

Clinical features

The patient may remain asymptomatic and the anaemia may be detected on routine examination or examination for some other illness. Alternatively patient may present with symptoms and signs of anaemia *e.g.*, pallor, weakness, lethargy, easy fatiguibility, dyspnoea on exertion, palpitation according to the degree and rapidity of development of anaemia. The disease is very uncommon in individuals younger than 50 years, except in patients in whom the disease occurs as a result of radiotherapy or chemotherapy of a malignant disease. The spleen is slightly increased in size in approximately 5 p.c. of patients. Splenic and hepatic enlargement does not necessarily occur together and more than slight enlargement is unusual.

Haematological findings on laboratory tests include macrocytic anaemia with hypochromic cells (dimorphic anaemia), anisocytosis, basophilic stippling and slight polikilocytosis are present. Total white cell count, platelet counts are usually normal, occasionally increased markedly. Nucleated red cells are present in the blood film. The reticulocyte count varies between 0.5 to 2 p.c. *i.e.*, count is low corresponding to the degree of anaemia. Several red cell changes like increased red cell enzyme activity. haemolysis in cases of pyruvate kinase deficiency, enhanced sensitivity of membrane complement, modification of red cell group antigen and acquired HbH disease have been reported Haemoglobin F may be increased slightly Morphology of red cells similar to that seen in thalassaemia has been seen in acquired HbH disease.

Bone Marrow changes

Marrow cellularity is increased or normal, and occasionally decreased resulting in aplastic anaemia. Islands of dysmorphic cells, especially atypical megakaryocytes usually are present. Dyserythopoiesis in the form of vacuolated small, large, or binucleate erythroblasts may be present. Prussian blue staining invariably shows pathological sideroblasts. Sideroblasts are erythroblsts with an increased number and size of siderosomes (cytoplsmic ferritin containing vacuoles), referred to as intermediate sideroblasts and erythroblasts with mitochondrial iron aggregates that take the form of a complete or partial circumscribed ring of iron globules, referred to as ring sideroblasts. Ring sideroblasts are uncommon or present in small numbers in clonal myeloid disorders than refractory anaemia. If the disease progresses to oligoblastic leukaemia, sideroblasts may become less promonemt. Granulopoiesis and thrombocytopoiesis are not altered significantly in two-third patients In the other third, acquired Pegler-Huet abnormality, hypersegmented nucleus, lobulated megakaryocytes are present. Marrow iron is often increased.

Changes in cell lines other than red cells

Neutropenia is found in 50% of cases at the time of diagnosis. Monocytosis per se may be dominant abnormality for months or years. Pegler-Huet abnormality in neutrophils *i.e.*, ring shaped or bilobed nuclei with very condensed chromatin and neutrophils in the process of apoptosis are common findings. Neutrophil alkaline phosphatase activity is low in some of the cases. Expression of normal antigens on neutrophils and monocytes is low. Defective primary granules of abnormal size and shape and low myeloperoxidase content of neutrophils is another common finding. Chemotactic, phagocytic and bactericidal capability of neutrophils and monocytes is impaired. These patients present with recurrent infection.

Approximately 25% patients have mild to moderate thrombocytopenia at the time of diagnosis. Mild thrombocytosis may be also seen. Platelets may be abnormally large, have large fused central granules. Abnormal platelet function *i.e.*, decreased aggregation to collagen or epinephrine is frequent. These patients may present with bleeding, either spontaneous or on trivial injury.

Decreased natural killer cells but no decrease in large granular lymphocytes, a decrease in helper T-cells and a decrease in Epstein Barr virus receptors on B lymphocytes are some other findings. Antibody dependent cellular cytotoxicity is normal. Thymidine incorporation after mitogenic stimulation and colony growth of T lymphocytes are decreased. The defect in lymphoid cells could reflect the level of somatic mutation in a primitive multipotential cell.

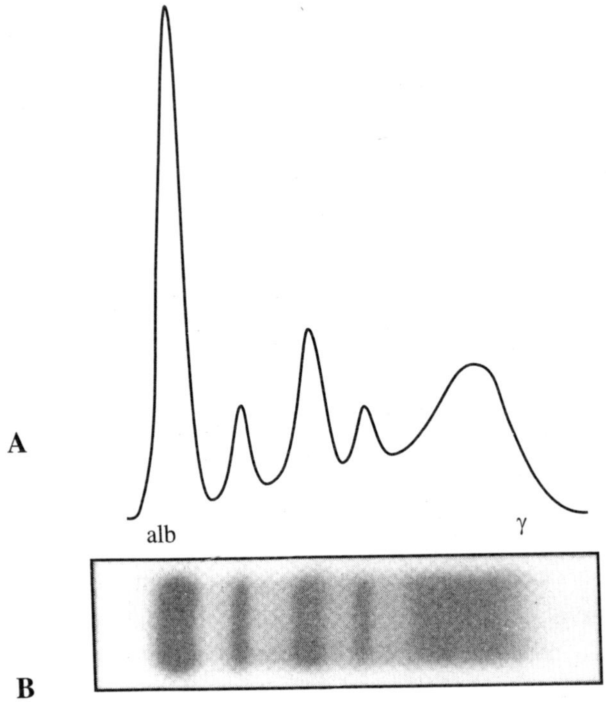

Fig. Pattern of monoclonal protein as seen in (A) demitometer tracing (B) electrophoresis on agarose gel

Changes in the serum

Serum iron, ferritin, transferring may be elevated. LDH and uric acid may be increased due to ineffective erythropoiesis and a high death rate of maturing marrow precursors. Frequently monoclonal gammopathy, hypogammaglobulinaemia, β microglobulinaemia, are in proportion to prognostic category.

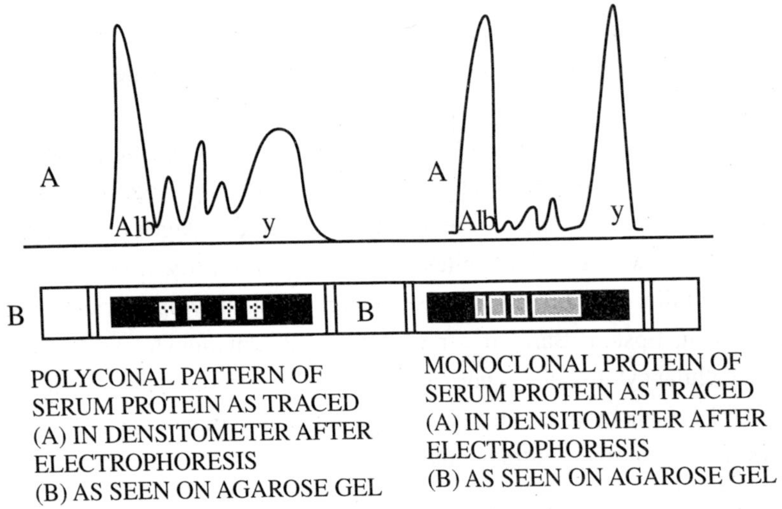

Fig. Pattern of polygonal protein (Left) and monoclonal protein (right) – schematic diagram

Other special clinical features

1. Patients with smouldering myeloid leukaemia (indolent phase) may develop diabetes insipidus. Hypothalamic involvement may occur, can lead to polyuria, polydipsia, and decreased libido. Hypothalamic-pituitary insufficiency in clonal myeloid states has been associated with monosomy 7. [18]
2. Hypodipsia may occur, in extensive thalamic involvement, due to the signal transmitted by thirst centre in cerebral cortex blocked.
3. Acute neutrophilic dermatoses characterized by erythematosus patches on arm, face, legs progressing to painful brown plaque, ulcerating to necrotizing lesions may occur. The condition is found in middle aged women, associated with dense neutrophilic infiltrate and blood neutrophilia. At least 10 p.c. of this syndrome (Sweet disease) progress to acute myeloid leukaemia. G-CSF and ATRA administration has been followed by Sweet disease in some cases. [19]
4. Symptom complex like SLE with fever, flushing, systemic arthritis, ANF and with hyperplastic marrow may precede AML. Several cases of LE cell phenomena are reported to precede AML. [20]
5. Bechet disease, glomerulonephritis, seronegative arthritis, polychronditis, polyneuropathy, paniculitis, inflammatory bowel disease have been reported. The incidence of other cancers may be higher in MDS.[21 (a), (b)]

Therapy

I. Supportive therapy

Some patients do not require active treatment. Occasional patients have low serum and red cell folate concentration. They may show improvement in haemoglobin concentration after administration of **folic acid** in a dose of 1 mg/day orally. Rare patients may benefit temporarily from pharmacologic doses of **pyridoxine** (200 mg/day orally for at least 3 months) or **danazol**. A therapeutic trial from folic acid-pyridoxine is worthwhile if the anaemia is symptomatic, though in a small p.c. of cases. **If anaemia is severe** or symptoms of heart failure or coronary insufficiency are present, **periodic transfusion of red cells** is required.

Recombinant erythropoietin (Epo) is not useful unless pretreatment level is low for haemoglobin level [22]. **Combination of Granulocyte-colony-stimulating factor (G-CSF) with erythropoietin** may increase the response rate to greater than 40 p.c. Erythropoietin 20,000 to 40,000 units SC once in a week and G-CSF 300 microgram SC 2–3 times per week in one regimen that can be used if cytopenia is not tolerated [23] Serum iron should be maintained at a normal level by oral supplementation, if needed to ensure an optimal response from erythropoietin administration. A controlled trial of Epo (20,000 units I.V) and G-CSF (105 microgram), each given SC three times per week, compared to supportive care show better improvement than the group receiving supportive care alone. However, no difference in quality of life is evident and no marked difference in improvement of blood haemoglobin concentration occurs in treated group. [23]

II. Therapy for pancytopenia

(a) In patients with pancytopenia and hyperplastic marrow, cytopenias which are not troublesome, should not be treated. Transfusion of blood components when necessary is the mainstay of treatment. Regular transfusion of red cells is used for patients who do not adapt to moderate anaemia or in whom medical conditions like angina pectoris require a higher packed cell concentration and may decrease transfusion frequency. If thrombocytopenic bleeding occurs, platelet transfusions should be used. Aminocaproic acid may be used as useful adjuvant to platelet transfusion/ IL-2 may increase platelet count in some patients.IL-3 and thrombopoietin are not approved for clinical use.

(b) Amifostine, an aminothiol agent, used for radioprotection, when used in doses of 100–200 mgm/m 2 three times per week, may increase blood counts in some patients.[24]

(c) Asymptomatic neutropenia should not be treated, but fever should be evaluated promptly and suspected infection should be treated with broad spectrum antibiotics until result of culture is known.

(d) Androgens have not been generally useful. Rare cases may show minor improvement but likelihood of substantial improvement is low. Danazol is an attenuated, synthetic, androgen that has been used in the treatment of immune-mediated thrombocytopenia. It may increase the platelet count in low-risk MDS patients who are thrombocytopenic. The mechanism of action is unclear. Danazol, 200 mg administered three times weekly orally, is generally well tolerated and associated with an increase in platelets in 10% to 40% of treated cases. The duration of response is variable, 2 to 26 plus months, and is maintained only when the drug is administered. [25]

(e) Resolution of myelofibrosis by glucocorticoids (prednisone 40 mg/m^2 per day orally to 60 mg qd) has been shown. Protracted glucocorticoid use may increase the risk of infection.[26]

III. Biologic agents and Immunotherapy

(a) For patients with severe symptomatic anaemia or severe symptomatic neutropenia, therapeutic trials of erythropoietin and/ GM-CSF, G-CSF or IL-3 have been found beneficial in increasing counts and occasionally neutrophil function. Cytokines have not been found to increase survival and can produce troubling side effects such as local skin reaction, rash, fever, bone pain and capillary leak syndrome. They also increase immature granulocytes, including blasts in blood and bone marrow. [27]

(b) Immunotherapy

(i) In uncommon cases with hypoplastic marrow, cyclosporine A and antithymocyte globulin (ATG) have been used. These are some cases of MDS in which T-lymphocyte-mediated inhibition of haemopoiesis contributes to cytopenia. [28] Some series have reported response to ATG 15 to 60 p.c. This finding is attributed to incomplete clonal expansion with ATG improving normal haemopoiesis by removing immunologic pressure on remainng normal progenitor cells. Others have postulated that responses may result from suppression of IFN-γ secretion by CD4+ T cells.

Idiopathic thrombocytopenic purpura complicating MDS can respond to cyclosporine. [29]

(ii) Responses to pulse methylprednisolone therapy have occurred in patients with normocellular and hypercellular marrow.

(iii) Mycophenolate mofetil-in cases of autoimmune haemolytic anaemia complicating MDS, haemolysis and undergoing clonal disorders responded.

(iv) Vaccine- Wilm tumor protein (WTI) is a tumor antigen for myelogenous leukaemia. Peptide extracted from this antigen when used for therapy, showed an increase of cytotoxic T cells followed by rapid reduction in leukaemic blast cells. Severe leucopenia has been also reported. [30]

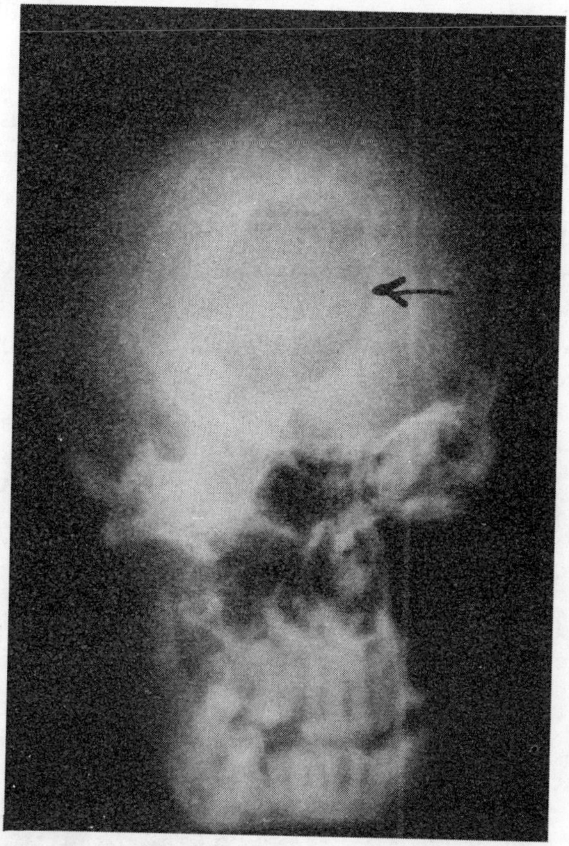

Fig. Large osteolytic levion of skull-view of a small plasmaeysoma on skull bone

IV. Chemotherapy

A series of chemotherapeutic agents have bee been used, especially when the disease evolves to oligoblastic to frank AML.

1. Patients with poor performance status, or of advanced age, or those who choose not to be treated by combined agent, are treated with cytarabarine, 5-azocytidine or dectibane, etposide, hydroxyurea, retinoid, butyrate or interferon coupled with transfusion therapy.
2. Patients younger than 50 years of age with a histocompatible donor are considered for allogenic transplant.
3. Other patients may be considered for non-myeloablative allogenic transplantation or, if in remission, intensive therapy and autologous stem cell transplantation.

Treatment depends on prognostic score which is further determined by

(a) three cytopenic subgroups

(b) number of cytopenias

(c) p.c. of marrow blasts

It has been observed in different studies, that, in MDS, frequency distribution of different risk groups is as follows:

Low risk-15–30% Intermediate risk-30–40% High risk-5–10%

Unexpected progression may necessitate change of treatment. In the cases of patients, who are candidates for stem cell transplantation, may prompt recommending the process.

If the patient is fit for therapy and progresses to cytopenia, haemorrhage, infection or polyblastic leukaemia, therapy for AML may be warranted.

If the patient's tolerance is reduced due to disease process or comorbid condition, attenuation of dose should be done. Cytarabine combined with anthracycline antibiotics or Etoposide has produced remission in approximately half of a group of selected patients. Recovery may be slow and remission is short however.

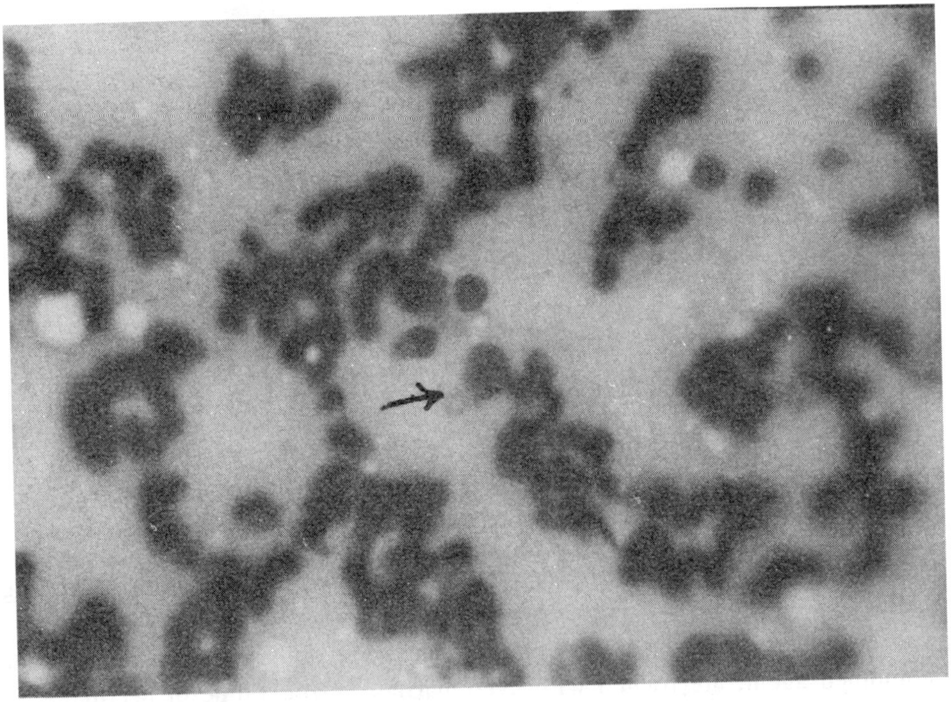

Fig. Plasma cell shown by an arrow in H-P picsure of FNAC of the solitary plasnacytoma on skull bone (in the same patient)

Low intensity single agent therapy is suitable for patients of intermediate risk category. Following agents have been used.

(a) Cytarabine: Low dose cytarabine show occasional remission and it is consistent with effect on leukaemic cell maturation. Most patients experience suppression of malignant stem cell clone alone leading to marrow exploitation with polyclonal haemopoiesis. Cytarabine, in a dose of 5 to 20 mg/m^2 /day by S.C. injection every 12 hours for up to 8 to 16 weeks or by continous IV infusion, when administered, remission in approximately 20 p.c. has been observed. Survival has not been influenced. Therapy is prone to produce marrow hypoplasa and cytopenia. Combination with growth factor does not show clear advantage. [31]

(b) 5-azacytidine: It is a pyrimidine analogue that inhibits DNA methyl transferase, reduces cystosine methylation and inhibits maturation of leukaemic cells. It inhibits release of concostatin-M, IL-6, IL-11 from mononuclear cells. In a dose of 75 mg/m^2 per day S.C. for 7 successive days, it provides significant more benefit than in those patients who are on supportive therapy only. A decrease in WBC count during initial cycle indicates response. [32]

(c) Amifostine: As a single agent given as 200 mg/m^2 IV thrice daily per week for 3 weeks did not result in reduction of transfusion but did some improvement in blood count. Combined with chemotherapy *e.g.*, idarubicin, it reduces toxicities and allows escalation of dose.

(d) Hydroxyurea and etoposide are useful in controlling leukaemic cell proliferation and usually produce only partial response. Etoposide in a dose of 50 mg as a 2 hour infusion 2 to 7 times weekly for 4 weeks or 100 μg per day orally for 3 days and then 50 mg thrice weekly has been found to be effective.[33]

(e) Low dose mephalan, a DNA topoisomerase I inhibitor and weekly doses of idarubicin each has resulted in response in some patients. [34]

Biologic agents

(a) Anti ANF-α therapy has produced mixed results especially eternecept. Infliximab results in two sustained erythroid responses. [35]

(b) Vitamin analogues: Vitamin A analogues (Retionic acid-ATRA) and vitamin D analogues (dihydroxycholecalciferol-Vit D3) when administered in low risk patients produce significant improvement. ATRA in a dose of 45 mg/m^2 daily or isoretinon 25 mg/m^2 and Dihydroxy vitamin D 2.5 mg/day orally for 8 weeks have been found to produce beneficial result in oligoblastic leukaemia. Toxic effects of vitamin A *e.g.*, dry skin, cheilitis, pruritus, lethargy, arthalgia are transitory. Hypercalcaemia is a dose limiting factor in cases of vitamin D administration. [36]

(c) Interferons have maturation effect on mouse and human leukaemic cells, IFN-α in a dose of 3×10^6 units to 1×10^6 units/ml three times a week, when administered, produce a median survival rate which is not better than in untreated group.

(d) Interleukins: IL-2 in a dose of 2.5 to 8 $\times 10^5$ IU twice daily for 30 days, enhaces NK cell activity and eliminate blasts in marrow. Phase II clinical trial failed to show improved blood count.

(e) Arsenic trioxide Trials with this drug in MDS are in progress. Whether the drug affects maturation or apoptosis or proliferation remains to be determined. [37]

Combination therapy

Low dose cytarabine, retinoic acid, 1, 25 dihydroxy vitamin D3, produce 50 p.c. response rate. Amifostine, pentoxyfylline, dexamethasone have been shown to be effective in prolonging survival in oligoblastic leukaemia.

Chapter 10

V. Antiangiogenic agents

Thalidomide in doses of 100–400 mg/day for 12 or more weeks of therapy showed haematologic improvement but no cytoogenetic or complete remission. Cytogenetic responses, in 5q or trisomy 7 syndrome and complex karyotypic abnormalities, have been found. Thalidomide also decreases vascular endothelial growth factor (VEGF) and basic fibroblast growth factor levels. Thromboembolic events have been reported. The drug may have a particular role in marrow fibrosis.

Thalidomide derivative CC-5013 (Revilimid) lowers level of pro-angiogenic cytokines, inhibits attachments of stromal cells, provides cell cycle arrest and apoptosis, affect functional natural killer and T-lymphocytes. In 5q syndrome response was noted in a dose of 25 mg/day. Unlike thalidomide, dose reduction for myelosuppression is required. [38]

VI. Signal inhibitors

(a) Tyrosine kinase inhibitor SU 5416 which also inhibits VEGF has minimal activity in MDS. RTK 474 and anti-VEGF antibody bevacizumab have entered clinical trial Imatinib mesylate is a tyrosine kinase inhibitor of c-abl, c-kit, platelet derived growth factor receptor has not resulted in clinical remission in MDS. [39]

(b) Inhibitor of raf protein kinase, and farsenyl transferase inhibitor, produced an overall response rate of 30 p.c. Statins that inhibit geranyl-geranyl-transferase are being studied for treatment of AML and MDS. [40]

(c) Progenitors involved in MDS rarely express fit-3 antigen. So fit-3 inhibitors doubtfully have an important role in the treatment of MDS. [41]

VII. Combination Chemotherapy

Chemotherapeutic agents, in combination are the choice of therapy in high risk group. Antracycline, cytaribine and/or etoposide result in remission in fewer than 20% of patients with oligoblastic leukaemia. Advanced age, high frequency of cardiac, renal, immunologic, and other system impairment in most patients with oligoblastic leukaemia are highly responsible for poor outcome. Patients, younger than 60, have higher remission rate. FLAG-IdA regime (fludaribine, cytabirine, idarubicin, G-CSF) produces 53% complete remission, 11% improvement in high risk myeloid malignancies. [41]

II. Haematopoietic stem cell transplantation

It remains the only treatment of MDS with curative potential. Conditioning regime consists of cyclophosphamide plus irradiation or busulphan plus cyclophosphamide.

An international bone marrow transplant registry report of 452 patients with MDS who received allogenic transplant, found that young age and platelet count greater than 100×10^9/litre prior to transplant were associated with lower transplant mortality, higher disease free interval and overall survival. Patients with higher percentage of blasts, high prognostic score have higher relapse rate. One report showed superior result with mobilised blood cells rather than bone marrow stem cells. [42].

VIII. Autologous stem cell infusion

Patients with oligoblatic leukaemia, treated with their own stem cells, after intensive chemotherapy, show significant improvement. There is limitation of the procedure in the form of contamination of stem cells with repopulating leukaemic cells, though there is absence of growth-versus-host reaction.

Peri-transplant mortality with intensive therapy and stem cell rescue has been estimated to be approximately 50% of selected patients with extended survival. [43]

The more advanced the disease at the time of treatment, the worse is the outcome. In patients younger than 20 years allogenic transplant may be the treatment of choice to decrease the rate of relapse.

To summarize, the manifestations of MDS are varied, the prognosis depends upon the degree of malignant change in bone marrow as well as cytogenetic type, therapy is different in different risk categories, therapy varies from supportive treatment with by periodic blood transfusion, different growth promoting factors to control pancytopenia in low risk category, single agent low dose therapy in intermediate risk patients to combination chemotherapy in high risk groups. Immunologic and biological agents are recently tried with variable success. Allogenic bone marrow transplant has only curative potential.

REFERENCES

1. Layton DM, Mufti GJ: Myelodysplastic syndromes: Their history, evolution and relation to acute myeloid leukaemia. Blut 53: 423, 1986.
2. Leitman MA: Myelodysplasia or myeloneoplasia: Thoughts on the nosology of the clonal myeloid disorders. Blood cell Mol Dis 26: 572, 2000.
3. Saarni ML, Linman JW: Preleukaemia. Am J Med 55: 38, 1973.
4. Aul C, Gatterman N, Schedirw. Age related incidence and other epidemiologic aspects of myelodysplastic syndromes. Brit J Haematol 82: 358, 1992.

5(a). Berger R, Le Cniat M, Schaison G: Chromosome abnormalities in bone marrow of Fanconi anaemia patients. Cancer Genet Cytogenes 65: 47, 1993.

5(b). Hayashi Y, Egushi M, Sugita K et al., Cytogenetic findings and clinical features in acute leukaemia and transient myeloproliferative disorders and Down's syndrome. Blood 72: 15, 1988.

6. Mimmeli A, Maserati E, Griedice G et al., Familial partial monosomy 7 and myelodysplasia: Different parental origin of monosomy 7 suggests action of a mutator gene. Cancer Genet cytogenet 124: 147, 2001.
7. Culligan DJ, Cachia P, Whittaker A et al., Clonal lymphocytes are detectable only in some cases of MDS. Brit J Haematol 81 : 346, 1992.
8. Brunning RD, Head D, Bernett JM, et al., Myelodysplastic syndromes, in World Health Organization. Classification of Tumors of Haemopoietic and Lymphoid tissues, Chap.2, edited by E Jaffe, NL Harris, H Stein, JN Vardiman, p 63, IARC Press, Lynon, 2003.
9. Bernstein SH, Brunetto VL, Davey FR, et al., Acute myeloid-type therapy for newly diagnosed patients without antecedent cytopenias having myelodysplastic syndrome as defined by French-American-British criteria: a cancer Leukaemia Group B study, J Clin Oncol 14 : 2486–2494, 1996.
10. West RR, Stafford DA, White DT, et al., Cytogenetic abnormalities in the myelodysplastic syndromes and occupational or environmental exposure. Blood 95 : 2003, 2001.
11. Greenber B, Cox C, Le Beau MM, et al., International scoring system for evaluating prognosis in myelodysplastic syndromes. Blood 91 : 1100–1110, 1998.

12. Ransking WH, Tirumali N, Jacobson R et al., Evidence of a multistep pathogenesis of myelodysplastic syndrome. Blood 63: 1318, 1984.

13. Giagonnidis AAN, Germing U, Hasse S et al., Clinical, Cytogenetic and prognostic features of patients with myelodysplastic syndrome and del (5q) including band q 31. Leukaemia 18 : 113, 2004.

14. Bartman CR: Molecular genetic aspects of myelodysplastic syndrome. Blood 82 : 590, 1993.

15. Gerristen WR, Donohue J, Bauman J et al., Clonal analysis of myelodysplastic syndrome: Monosomy 7 is expressed in myeloid lineage as detected by fluorescent in situ hybridization Blood 80 : 217, 1992.

16. Sasaki H, Manalk A, Kojima S et al., Myelodysplastic syndromes in childhood leukaemia. Leukaemia15 : 713, 2001.

17. Perk DJ, Koeffler HP: Therapy related myelodysplastic syndromes. Semin Haematol 338 : 256, 1996.

18. De La Chapelle A, Lahitnn R: Monosomy 7 predisposes to Diabetes insipidus in leukaemia and myelodysplastic syndrome. Eur J Haematol 75 : 8213, 2004.

19. Arbetter KR, Hubbard KW, Germing U, Hassi S et al., Case of granulocyte colony-stimulating factor-induced Sweet's syndrome. Am J Haematol 616 : 126, 1999.

20. Saif MW, Hopkins JL, Gore SD: Autoimmune phenomena in patients with myelodysplastic syndromes and myelomonocytic leukaemia. Leukaemia Lymphoma 43 : 2409, 2002.

21(a). Ohio-E, Ohtasuka E, Watanbe K et al., Bechet's disease associated with myelodysplastic syndromes. A case report and a review of literature Cancer 79 : 262, 1997.

21(b). Harewood GC, Lotust EV Jr, Tefferi A et al., Concurrent inflammatory bowel disease and myelodysplastic syndromes. Inflmn Bowel Dis 5 : 98, 1999.

22. Stein RS, Abibs RI, Krantz S: Pharmacologic dosage of recombinant human erythropoietin in the treatment of myelodysplastic syndromes. Blood 78 : 1658, 1991.

23. Negrin RS, Haeuber DH, Nagber A et al., Maintainance treatment of patients with myelodysplastic syndromes using recombinant human granulocytic colony-stimulating factor. Blood 76 : 36, 1990.

24. List AF, Brasfield F, Heaton R, et al., Stimulation of Haeematopoiesis by Amifostine in patients with myelodysplastic syndrome. Blood 90 : 3364, 1997.

25. Naean Y, Pecking A: Refractory anaemia with excess of myeloblasts in the bone marrow. A clinical trial of androgens in 90 cases. Brit J Haematol 37 : 23, 1977.

26. Watts EJ, Majer RV, Green PJ: Hyperfibrotic myelodysplasia: A report of three cases showing haematological remission following treatment with prednisone. Brit J Haematol 78 : 129, 1991.

27. Schuster Mw: Will cytokines alter the treatment of myelodysplastic syndrome? Am J Med Sci 305: 72,1993.

28. Moliderm JJ, Jiang YZ, Stevenson M et al., Haematologic response of patients with myelodysplastic syndrome to Antithymocyte globulin is associated with lymphocyte-mediated inhibition of CFU-GM and alterations in T-cell receptor V-beta profile. Brit J Haematol 102 : 1314, 1996.

29. Janasova A, Newirdova R, Cermark J et al., Cyclosporin A therapy in hypoplastic MDS and certain refractory anaemia without hypoplastic bone marrow. Brit J Haematol 100 : 304, 1998.

30. Oka Y, Tsuboi A, Murakami M, et al., Wilm's tumor gene peptide-based immunotherapy for patients with overt leukaemia from MDS or MDS with myelofibrosis. Int J Haematol 78 : 56, 2003.

31. Cherson BD: Standard and low dose chemotherapy for the treatment of myelodysplastic syndromes. Leuk Res 22 (Supl 1): 517, 1998.

32. Silverman LF, Holland JF, Weinberg EP, et al., 5-azacytidine on the in-vivo and in-vitro haematopoiesis in patients with myelodysplastic syndrome. Leukaemia 7 (Supl 1): 21, 1993.

33. Ogawa K, Yamada T, Ito T et al., Low dose etoposide: A potential therapy for myelodysplastic syndrome. Brit J Haematol 82: 354, 1992.

34. Invernizzi R, Pecci A, Rossi G et al., Idarubicin and cystosine arabinoside in the induction and maintainance therapy of high risk myelodysplastic syndromes. Haematologica 82: 660, 1997.

35. Gersuk GM, Beckham C, Loken MR, et al., A role for tumor necrosis factor alpha, Fas and Fas-ligand in marrow failure associated with myelodysplastic syndrome. Brit J Haematol 103: 176, 1996.

36. Nagler A, Rikills I, Tartasky I Fabian I: Effect of 1, 25 dihydroxy vitamin D, and cis-retinoic acid and low dose prednisone. Am J Haematol 78: 56, 2003.

37. Miller WH Jr: Molecular targets of Arsenic trioxide in malignant cells. Oncologist (Supl 1): 14, 2002.

38. Strupp C, Germing U, Aivado M, t al., Thalidomide for the treatment of patients of myelodysplastic syndromes with fibrosis. Leuk Res 26: 965, 2002.

39. Drummond MW, Lush CI, Vickers MA, et al., Imatinib mesylate- induced- molecular remission of Philadelphia chromosome positive myelodysplastic syndrome. Leukaemia 17: 463, 2003.

40. Kurzrock R, Kuntarjian H, Cortes J: Farnesyl transferase inhibitor R 11577, in myelodysplastic syndromes: Clinical and biological activities in the phase I setting Blood 192: 4527, 2003.

41. Sawyears CL: Finding the next gleeve. FIT_3 targeted kinase inhibitor therapy for acute myeloid leukaemia. Cancer cell 1: 413, 2002.

42. Estey EH, Thall PF, Pierce S, et al., Randomized Phase II study of fludarabine,+/– cystosine arabinoside + idarubicin +/– all trans retinoic acid +/– granulocyte-colony-stimulating factor in poor prognosis newly diagnosed acute myeloid leukaemia and myelodysplastic syndrome. Blood 93 : 2478, 1999.

43. Appelbaum FR, Anderson J: Allogenic bone marrow transplantation for myelodysplastic syndrome: Outcome analysis according to IPSS score for myelodysplastic syndrome. Leukaema 12 (Supl 1): 525, 1998.

44. Wathel E, Solary E, Lelen X, et al., A prospective study of autologous bone marrow or peripheral stem cell transplantation after intensive chemotherapy in myelodysplastic syndromes. Leukaemia 13 : 5211, 1999.

Chapter 10

CHAPTER

11

Multiple Myeloma and Monoclonal Gammopathies

11.1 INTRODUCTION

A spectrum of disorders characterized by bone pain, osteolytic bone lesion, progressive anaemia, unexplained fatigue, elevation of erythrocyte sedimentation rate, and hypercalcaemia, is designated as Multiple Myeloma and Monoclonal gammopathies. The basic pathology of the disease is the secretion of an abnormal protein (paraprotein), called M protein, by the malignant plasma cells of the bone marrow.

Each monoclonal protein consists of two heavy chain polypeptides of same class and subclass and two light chain polypeptides of same type. The different monoclonal proteins are designated by capital letters that correspond to the class of their heavy chains, the chains being represented by Greek letters, e.g. γ in IgG, α in IgA, μ in IgM, δ in IgD, μ in IgM, e in IgE, and their light chain types are designated as kappa (κ) and lambda (λ).

A monoclonal protein is characterized by a narrow peak (like a church spire) or a localized band on electrophoresis or by a localized band on immunofixation. In contrast, a polyclonal protein consists of one or more heavy chain polypeptides and both light chain classes. A polyclonal protein is characterized by a broad peak or band, usually of γ mobility on electrophoresis and by the absence of a localized band with appropriate anti-sera on immunofixation. The differential diagnosis of monoclonal increase from polyclonal increase in immunoglobulin is essential because the former is associated with a neoplastic or potentially neoplastic process, whereas the latter is associated with an inflammatory or reactive process.

11.2 MONOCLONAL PROTEINS

Monoclonal proteins have long been considered as abnormal proteins, but studies during past several years indicate that they are only excessive quantities of normal immunoglobulins. Monoclonal proteins are individual antibodies and are products of a single clone of plasma cells. Although some monoclonal proteins represent known antibodies, most do not. The one-cell one-immunoglobulin concept is supported by the fact that nearly all individual plasma cells contain either κ or λ light chains but not both.

Monoclonal proteins are best examples of tumor specific antigens. Malignant B cells may express both early and late B cell antigens. Multiple Myeloma is a disease in which transferring event occurs in mature plasma cells. Cells resembling small lymphocytes may have the same immunoblastic gene arrangement, same immunoblastic idiotypes and surface antigens as all malignant plasma cells. As such, these neoplasms consist of transformed B cells that have retained the ability to mature into plasma cells. Thus myeloma contrasts with chronic lymphocytic leukaemia, in which there is not production of significant number of plasma cells. Since Bence Jones first described what termed out to be monoclonal light chains in the urine of myeloma patients, the protein goes by his name. This along with M protein (which stands for Myeloma, Monoclonal, or Malignant) is the cell marker of this disease. The spectrum of the disorder, producing M protein, includes tumours of small lymphocytes e.g., Chronic lymphocytic lukaemia and tumours of plasmacytoid cells e.g., Waldestrom macroglobulinaemia. These types of tumours usually produce IgM, whereas plasmacytomas usually produce IgG or IgA.

11.3 DETECTION OF MONOCLONAL PROTEIN

Serum Electrophoresis: The most common screening test for M protein is electrophoresis.

Method: A few microlitre of serum are spotted on a support medium e.g., cellulose acetate that has been equilibrated at a basic pH. The proteins in the serum migrate toward anode at a velocity proportional of their negative charge to their molecular weight, when current is applied across the medium. After a migration period of approximately 30 minutes, the cellulose acetate is taken up and dried, stained for proteins and examined by densitometry.

Interpretation: Albumin is the most abundant protein of the serum and migrates as a sharp peak. They have the same amino acid sequence, but γ globulins have millions of different amino acid sequences and varying carbohydrate side chains. Consequently they migrate in a very broad band that typically consists of IgA and IgM from the front (towards β globulin) and IgG spread through the entire spread of globulins. IgD and IgE are normally secreted at a low level and not detected by this method. M protein migrates anywhere in the globulin-occupying compartment, IgM and IgA tend to migrate faster than most IgG molecule.

Normal Serum Electrophoresis Pattern

Anode + ⟷ Cathode –

Albumin	α_1 globulin	α_2 globulin	β globulin	γ globulin
Albumin	α_1 antitrypsin	α_2 Macroglobulin	β_2 Lipoprotein	IgG
	α_1 Lipoprotein	α_2 lipoprotein	Transferrin	IgA
	α_1 Acid Glycoprotein (orosomucoid)	Haptoglobin	Plasminogen	IgM
		Ceruloplasmin	Complement	IgD
		Erythropoietin	Haemopexin	IgE

To distinguish these immunoglobulin classes, immunofixation is necessary.

Pitfalls in the diagnosis by electrophoresis:

(1) A monoclonal protein may be present even when the total serum protein concentration, β and γ globulin peaks and quantitative immunoglobulins are all normal.

(2) The agarose gel must be examined visually because the densitometer tracing may not detect a small monoclonal protein.

(3) A small monoclonal protein may also be concealed among the γ or β region.

(4) A monoclonal light chain (Bence Jones proteinaemia) is rarely seen on agarose gel.

(5) A localized band is occasionally seen in μ heavy chain disease, but it is never seen in α heavy chain disease.

(6) In γ heavy chain disease a broad band rather than a sharp, localized band is often seen on electrophoresis.

(7) A monoclonal protein may appear as broad band and may be mistaken for a polyclonal increase in immunoglobulin. Hence, immunofixation is necessary for identification.

11.4 INDICATIONS OF ELECTROPHORESIS

This test should be done in all suspected cases of multiple myeloma, macroglobulinaemia, or amyloidosis. This is also indicated in any patient with unexplained fatigue or anaemia, persistent elevation of ESR without any obvious reason, osteoporosis, osteolytic lesion, or non-traumatic fractures, immunoglobulin deficiency, unexplained renal insufficiency or hypercalcaemia.

Because the presence of a localized band or spike is strongly suggestive of primary amyloidosis, serum protein electrophoresis should be also performed in unexplained peripheral neuropathy, carpal tunnel syndrome, refractory congestive failure, nephrotic syndrome, orthostatic hypotension or malabsorption syndrome. A densitometer tracing is preferred to other methods, for following the size of a monoclonal protein, to judge the effect of therapy.

11.5 IMMUNOFIXATION Vs NEPHELOMETRY

Immunofixation should be done in all sera showing a sharp peak or a localized band on electrophoresis and in all sera with monoclonal free light chain for IgD or IgE monoclonal proteins, or in clinically suspected cases of myeloma, macroglobulinaemia or primary amyloidosis. Immunofixation may detect a small monoclonal protein in suspected primary amyloidosis, apparently solitary plasmacytoma or extramedullary plasmacytoma, treated myeloma or macroglobulinaemia when the localized band has disappeared on electrophoresis. It can also detect polyclonal increase in immunoglobulin and is especially helpful in detection of biclonal gammopathy.

Rate nephelometry is the preferred method for quantification of immunoglobulin because it is not affected by the molecular size of the antigen. The degree of turbidity is measured near the ultraviolet region. The $\kappa : \lambda$ ratio obtained by nephelometry has been used for detection of light chain type of large monoclonal gammopathies, but small monoclonal proteins have a normal ratio and are not recognized. Immunofixation is necessary in these cases. Nephelometry measures accurately 7S IgM, polymers of IgA, or aggregates of IgG, unlike radial immunodiffusion, which is not recommended. Quantification of immunoglobulins is more useful than immunofixation for the demonstration of hypogammaglobulinaemia. [1]

Method of Nephelometry: Varying dilutions of the test fluid are incubated with antibodies specific for anyone of the different immunoglobulin light and heavy chains. After precipitates form, the amount of precipitate is determined by comparing with standard curves produced by precipitating immunoglobulins. This new automated technique has replaced the slow, laborious, semi-quantitative technique of radial immunodiffusion.

Immunoglobulins in serum, urine or CSF are measured by nephelometry. This technique is based on the observation that antigen-antibody complexes form cloudy precipitate. The precipitate can be detected photo-electrically.

11.6 DETECTION OF MONOCLONAL PROTEIN IN URINE

Free light chains that appear in the urine of myeloma patients can be detected by sulfosalicylic acid precipitation, electrophoresis of concentrated urine, immunoelectrophoresis or immunofixation. Common urine dipsticks rely on bromophenol blue, a dye that binds specifically to albumin. These dipsticks are not reliable screening tests for Bence Jones proteinuria and sulphosalicylic acid should be used. The heat test is not worthwhile for detection of Bence Jones protein. When the immunoglobulin light chains filtered through the glomeruli exceeds the resorption capacity of the proximal tubule, free light chains are excreted in the urine and this is again proportional to the number of plasma cells. Serial measurement is, therefore, a convenient way of estimating the effect of therapy. As renal damage progresses light chain excreted in the urine increases. For this reason, the best estimate of tumour mass is by estimating M protein in the serum.

Electrophoresis of urine must be preceded by a 24 hour collection for estimation of total protein excreted each day. A urinary monoclonal protein is seen as a dense, localized band on agarose gel or as a tall, narrow, homogenous peak on densitometer tracing. The amount of Bence Jones protein is calculated from the size of the spike on the densitometer tracing and the total 24 hour urine protein content.

Immunofixation should be performed in the urine of patients with monoclonal gammopathy of undetermined significance, who have a serum monoclonal protein in urine of greater than 1.5 g per dl, in every adult with nephrotic syndrome of unknown cause, in patients with known or suspected cases of myeloma, plasmacytoma or amyloidosis.

11.7 HISTOPATHOLOGICAL EXAMINATION OF BONE MARROW

On histologic sections of bone marrow from multiple myeloma patients, many plasma cells have nuclei with an immature chromatin network rather than the highly condensed pattern of normal plasma cells. An increased frequency of binucleate or multinucleate cells is also observed. The abilities to divide and to incorporate tritiated thymidine into DNA are criteria that are useful in distinguishing "malignant" from "benign" plasma cells. These criteria are not routinely used in the clinical laboratory, as less expensive tests yield similar information.

Plasma cell labelling index (PCLI)

A monoclonal antibody to 5-bromo-2-deoxyuridine is used which is helpful for differentiating patients with monoclonal gammopathy (MGUS) and smouldering multiple myeloma (SMM) from those with multiple myeloma. Patients whose plasma cells have a high labelling index (> 1%) most likely have to develop multiple myeloma in near future.

Phenotype determination: The typical phenotype of multiple myeloma cells as determined by flow cytometry is found to be, CD45-, HLA DR-, CD19-, P CAL+, CD 38+, CD138+, Ki67 in variable proportions, and monoclonal cytoplasmic Ig+ ($\gamma > \alpha > \mu$; $\kappa > \lambda$).

11.8 GENETIC ABNORMALITIES OBSERVED IN MYELOMA CELLS

Malignant transformation occurs in a B-cell during its differentiation in germinal centre. The presence of clonotypic cells in the blood even at diagnosis, underscores the haematogenous spread as the way for disease dissemination. Interphase fluorescence in situ hybridization (FISH) and other molecular genetic studies identified five primary recurrent chromosomal rearrangements involving IgH translocations. Complex unbalanced translocations or insertions often involving multiple chromosomes represent secondary genetic alterations.

Hyperproliferative nature of myeloma and its stromal dependence for growth account for high frequency of normal diploid metaphase karyotype (originating in normal haemopoietic cells) observed in untreated patients. The remaining myeloma patients have complex cytogenetics abnormalities involving, on average 11 different chromosomes. A major breakthrough in myeloma genetics was the successful application of gene expression profiling highly purified CD 38+ plasma cells Cyclin D3 is a newly recognized translocation product found to be associated with primary gene expression in myeloma. [2]

11.9 ANALYSIS OF GENE REARRANGEMENT

The most specific means to determine whether a myelo- or lympho-proliferative disorder is monoclonal or not, is by analysing gene rearrangement. The most common technique is the flow cystometry looking for light chains (κ or λ) on tumor cells. Because B-cells rearrange both heavy and light chains of immunoglobulin on non-germ line, immunoglobulin gene fragments, following digestion by restriction endonucleases, when studied, show that genomic DNA sequences are of different length on non-germ line B-cells, when compared to DNA sequences of germ-line B-cells. Myelomatous and normal bone marrow plasma cells, can be readily distinguished, but not the myeloma cells and cells of monoclonal gammopathy.

11.10 MOLECULAR PATHOGENESIS OF MULTIPLE MYELOMA

Myeloma arises from a normal germinal centre B-cell. At least 30–60% of cases are benign plasma cell monoclonal gammopathy. It does not always pass through the stage of smouldering myeloma. Initially the myeloma is confined to the marrow (intramedullary) but with time, the tumor may acquire the ability to grow in extramedullary sites (e.g., blood, pleural fluid, skin). Some of the extramedullary myeloma can establish immortalized cell lines in vitro. The transition of monoclonal gammopathy to myeloma may be manifested by increased number of myeloma cells at multiple foci and is associated with angiogenesis and osteolytic lesion. [3]

Milestones in myeloma biologic research are linked to the discovery of IL-6 as a myeloma growth and survival factor and to the recognition of stromal cell dependence. [4]

A critical cell adhesion-mediated cross-reaction exists between myeloma plasma cells and different cytokines and chemokines, especially Il-6 and IL-15. Insulin like growth factor (IGF), hepatocyte growth factor, the receptors of which are endowed with surfaces of plasma cells. [5]

A hallmark of plasma cell stage of B-cell differentiation is CD 138 antigen (syndecan-1). It is shed and often deposited in the cellular matrix, trapping growth-promoting factors and pro-angiogenic cytokines, thus contributing to myeloma progression and invasion. [6]

Growth and survival signals are mediated via PI3/AKT, STA3, RAS/MAPK and nuclear factor (NF)-kB pathways. Thus myeloma/microenvironment interaction holds important clues to the understanding of the disease progression or drug resistance and opens new venues for novel therapeutic interventions. [7]

DKK1 antigen expression can be detected in plasma cells that grow interstitially, however expression is dramatically reduced or undetectable in cells within focal lesions. During progression myeloma cells shift from DKK1 positive interstitial growth pattern to DKK1 negative nodular growth pattern. Down regulation of DKK1 expression accompanies the shift. At terminal stage, plasma cell growth occur in extramedullary foci, which are DKK1 negative.

The two main features of this disease are osteolytic lesions and anaemia.

Osteolytic lesions result from an imbalance of osteoblast and osteoclast number and function. The underlying mechanism is osteoclast activation through the Receptor Activation of NF-kB ligand (RANKL), the Macrophage Inflammatory Protein (MIP), α/β chemokine and IL-3 axes. Expression of RANKL by stromal cells is drastically increased by contact with myeloma cells whereas its decoy receptor osteoprotegerin (OPG) is suppressed and additionally inactivated by syndecan-mediated internalization into myeloma cells and by MIPα, which originates in myeloma cell. [8]

Osteoblast progenitor cells in the mesenchyme and not the mature osteoblasts are rich sources of RANKL. Bone destruction is caused by activation of osteoclasts and block of differentiation of mesenchymal precursor cells to mature osteoblasts. Myeloma plasma cells ordinarily do not express DKK-1 antigen, but do so during disease progression. The antigen is a potent inhibitor of signalling process of the cell and thereby blocks the terminal differentiation of mesechymal cells to osteoblasts Mechanism of activation of the antigen is unknown. [9]

A relevant aspect of myeloma biology is the resistance to apoptosis, an important mechanism of increasing tumor burden in this hyper-proliferative malignancy. Bcl-2, Bcl-XL and especially mcl-1 are expressed in myeloma cell lines. Through intrinsic pathway they release mitochondrial constituents (cytochromeC, SMAC, [second mitochondrial activator of catepases] and activate catepase-9 leading to apoptosis. The extrinsic apoptosis pathway comprises of the tumor necrosis factor (TNF), FAS ligand, Tumor-necrosis-factor-related-apoptosis-inducing ligand (TRAIL). Death receptor 4 & 5 expressed on myeloma cell lines may be activated by TRAIL. This activation may be blocked by expression of TRAIL decoy receptors. Sequestration of OPG by soluble Syndecan1 may also protect myeloma cells from TRAIL activation. The outcome depends on relative levels of proapoptotic and antiapoptotic molecules and cell adhesion molecules, which may be exploited therapeutically and may be the cause of drug resistance. [10]

The continued and chronic exposure of marrow to DKK-1 antigen results in overproduction of RANKL and IL-6 by immature osteoblasts and mesechymal cells, which, in turn, lead to differentiation into bone-resorbing osteoclasts which also produce IL-6.

Chapter 11

11.11 SPECTRUM OF MONOCLONAL GAMMOPATHIES

A. Malignant Monoclonal Gammopathies

Multiple Myeloma (IgA, IgD, IgE, IgG and free light chains)

1. Overt Multiple Myeloma
2. Smouldering multiple myeloma
3. Plasma cell leukaemia
4. Non-secretory multiple myeloma
5. Osteosclerotic multiple myeloma (POEMS syndrome)

B. Plasmacytoma

1. Solitary plasmacytoma of bone
2. Extramedullary plasmacytoma

C. Malignant lymphoproliferative disease

1. Waldenstrom Macroglobulinaemia
2. Malignant Lymphoma

D. Heavy Chain Disease (HCDs)

1. α-HCD 2. γ- HCD 3. μ-HCD

E. Amyloidosis

1. Primary
2. With Myeloma (secondary, localized, familial, having no monoclonal protein)

F. Monoclonal gammopathies of undetermined significance (MGUS)

1. Benign (IgG, IgA, IgD, IgM, and rarely, free light chains)
2. Biclonal gammopathies
3. Idiopathic Bence Jones proteinuria

11.12 MULTIPLE MYELOMA (PLASMA CELL MYELOMA, MYELOMATOSIS, OR KAHLER DISEASE)

The disease is characterized by a neoplastic proliferation of a single clone of plasma cells engaged in the production of a monoclonal protein (IgG κ, IgG λ, IgA κ. IgA λ, IgD κ, IgD λ, IgE κ, IgE λ, free κ, and free λ). Multiple myeloma consists of 1% of all malignancies and more than 10% of haematological malignancies. The incidence is approximately 4 per 100,000 of population. The cause of multiple myeloma is unknown. Radiation, exposure to industrial or agricultural toxin or a genetic material, all seem to be related.

Human Herpes Virus 8 (KSHV) is involved in pathogenesis of pleural cavity lymphoma. Some investigators have identified HHV-8 in marrow dendritic cells in myeloma patients. Current researches focus on inflammatory reaction of the marrow microenvironment which may contribute to the transition from essential gammopathy to myeloma.

11.13 CLINICAL PICTURE

The peak incidence is in the seventh decade of life and a male preponderance is seen. Only 2% of patients are below 40 years. Bone pain, particularly in the back or chest, aggravated by movement is the commonest presenting feature, which occurs in about two-thirds of patients at diagnosis. Next common presenting feature is the renal insufficiency, which occurs in half of the cases. This is often due to so called myeloma kidney, in which the distal and collecting tubules become obstructed with large laminated casts consisting mainly of Bence Jones protein. Hypercalcaemia is also a common and preventable cause of renal insufficiency.

Neurologic manifestations may be also presenting feature. This occurs in the form of root pain or compression of spinal cord or cauda eqina, as a result of bone lesion or myelomatous deposit. Leptomeningeal infiltration by myeloma cells is quite infrequent and found in only 5% of cases. Bacterial infection, recurrent and protracted, particularly gram negative ones, viral infection like herpes zoster are quite common in multiple myeloma.

Bleeding from different sites may be an associated feature. This may result from thrombocytopenia, platelet abnormalities or inhibition of coagulation factors from the monoclonal protein. Physical findings include pallor which is the most frequent finding and hepatomegaly in 20% of patients, associated with splenomegaly in 5% of cases. Extramedullary plasmacytomas are more common in the late stages of the disease.

Anaemia in multiple myeloma is believed to be due to a combination of factors:

1. Overproduction of FAS ligand, MIPα, and TRAIL, (produced by myeloma cells, which, together, trigger death signals in immature erythroblasts.
2. Most patients have an inappropriate erythopoietin response on lowering of haemoglobin. Blunted erythropoietin response may emerge from abundant production of cytokines, IL-1, TNF-β or increased serum viscosity level. [11]
3. Overproduction of IL-6 by marrow stroma, normal accessory cells or tumor cells may contribute to anaemia in myeloma. [12]
4. Anaemia is further accentuated by presence of renal failure in cases of myeloma kidney.

Anaemia is of variable severity and of normocytic, normochromic in character.

Possibly due to thrombopoietic activity of cytokines, myeloma patients do not usually manifest thrombocytopenia.

Pain at different sites of the body results from different aetiologies related to plasma cell proliferation.

1. It frequently occurs due to vertebral osteoporosis or more typically lytic lesion of bone, as a consequence of, excessive osteoclast activation and inhibition of compensatory osteoblastic activity.
2. Localized pain may result from regional tumor growth towards the spinal cord and nerve roots.
3. Painful mass effect may be produced by amyloid deposit.

11.14 NEPHROPATHY

Abnormalities of renal function occur when the tubular absorptive capacity for the light chains is exhausted resulting in interstitial nephritis because of light chain casts. The second most common cause of nephropathy is hypercalcaemia with hypercalciuria, leading to volume depletion and pre-renal azotaemia. In addition, hypercalcaemia is conductive to calcium deposits in the renal tubules, also producing interstitial nephritis. Amyloidosis (described in detail in separate chapter) is associated with light chain proteinuria usually present with nephrotic syndrome but with passage of time, lead to renal failure. Amyloidosis is more common in patients with λ light chain myeloma than with κ light chain myeloma, especially those with λ light chain proteins that have Ig variable region belonging to λ V1 subgroup. Probably underestimated, however, is the frequency of Ig light chain, in Immunoglobulin disease D, a disease more commonly associated with light chain myeloma often at barely detectable level. This condition leads to impaired glomerular filtration. [13]

The following points should be considered in development of renal failure in myeloma patients:

(1) Tumor cell involvement occurs especially in cases of enlarged kidneys, though it more often results from amyloidosis.

(2) Frequent use of non-steroidal anti-inflammatory drugs for relieving pain, may cause it.

(3) Experimental studies show that high level expression of IL-6 transgene under the control of metallothiocin-1 promoter, can induce dysproteinaemia and protracted acute phase response leading to renal damage.

(4) An important reason for renal function impairment is the liberal administration of biphosphonates, especially when administered rapidly.(< 2 hrs for Pamidronate and < 30 minutes for Zolandroate).

11.15 INFECTIONS

Deficiencies of cellular immune function account for recurrent infections commonly seen in myeloma. The mechanism of immunosuppression is obscure, though myeloma cell expression of transforming growth factor β (TGFβ) and FAS ligand have been implicated. In addition patients have impaired ability to mount a humoral response to antigen and low levels of polyclonal serum Igs. As a result myeloma patients are highly susceptible to serious infections from bacteria, such as Streptococcus pneumoniae, which ordinarily may be opsonized by a specific antibody.

11.16 NEUROPATHY

This is generally caused by regional tumor growth, compressing the spinal cord, or cranial nerves. Polyneuropathies are observed with perineuronal or perivascular (vasa nervorum), amyloid deposition, but can also be seen in osteosclerotic myeloma, sometimes as a part of POEM syndrome. The humoral and cellular mechanisms underlying the syndrome are unknown.

11.17 HYPERVISCOSITY

It occurs in fewer than 10% of cases. Although it is found in higher percentages of patients with Waldenstrom Macroglobulinaemia, it is seen commonly associated with myeloma with 10-fold higher incidence. Symptoms arise from circulatory problems leading to cerebral, pulmonary, renal and other organ dysfunction. Hyperviscosity is often associated with bleeding. Because of greater tendency to form polymers with IgA molecules, IgA myeloma have greater tendency to have hyperviscosity.

11.18 BLEEDING AND THROMBOSIS

Bleeding has been reported in 15% of cases and in more than 30% of patients with IgA myeloma. The bleeding may result from anoxia, and thrombosis in capillary circulation, perivascular amyloid and/or acquired coagulopathy, such as factor X deficiency.

Thrombocytopenia is, however, rare in early phase of myeloma, even with extensive marrow involvement.

A new syndrome of thromboembolic disease has been linked to thalidomide, especially in combination with doxorubicin. Use of low molecular weight heparin has been an effective method of preventing such complication, especially in early phases of myeloma, even with extensive marrow involvement, when a high burden of myeloma cells is present.

11.19 EXTRAMEDULLARY DISEASE

Plasma cell leukaemia (> 2000/μl) is rare at presentation. But can develop in 5% of patients at terminal disease presentation. Using appropriate tools (Flow cystometry) low levels of plasma cells can be detected in majority of patients. Extramedullary disease presentation is found in higher frequency as duration of survival is extended by current therapy. Organ involvement of liver, spleen, lymph node, kidney, pleura, breast, meninges, and cutaneous sites should be suspected in cases of elevated LDH. Recently CT scanning or PET scanning may confirm such cases. Usually extramedullary features are associated with complex cytogenetics abnormalities, high PCLI, high grade immunoblastic morphology of plasma cells. [14]

11.20 LABORATORY FEATURES

Anaemia— A normocytic, normochromic anaemia is present in two-thirds of patients at diagnosis. Increased plasma volume from osmotic effect of large amounts of monoclonal protein may produce a spurious decrease of haematocrit values.

Monoclonal protein- Serum electrophoresis reveals a tall, sharp, peak or localised band in 80% of patients, hypogammaglobulinaemia in 10%, and no apparent abnormality in the remainder. A monoclonal protein is detected in the serum in 90% of cases. Approximately 60% are IgG, 20% are IgA, 10% are light chains only (Bence Jones proteinaemia), and 1% IgD.

Immunofixation of the urine reveals a monoclonal protein in 75% of patients. Almost all patients of multiple myeloma have a monoclonal protein in the serum or urine at diagnosis.

The serum creatinine level is increased in about half of the cases.

Hypercalcaemia is present in 20% of cases at diagnosis.

Skeletal changes— Conventional radiographs reveal abnormalities like, punched out lytic lesion, osteoporosis, or fractures in 75% of patients. The vertebrae, skull, thoracic cage, pelvis, and proximal humerus and femur are the most frequent sites of involvement. Technetium-99 m bone scans are inferior to conventional radiographs for detecting lesions in myeloma. Magnetic resonance imaging is too expensive for routine use.

Peripheral blood lymphocytes show an increased number of CD4+ helper cells and a diminished number of CD 8+ suppressor lymphocytes. The demonstration of monoclonal protein idiotype and the production of monoclonal protein by peripheral blood lymphocytes indicate that these cells are part of malignant clone.

11.21 CRITERIA FOR DIAGNOSIS OF MULTIPLE MYELOMA

Major Criteria

Plasmacytoma on tissue biopsy

Marrow Plasmacytosis with > 30% of plasma cells

Monoclonal globulin spike on serum electrophoresis: > 3.5 g/dl for IgG or > 2.0 g/dl for IgA, 1.0 g/24 hrs κ or λ light chain excretion in urine in absence of amyloidosis.

Minor Criteria

Marrow plasmacytosis 10–30%

Monoclonal globin spike on serum electrophoresis is present but less than the level defined above

Lytic bone lesion

Normal IgM < 0.05 g/dl, IgG < 0.6 g/dl

11.22 MYELOMA RELATED ORGAN DYSFUNCTION

Calcium induced renal dysfunction occurs when Serum Calcium > 0.25 m mol/l above upper limit of normal or > 2.75 m mol/l

Renal insufficiency is evident when serum creatinine exceeds >173 m mol/l

Bone lytic lesion evident on CT or MRI scan

Symptomatic Hyperviscosity

Symptoms of anaemia when Hb level 2 g/dl or less than lower limit of normal or > 10 g/dl

Recurrent bacterial infection

Amyloidosis

11.23 CLINICAL VARIANTS OF MULTIPLE MYELOMA AND MONOCLONAL GAMMOPATHIES

(1) Smouldering Multiple Myeloma

The diagnosis of this disease depends on

(*a*) demonstration of monoclonal protein > 3 g/dl in the serum

(*b*) > 10% atypical plasma cells in the bone marrow

BUT NO

(*c*) skeletal lesion

(*d*) anaemia

(*e*) renal insufficiency

Only a small amount of monoclonal protein is found in the urine. Uninvolved immunoglobulins are found to be reduced in the serum. Clusters of plasma cells are often seen on the bone marrow biopsy specimen. Plasma cell labelling index is low in these patients. It is important to recognize these patients as they should not be treated unless there is progression. In some patients, symptomatic multiple myeloma does not develop for years. [15]

(2) Plasma Cell Leukaemia

Patients of this group have > 20% of plasma cells in the peripheral blood and an absolute plasma cell content of at least 2000 per microlitre. Plasma cell leukaemia can be termed as primary when it is diagnosed in the leukaemia phase or as secondary when leukaemic transformation occurs in a case of a previously diagnosed multiple myeloma. Approximately 60% of patients with plasma cell leukaemia are younger and have a greater incidence of hepatosplenomegaly lymphadenopathy, a higher platelet count, fewer lytic bone lesions, a smaller serum monoclonal protein peak, and longer survival than do patients with secondary plasma cell leukaemia. [16]

(3) Nonsecretory Myeloma

Patients with this type of myeloma have no monoclonal protein in either the serum or in the urine, and this condition occurs in 2% of cases of multiple myeloma. For definitive diagnosis, a monoclonal protein should be identified in the plasma cells by immunoperoxidase or immunofluorescence method. In some cases there is no evidence of monoclonal protein within the plasma cells, suggesting that no such protein is synthesised. The more carefully serum or urine is examined for evidence of monoclonal protein, fewer cases of nonsecretory myeloma are found. [17]

(4) Immunoglobulin D Myeloma

This is different from IgA and IgM myeloma. The monoclonal spike is smaller. Bence Jones priteinuria of λ type is more common. Extramedullry plasmacytomas, plasma cell leukaemia, and amyloidosis are more frequent. Survival is generally shorter than other types. IgD myeloma is often not diagnosed until late in the course of the disease. [17]

(5) Osteosclerotic Myeloma

This often presents with a chronic inflammatory demyelinating polyneuropathy with predominantly motor disability. Single or multiple bone lesions are common. In contrast to multiple myeloma, haemoglobin level is often normal and erythrocytosis occurs in some patients. Thrombocytosis is common. The bone marrow aspirate usually contains < 5% plasma cells, whereas hypercalcaemia and renal insufficiency rarely occur. Most patients have λ monoclonal protein, the protein level of CSF is high and slow motor nerve conduction velocity is found. Hepatosplenomegaly, hyperpigmentation, gynaecomastia, oedema, digital clubbing, hypertrichiosis, atrophic testis and impotence may occur. The diagnosis is confirmed by biopsy of an osteosclertic lesion. The acronym POEMS (P = polyneuropathy, O = Organomegaly, E = Endicrinopathy, M = M protein, S = skin changes) is used to describe the complete syndrome. [18]

(6) Solitary Plasmacytoma of Bone

The diagnosis depends on demonstration of plasma cells in histologic swelling of bony lesion. In addition, complete skeletal radiograph must show no other lesion, the bone marrow aspirate must not show evidence of multiple myeloma, and immunofixation of serum and concentrated urine usually does not show monoclonal protein. Some exceptions to last named criterion may occur. But therapy of the solitary lesion should result in disappearance of monoclonal protein. [19]

(7) Extramedullary Plasmacytosis

The plasma cell tumour arises outside the bone marrow. The upper respiratory tract, the nasal cavity and paranasal sinuses, nasopharynx, the larynx, are most common sites of tumour. Epistaxis, rhinorrhoea, nasal obstructions are frequent features. Solitatry extramedullary plasmacytoma may virtually occur in any organ and spread locally or develop into multiple myeloma. There is predominance of IgA monoclonal protein. The diagnosis is based on finding of plasma cell tumour in extramedullary sites, absence of evidence of multiple myeloma by examination of bone marrow and absence of monoclonal protein in serum or urine by immunofixation, also absence of plasmacytoma in bones. Extramedullary plasmacytoma develops into overt multiple myeloma in 15% of cases, in contrast to solitary plasmacytoma. [20]

(8) Waldenstrom Macroglobulinaemia

This is a malignant lympho-plasma- proliferative disorder, characterized by formation of IgM monoclonal protein. The disease has got similarities to multiple myeloma. The lymphoid cells express CD 19, CD 20 and CD 22 antigens on their surface membranes CD5 is expressed in about 15% of cases, whereas CD 19 and CD 23 expressions are absent.

The disease has a predilection for elderly men. Onset is insidious with weakness, fatigue, bleeding (often in the form of oozing from oral cavity, nasal tract or gasrointestinal tract). In contrast to multiple myeloma, bone pain is rare, .In addition, headache, vertgo, paraesthesia, nystagmus, somnolence, coma or blurred vision may occur due to hypervoscosity. Pallor, hepatosplenomegaly, lymphadenopathy are the most frequent features. Retinal lesions, including haemorrhages, exudates, venous congestion, vascular segmentation (sausage formation) may be impressive. [21]

Peripheral neuropathy may be the initial symptom and may involve both the motor and the sensory nerve functions, Sudden deafness, progressive spinal muscular atrophy, and multifocal leukoencephalopthy, all have been reported. Pulmonary involvement may occur as diffuse infiltrate, solitary masses, and pleural effusion. Renal failure rarely occurs. The skin may be infiltrated with plasmacytoid lymphocytes or deposits of IgM. Systemic amyloidosis has been also found.

Laboratory Features

1. Almost all patients have normocytic, normochromic anaemia.
2. Occasionally there is Coomb positive haemolytic anaemia.
3. Haemoglobin and haematocrit values are spuriously reduced due to rise of plasma volume.
4. A tall, narrow peak or dense band of γ motility constituting the IgM is seen.
5. The urine contains a monoclonal light chain in 70% to 80% of cases.
6. Rouleux formation (in PBS) is striking and erythrocyte sedimentation rate is greatly increased
7. The serum creatinine level is nearly normal.
8. The bone marrow is usually hypocellular and infiltrated with lymphoid and plasma cells. The number of plasma cells is greater than normal. The number of mast cells is increased, and this finding differentiates macroglobulinaemia from myeloma and lymphoma.

11.24 DIFFERENTIAL DIAGNOSIS AMONG CLINICAL VARIANTS

This is important from the treatment point of view. The major problem in the differential diagnosis centre around the distinction from multiple myeloma, and MGUS of the IgM type. Patients with typical symptoms and physical findings just dercribed, and IgM monoclonal protein of more than 3 g/dl are classified as Waldenstrom Macroglobulinaemia. Patients with a malignant lymphoproliferative process manifested by an increase in lymphocytes and plasmacytoid lymphocytes in the bone marrow, anaemia, constitutional symptoms requiring therapy, and a serum M spike of less than 3 g per decilitre should be classified as having Waldenstrom Macroglobulinaemia, progressing to multiple myeloma. A concentration of monoclonal protein less than 1 g/decilitre, an absence of anaemia and organomegaly, mild lymphocytosis of the bone marrow, and absence of clinical symptoms are suggestive of MGUS.

11.25 HEAVY CHAIN DISEASE

The heavy chain diseases (HCDs) are lymphoplasma cell proliferative syndrome characterized by the production of monoclonal protein consisting of an incomplete heavy chain devoid of light chains. There are three major varieties: α, δ, μ.

The lymphoplasma cell proliferative syndrome produces a monoclonal γ heavy chain in the serum or urine or both. In all instances, the abnormal protein consists of a monoclonal γ chain with significant amino acid deletions, including deletion of the HC1 domain, and a portion of VH 1 constant (C) region. The median age at diagnosis is 60 years, although the condition has been noted in persons younger than 20 years.

Patients with γ HCD usually present with lymphoma-like syndrome, but the clinical findings are diverse and range from an aggressive lymphoproliferative disorder to an asymptomatic state. Weakness, fatigue and fever are common, but other features like parotid swelling, severe soreness of tongue, nodular infiltration of skin, extranodal non-Hodgkin lymphoma, autoimmune haemolytic anaemia, idiopathic thrombocytopenic purpura, rapid enlargement of thyroid are also found. Neutropenia from hypersplenism, and an atypical lymphoproliferative process have all been recognized. Hepatosplenomegaly is found in 60% of cases. The histopathological findings are non-specific and usually include generalized or localized lymphoma, myeloma, or macroglobulinaemia, but there may be no evidence of a lymphoplasmacytic proliferative process. [22]

Anaemia occurs in about 80% of cases. The serum protein electrophoresis pattern is variable and often does not suggest monoclonal gammopathy. It may appear as broad band increase of γ globulin or dicrete localized band. The urinary heavy chain protein concentration ranges from traces to 20 g in 24 hours. More than half of patients excrete less than 1 g in that time. Bence Jones proteinuria is not found. Osteolytic lesions are rare.

Alpha Heavy Chain Disease

This is the most common type of this disease which is characterized by the presence of a monoclonal α chain with extensive terminal deletion encompassing the VH region and the entire first constant domain.

Most patients with this disease are from Mediterranean area and have involvement of the digestive tract with severe malabsorption, loss of weight, diarrhoea and steatorrhoea. The term

Immunoproliferative Small Intestinal Disease (IPSID) is restricted to patients with small intestinal lesions that have the same pathologic pattern as that of α HCD, but these patients do not synthesize α heavy chains. Infrequently the respiratory tract is involved. Patients in their second or third decade of life, most often, and 60% of patients are men. Poor hygiene and low socioeconomic status are important risk factors.

The serum protein electrophoretic pattern is normal in half of the patients; in the remainder, an unimpressive broad band may appear in the α2 or β regions. Bence Jones proteinuria does not occur. The bone marrow is normal. The small bowel is infiltrated with mature plasma cells or lymphoplasmacytic cells. The mesenteric lymph nodes are usually affected but involvement of liver, spleen, peripheral lymph nodes is uncommon. The stomach and colon may be affected. The diagnosis depends on the recognition of a monoclonal α heavy chain that is not associated with α light chain.

μ Heavy Chain Disease

It is characterized by a μ-heavy chain in which the VH domain is absent. Other deletions also may occur. In this disease chronic lymphocytic leukaemia or lymphoma like pattern is most common. A stable asymptomatic state has been noted. The clinical spectrum of μ heavy chain disease should broaden, as it has no γ –HCD. Serum electrophoresis usually reveals hypogammaglobulinaemia. A localized peak or band occurs in 40% of case. Bence Jones proteinuria occurs in two-thirds of patients. The presence of vacuolated plasma cells in the bone marrow aids in the diagnosis. Demonstration of a monoclonal μ heavy chain in the serum is necessary for diagnosis. [23]

11.26 MONOCLONAL GAMMOPATHY OF UNDETERMINED SIGNIFICANCE (MGUS)

Due to its benign nature, it has been described as benign monoclonal gammopathy. Patients have a monoclonal protein in the urine without clinical evidences of multiple myeloma, macroglobulinaemia, amyloidosis, or related disease. Frequency is approximately 3% of persons older than 70 years. Of the patients with monoclonal protein, 65% have MGUS, 13% have multiple myeloma, and 11 % amyloidosis.

Criteria for diagnosis are:

1. The monoclonal protein value in the serum is less than 3 g/dl.
2. Either no Bence Jones proteinuria is present or small amounts are present.
3. Anaemia is absent.
4. Renal function is normal.
5. Hypercalcaemia is absent.
6. Osteolytic lesions are not present unless caused by other diseases.
7. No progressive increase of the monoclonal protein or development of a plasmalympho-proliferative process occurs during long term follow-up.
8. Bone marrow contains less than 10% of plasma cells.

Differentiation of this benign condition from multiple myeloma or macroglobulinaemia is important from the treatment of view, but it is not so easy, however, certain points may help as follows: [24]

1. More than 3 g per dl of monoclonal protein usually indicates overt myeloma or macro-globulinaemia, but some exceptions (e.g. smouldering leukaemia) do exist.

2. Level of immunoglobulin, not associated with the monoclonal protein (normal polyclonal or background immunoglobulin), are reduced in most patients with myeloma, but a reduction also occurs in more than one-third of patients with MGUS.
3. The association of significant Bence Jones proteinuria with a serum monoclonal protein usually indicates a neoplastic process.
4. More than 10% of plasma cells in the bone marrow is indicative of myeloma, but in some patients with more pronounced plasmacytosis, the disease has remained stable for long periods.
5. The atypical morphological changes in plasma cells may also appear in MGUS and smouldering myeloma.
6. The presence of osteolytic lesion is suggestive of multiple myeloma.
7. Monoclonal plasma cells can be detected in peripheral blood of 80% of cases of active multiple myeloma, but patients with MGUS or smouldering multiple myeloma have very few or no circulating plasma cells.
8. Patients with MGUS or smouldering multiple myeloma have a low plasma cell labeling index.

During follow-up period for more than 20 years, the patients are classified to have following groups of the disease. [25]

Group I: Patients alive and without increase in serunm monoclonal protein during follow-up (benign) (10%).

Group II: Patients with monoclonal protein of more than 3 g/dl and they did not require therapy.

Group III: Stage IV patients who died of unrelated causes (53%).

Group IV: Patients in whom myeloma, macroglobulinaemia, amyloidosis or related disease develop.

11.27 PROGRESS OF BENIGN MONOCLONAL GAMMOPATHY TO MULTIPLE MYELOMA

The initial clinical features (e.g., age, sex, initial haemoglobin level, level of monoclonal protein in serum or urine, level of normal immunoglobulin, number of plasma cells in the bone marrow, IgG subclass etc.) did not help in identifying the group of patients with benign monoclonal gammopathy, who will develop various types of diseases. Various studies show that Multiple Myeloma develops in 68% of cases, the interval from recognition of monoclonal gammopathy to multiple myeloma ranging 2 to 29 years with a median of 10 years, median survival being 33 years after detection to multiple myeloma.

Waldenstrom Macroglobulinaemia occurred in 7 patients, 4 to 20 years (median 8.5 years) after recognition of monoclonal protein, systemic amyloidosis developed in 8 cases after 6 to 19 years (median 9 years) after recognition, malignant lymphoma in 3 patients, chronic lymphocytic leukaemia in 1 and a malignant lymphoproliferative disorder in 1 patient out of 63 patients, who progressed to overt disease.

Though MGUS should not be treated and the condition exists without any other disease, the clinician must periodically reexamine the patients to determine whether the condition is really benign or initial manifestation of multiple myeloma, macroglobulinaemia, amyloidosis or malignant lymphoproliferative disorder. Monoclonal protein may be found in lymphoma, leukaemia, and a wide variety of haematological conditions. So association of any disease with MGUS must be properly evaluated whether this is a mere association or not.

11.28 BICLONAL GAMMOPATHY

Biclonal gammopathies occur in 8–9% of cases with monoclonal gammopathy IgG and IgA are the most frequent combinations, followed by IgG and IgM monoclonal immunoglobulins. The similar findings are similar to those of monoclonal gammopathies. In two-thirds of patients, the biclonal gammopathies are of undetermined significance. The remainders have multiple myeloma, amyloidosis, macroglobulinaemia or other lymphoproliferative disorders. In many cases, the serum electrophoresis pattern shows only a single band, the biclonal gammopathy is unrecognized until immunofixation is performed. More than 20 patients with triclonal gammopathy have been reported. [26]

11.29 IDIOPATHIC BENCE JONES PROTEINURIA

Although Bence Jones proteinuria is frequently associated with multiple myeloma, primary amyloidosis, Wadenstrom macroglobulinaemia or other malignant lymphoproliferative disorder, it may be benign. Small amounts of monoclonal light chains are not uncommon. Most patients who excrete more than 1g of Bence Jones protein in 24 hours and have no evidence of malignant plasma cell proliferation, eventually develops multiple myeloma or amyloidosis. This may not occur for 20 years, however. Therefore, patients with such idiopathic Bence Jones proteinuria should be observed indefinitely. [27]

REFERENCES

1. Kyle RA et al. (2000). *Clinical indications and applications of electrophoresis and immunofixation.* In: Rose NR, ed., Manual of clinical laboratory immunology, 6th ed, Washington, D.C. American Society of Microbiology (In Press).
2. Jansen JW, Vaadrager JW, Henser T, et al. (2000). *Concurrent activation of a novel putative gene mycov, and cyclin D1 in a subset of multiple myeloma cell lines with t (11:14) (q13:q32).* Blood 95:2691.
3. Hidishi T, Nakamura N, Chauhan D, et al. (2001). *Biologic sequalae of Interleulin-6 inducedP-13-k-Akt signalling in multiple myeloma.* Oncogene 20:5991.
4. Yacchobi S, Pearse RN, Johnson CL, et al. (2002). *Myeloma interacts with microenvironment to induce osteoclastogenesis and is dependent on osteoclastic activity.* Brit J Haematol 116: 278.
5. Ge NL, Rudikoff S (2000). *Insulin-like growth factor I is a dual effector of multiple myeloma cell growth.* Blood 96:2856.
6. Seidel C, Sundan A, Hjorth M, et al. (2000). *Serum syndecan-1: a new independent prognostic marker in multiple myeloma.* Therapeutic applications. Blood 95:338.
7. Mitslades N, Mitisides CS, Poulaki V et al. (2002). *Biologic sequelae of the nuclear factor-kappa X blockade in multiple myeloma.* Therapeutic applications. Blood 99:4079.

8. Choi SJ, Cruz JC, Craig F, et al. (2002). *Role of Macrophage inflammatory protein: protein -1-α is a potential osteoclast stimulatory factor in multiple myeloma*. Blood 100 :: 3002.
9. Bataille R, Chappard D, Marcelli C, et al. (1989). *Mechanism of bone destruction in multiple myeloma: The importance of an unbalanced process in determining the severity of lytic bone disease*. J Clin Oncol 7:1909.
10. Deamiano JS, Cress AE, Hazlaharst LA et al. (1999). *Cell adhesion mediated drug resistance (CAM-DR). Role of integrins and resistance to apoptosis in human myeloma cell lines*. Blood 93 : 1658.
11. Silvestris F, Cafforio P, Tucci M et al. ((2002). *Negative regulation of erythroblast maturation by FAS-L(+) TRAIL(+) highly malignant plasma cells. A major pathogenetic mechanism of anaemia in multiple myeloma*. Blood 95: 1305.
12. Singh A, Eckardt KV, Zimmerman A et al. (1993). *Increased plasma viscosity as a reason for inappropriate erythropoietin formation*. J Clin Invest 91 : 251.
13. Solomon A, Weiss DT: (1988). *Clinical implications of monoclonal light chains in renal disease, in the kidney in plasma cell dyscrasia*, edited by G. Minetti, GD Amico, C. Ponticell, p3 Kluwer, Dordrechi, Netherlands1988.
14. Alexion C et al. (1999). *Extramedullary plasmacytoma: tumor occurrence and therapeutic concepts*. Cancer 85:2305.
15. Kyle RA, Griepp PR (1980). *Smouldering multiple myeloma*. NEngl J Med 302:1347.
16. Garcia-Sanz R, et al. (1999). *Primary plasma cell leukaemia: clinical, immunohaemotypic, DNA ploidy, and cytogenetics characteristics*. Blood 93:1032.
17. Blade J, Kyle RA. (1999). *Non-secretory myeloma, immunoglobulin D myeloma, and plasma cell leukaemia*. Haematol Oncol Clin North 13 : 1259.
18. Waldenstrom JG (1992). *POEMS: a multifactorial syndrome [Editorial]*. Haematologica 77:197.
19. Frassica DA, et al. (1989). *Solitary plasmacytoma of bone: Mayo clinic experience*. Int J Radiat Oncol Biol Phys 16:43.
20. Soesan M et al. (1992). *Extramedullary plasmacytoma: clinical behaviour andresponse to treatment*. Ann Oncol 3:51.
21. Dimopoulus MA, et al. (2000). *Waldenstrom Macroglobulinaemia: clinical features, complications and management*. J Clin Oncol 18:214
22. Wahner-Roedler DL, Kyle RA (1998). *Heavy chain diseases*. In: Malpas JS, Bergsagel DE, Kyle RA, et al. eds. Myeloma: biology and management, 2nd ed. New York Oxford University Press, 1998: 604–638.
23. Wahner-Roedler DL, Kyle RA (1992). *Mu-heavy chain disease: presentation as a benign monoclonal gammopathy*. Am J Haematol 40 : 56.
24. Kyle RA, Rajkumar SV(1999). *Monoclonal gammopathies of undetermined significance*. Haematol Oncol Clin North Am 13 : 1181.
25. Kyle RA (1993). *"Benign monoclonal gammopathy"- after 20 to 35 years of follow-up*. Mayo clinic Proc 1993; 68:26.
26. Kyle RA, Robinson RA, Katzman JA (1981). *The clinical aspects of biclonal gammopathies: review of 57 cases*. Am J Med 71:999.
27. Kyle RA, Griepp PR, (1982). *'Idiopathic' Bence Jones Proteinuria: long term follow-up in seven patients*. N Engl J Med 306:564.

CHAPTER

12 Management of Multiple Myeloma

12.1 INTRODUCTION

Multiple Myeloma is a malignant condition primarily involving the bone marrow and with multi-system effect and varied clinical manifestations. The clinical spectrum may vary, starting from smoldering myeloma, developing into solitary myeloma, and expressing as overt multiple myeloma. On the other hand myeloma may present with some very non-specific symptoms like anemia, renal insufficiency, proteinuria, or neurologic manifestations e.g., cord compression or neuropathy. Certain clinical signs are sometimes important clue to the diagnosis e.g., bone pain and high ESR (> 100 mm/hr). However, these things may be present in other clinical conditions like metastatic bone disease, other malignancies and inflammatory diseases. Only the lytic lesions in the bones, detected on plain X-Ray is not also sufficient to confirm the diagnosis of multiple myeloma. Only special tests, guided by clinical observations, are necessary to detect Multiple Myeloma. The treatment of Multiple Myeloma is therefore, multidimensional, not only eradicating malignant cells but also controlling the perpetuating process in the body and the symptoms thereby.

12.2 GOALS OF THERAPY

1. To reduce the tumor burden by chemotherapy and radiotherapy.
2. To eradicate the tumor cells and to prevent its micrometastasis by new biologic therapy e.g., Interferon, Interleukin and Monoclonal antibody against vascular endothelial growth factor (VEGF) or chemical agent like thalidomide.
3. To promote normal cell proliferation by Stem cell transplantation.
4. To prevent further abnormal cell proliferation- newer agents e.g., thalidomide, arsenic trioxide.
5. To control troublesome symptoms, related to disease process or its complications e.g., bone pain or hyper viscosity syndrome.

12.3 SYMPTOM RELATED THERAPEUTIC MODALITIES

1. To handle kidney problems adequate hydration, avoidance of NSAID and IV contrast media are necessary. Acute renal failure may be precipitated by dehydration, infection, NSAID and contrast media.

2. Hypercalcaemia should be suspected when patient has got anorexia, nausea, vomiting, constipation, weakness, confusion, stupor or coma. Intravenous isotonic saline, an initial dose of prednisone 25 mg four times daily should be given, which should be reduced and ultimately discontinued. If these measures fail, IV Pamidronate disodium or etidronate disodium should be given in a dose of 90 mg over 2 hours every 4 weeks. [1]
3. Anaemia usually responds to erythropoietin, especially if serum erythropoietin is low.
4. Hyper viscosity syndrome should be suspected if there is oro-nasal bleeding, blurred vision, neurological symptoms. Most patients develop symptoms when viscosity is 7 or 8 centipoises (normal being > 1.8). Vigorous plasmapheresis with cell separator relieves the symptoms, though simultaneous chemotherapy is necessary to prolong the effect.
5. For skeletal pain and to prevent lysis bisphosphonates are used as it reduces osteoclastic activity and also has antitumour effect. It can be given safely for a long period but should not be used in severe renal failure (Cr. Clearance < 35 ml/min). [2]
6. To prevent bacterial pneumonia prophylactic daily oral penicillin is preferred to IV gammaglobulin which is very expensive and inconvenient.
7. The nephrotic syndrome should be managed with salt restriction and diuretics. Furesomide is usually unsatisfactory. The addition of metalozone is helpful Albumin infusions have only transient benefit and are not useful for long term treatment of oedema. If symptomatic azotaemia develops, chronic renal dialysis is necessary. Peritonitis may occur with peritoneal dialysis, whereas hypotension may lead to difficulties in haemodialysis.

12.4 MODALITIES OF THERAPY USED IN MULTIPLE MYELOMA

Radiation Therapy

Radiation therapy is indicated in

1. Solitary plasmacytoma
2. Progressive skeletal disease
3. Spinal cord compression
4. Demyelinating neuropathy associated with osteosclerotic lesions, (radiation of solitary bony lesion may cause regression of neuropathy).

Radiation usually consists of 3000c Gy and should be accompanied by dexamethasone daily to reduce oedema.

Chemotherapy

Chemotherapy is the use of drugs that kill rapidly dividing cells. Chemotherapeutic drugs are toxic not only to cancer cells but also to the cells that are actively multiplying. Cells of the bone marrow, the lining of the stomach and intestines, and the hair follicles are, therefore, vulnerable. Toxic effect of chemotherapy may result in a decrease in blood cell counts, nausea, vomiting, diarrhea, and loss of hair.

12.5 CLINICAL STAGING

Clinical staging is needed for institution of chemotherapy. [3]

Stage I

Hb > 10 g/dl, normal serum calcium, serum IgG < 5 g/dl or IgA < 3 g/dl, Bence Jones proteinuria <4 g and no generalized lytic lesion.

Stage II

In between limits specified for stage I and stage III.

Stage III

Hb < 8.5 g/dl, serum calcium > 12 mg/dl, IgG > 7 g/dl, IgA > 5 g/dl, Bence Jones protein > 12 g/day or advanced lytic bone lesion.

Monoclonal gammopathy of undetermined significance (MGUS) and smoldering multiple myeloma (SMM) must be differentiated from overt multiple myeloma before initiation of treatment.

These two conditions fall short of clinical criteria required for confirmation of multiple myeloma. The first condition is characterized by < 10% plasma cells in the bone marrow, < 3 g/dl monoclonal protein in the serum and no anaemia or osteolytic lesion, no or small amount of monoclonal protein in the urine. The second one is manifested by > 10% atypical plasma cells in the bone marrow, >3 g/l monoclonal protein in the serum, a reduction of uninvolved immunoglobulin in the serum, but no anaemia, renal insufficiency or osteolytic bone lesion and a small amount of monoclonal protein in the urine. These conditions should not be treated and second one should not be treated until sufficient clinical or laboratory features of myeloma develop.

Plasma cell labelling index, is of value in differentiating the conditions. A labelling index of > 1% indicates that the patient most likely will develop overt multiple myeloma. [4]

Another dependable means of differentiating benign from malignant disease is serial measurement of monoclonal protein in the serum either by electrophoresis or by immunofixation and the same method should be repeated each time. [5]

Chemotherapy in Multiple Myeloma may include one or several drugs in different combinations and toxicity may, therefore, vary. According to the goal achieved chemotherapy may be of following types:

- Conventional chemotherapy
- High dose chemotherapy with stem cell transplantation
- Salvage chemotherapy.

Conventional Chemotherapy

Conventional chemotherapy is also known as standard-dose chemotherapy. Conventional chemotherapy is typically the primary or initial treatment for most patients with myeloma. Patients may receive conventional chemotherapy as their only therapy, or they may receive it in preparation for high-dose chemotherapy and stem cell transplant.

Commonly used chemotherapeutic agents and regimens suitable for induction therapy for myeloma include VAD (Vincristine, Adriamycin [doxorubicin], and Dexamethasone), and DVd (Doxil [pegylated doxorubicin], vincristine, and reduced schedule dexamethasone).

Certain chemotherapeutic drugs are less suitable for use as induction therapy for myeloma. These include alkylating agents, which cross-link to a tumor cell's DNA and ultimately prevent the cell from dividing. Examples of alkylating agents that are less suitable for induction therapy include melphalan and carmustine (BCNU). Although the chemotherapeutic agent cyclophosphamide is also an alkylating agent, it is suitable for use as induction therapy.

When used as induction therapy, usually 3 or 4 cycles are given prior to collection of stem cells. After collection, patients may go straight to a transplant (early transplantation) or continue to receive chemotherapy until ((maligant cells) reach a plateau. In the latter case, the transplant is reserved for when the myeloma relapses (late transplantation).

The most common chemotherapeutic agent used in myeloma is an oral drug called melphalan. Melphalan is typically given in combination with prednisone, a potent corticosteroid drug with anti-myeloma activity. This combination has been a standard treatment for myeloma for the past 30 years and results in a response rate of 50%. Unfortunately, this alkylating agent is less suitable for use as induction therapy. [6]

Corticosteroids are sometimes used alone as myeloma therapy, especially in older patients and those who cannot tolerate chemotherapy. The most commonly used corticosteroid in this instance is dexamethasone. Corticosteroids may reduce the M protein in approximately 40% of previously untreated patients, and in 20% to 40% of patients who have not responded to primary therapy. Dexamethasone is also used as a form of induction therapy, alone or in combination with other agents, as stated above. [7]

New therapies with a new formulation of doxorubicin (pegylated liposomal doxorubicin, vincristine, and reduced-dose dexamethasone (DVd) has recently been shown to provide a slow release of the drug, thus exposing myeloma cells to the drug for a longer period of time. It may also result in an improved toxicity profile due to the potential for use of lower doses of doxorubicin, preferential accumulation of the drug at the tumor site and less exposure to the rest of the body, a shorter infusion time, and less damage to heart muscle.

Substituting this new formulation of doxorubicin for doxorubicin in the VAD regimen and reducing the schedule of dexamethasone appears to improve the safety profile and convenience of the induction regimen without compromising efficacy. In a Phase II study in 33 newly diagnosed patients, 67% of patients achieved at least a 50% reduction in M protein and the patient survival rate at 3 years was 67%. No patients required discontinuation of treatment due to side effects and only one patient experienced damage to heart muscle. The most common severe (Grade 3) toxicities were swelling, itching, and peeling skin on the hands and feet (a disorder known as palmar-plantar erythrodysesthesia or PPE, a common side effect of certain types of chemotherapy), mouth sores, and neutropenia.

High-Dose Chemotherapy with Stem Cell Transplantation

The administration of chemotherapy at doses higher than that used with conventional chemotherapy are often used in the treatment of myeloma. This type of chemotherapy is referred to as high-dose chemotherapy. Though more effective in killing myeloma cells than conventional chemotherapy, high-dose chemotherapy also destroys normal blood-forming cells in the bone marrow. Because a person cannot survive without these blood-forming cells, high-dose chemotherapy is always administered in conjunction with a stem cell transplant, which replaces these important cells. [8]

High-dose chemotherapy with stem cell transplantation is used after a patient receives induction therapy (conventional chemotherapy) to reduce the tumor burden. It is often used in younger patients with a good prognosis. Depending on the type of cancer and other factors, some patients may receive one or more treatments of high-dose chemotherapy, possibly in combination with radiation therapy, over a period of several days. This combination of treatments is also referred to as a conditioning regimen. Because this regimen is more intensive than conventional chemotherapy, it is used less frequently in patients over the age of 70, and may not be suitable for patients who have significantly impaired kidney function or performance status, or other coexisting conditions. [8]

Salvage Therapy

Chemotherapy may be used as salvage therapy, that is, treatment for patients who have not responded to primary or subsequent therapy or who experience relapsed disease after an initial response to therapy. A number of regimens are currently used as salvage therapy or are being investigated for this use. If longer than 6 months has passed since a patient had initially responded to primary conventional therapy, the primary therapy can be repeated as salvage therapy following relapse. Various combination therapies are also used. Thalidomide, an oral agent, is also often used as salvage therapy for myeloma patients alone, or in combination with dexamethasone or melphalan and dexamethasone. Velcade (bortezomib), a proteasome inhibitor, was approved in the US in May 2003 for the treatment of myeloma patients who have received at least two prior therapies and have demonstrated disease progression on the last therapy.

Names of Drugs Used in the Treatment of Myeloma

Many times a drug may be referred to its common (generic) name, while other times it may be referred to by a brand name or an abbreviation. It may be hard to determine the exact medication being discussed. The following table lists some of the common drugs used in the treatment of myeloma as well as brand names and abbreviations for each.

TABLE 12.1: Drugs for Myeloma, Brand names and Abbreviations

Drug Name	Brand Names	Abbreviations and Other Names
Ara-C (cytarabine)	Cytosar®	Ara-C
BCNU (carmustine)	BiCNU®	BCNU
Bortezomib	Velcade®	PS-341
Cyclophosphamide	Cytoxan®, Neosar®	C, CTX, CY
Dexamethasone	Decadron® and others	D, dex
Doxorubicin	Adriamycin®, Rubex®	A, D, Dox
Doxorubicin, liposomal	Doxil®, Caelyx®	D
Melphalan	Alkeran®	M, Mel
Prednisone	Various names	P, Pred
Thalidomide	Thalomid®	T, Thal
Vincristine	Oncovin®, Vincasar®, Vincrex®	V, VP-16

12.6 NEW ADDITIONS

1. Thalidomide

The drug was originally developed as a treatment for insomnia and morning sickness and abandoned thereafter for its teratogenic effect. After several years it is reintroduced in Medicine for its anti-myeloma activity.

Mechanism of action of thalidomide is multiple.

1. Inhibition of angiogenesis by blocking basic fibroblast growth factor (bFGF) and vascular endothelial growth factor (VEGF)
2. Altering production/ inhibition of cytokines involved in growth and and survival of myeloma cells.
3. Altering expression of Adhesion molecules located on surface of tumor cells, stromal cells, which trigger the release of tumor cell growth.
4. Stimulation of T-cells which help the immune cells to attack the tumor cells directly.

So the effect of thalidomide is a combined effect of chemotherapeutic agent and biologic agent.

Thalidomide is of choice in:

1. Initial therapy in patients with stage II or stage III disease
2. Patients who relapse after transplantation.
3. Patients who can not tolerate steroid.

In combination with Dexamethasone, Thalidomide is used in:

- Patients with more aggressive disease
- Newly diagnosed cases (both transplant-eligible or transplant-noneligible)
- Dose and Administration:
- Starting Dose is 100–200 mg/day.
- Starting dose is lowered in elderly or in case of other systemie diseases
- Dose is increased 50–100 mg/day every1-2 weeks
- In aggressive diseases higher starting dose of 200 mg/day is used.
- Target therapeutic dose is 200 mg/day with further dose escalation with tolerance.

Toxicities are managed by timing the dose at 7–10 PM and stopping and restarting the dose at lower level in case of neuropathy.

Drug is continued till there is response, the disease is stable and toxicities are manageable. In case of disease progression Dexamethasone is added or a second regime is considered.[9]

2. Arsenic Trioxide

Mechanism of action

Inorganic arsenic trioxide (ATO) and the organic arsenical, melarsoprol, are shown to inhibit growth and induce apoptosis in a variety of leukemic cell lines of lymphoid or myeloid origin. Similarly, ATO inhibits the growth and induces apoptosis in a variety of myeloma cell lines.

ATO also reduces plasma cell differentiation in normal B cells. Melarsoprol causes a dose and time-dependent inhibition of growth and survival in the myeloma cell lines. ATO and Melarsoprol inhibit viability and growth and induce apoptosis in plasma cell enriched preparations from the bone marrow or blood of patients in either the intramedullary or extramedullary stage of myeloma.

Multiple myeloma cells can be refractory to presently available treatments. The expression of a 170,000 P-glycoprotein encoded by a multiple drug resistant (MDR) gene is associated with drug resistance. Preliminary data showed that arsenic may be active against MDR-expressing cells, as evidenced by increased cell death in doxorubicin-resistant human leukemia and myeloma cells exposed to ATO and melarsoprol.

Treatment plan for arsenic trioxide

Trisenoxä (arsenic trioxide) injection (ATO) is to be administered intravenously over 1–4 hours. The treatment cycle is repeated every four weeks, with treatments 5 days a week during the first 2 weeks, and no study treatment during the last 2 weeks of each cycle. Up to 6 cycles of treatment may be administered.

Indications

1. Confirmed diagnosis of multiple myeloma of Durie-Salmon stage II or III (i.e., excluding monoclonal gammopathy, indolent or smoldering myeloma).
2. Current measurable disease based on serum and urine M protein and/or measurable plasmacytoma.
3. History of less than or equal to 3 prior treatment regimens (excluding focal radiation for symptom control). These prior regimens must have been completed at least 28 days before this regimen.
4. Failure of
   (*i*) 3 cytotoxic regimens
   (*ii*) 1 high-dose cytotoxic regimen as part of stem cell transplant

Patient selection

Age $\geq$ 18 years.
Karnofsky performance status of at least 70%.
Serum creatinine of $\leq$ 2.5 mg/dL.
Serum bilirubin, SGPT, and SGOT $\leq$ 2 times the upper limit of normal
Absence of other serious systemic diseases so that life expectancy is > 3 months.
Negative pregnancy test in women of child bearing age.

Contraindications

1. Pregnant or lactating women
2. Pre-existing neurotoxicity/neuropathy
3. Absolute QT interval > 460 msec in the presence of serum potassium and magnesium values within normal ranges.
4. Reduced hematology values that are not secondary to multiple myeloma.
5. Concurrent treatment with cytotoxic chemotherapy, high-dose corticosteroids, broad field radiation, or any other investigational agents.
6. Significant cardiac dysfunction
7. Prior malignancy in the 5 years before treatment
8. Uncontrolled diabetes.

9. History of seizures (other than infantile febrile seizures)
10. Active, serious infections not controlled by antibiotics.

Immunomodulatory therapies

Immunomodulatory therapies that induce cell apoptosis and inhibit angiogenesis are now being investigated in newly diagnosed patients as well as in those who have failed previous therapies. Additionally, several new agents that target receptors for vascular endothelial growth factor (VEGF) are in early trial stages.

The table below shows the newer agents that are under phase I/phase II clinical trial.

TABLE 12.2: Newer Agents under Trial for Multiple Myeloma

Clinical Trial	Agent	Action
PhaseII (in Europe)	Actimid	Immunomodulatory drug
Phase II	Amifostine	Cytoprotective agent in Combination with Mephalan
Phase II	Apiliolin	Marine derived anti-tumor agent that induces rapid apoptosis
Phase I (Europe) PhaseII (France)	Atizumab	Humanized antibody against IL-6 receptor
Phase II	AP 23573	Agent that blocks a critical cell signaling protein known as m TOR; shrinks tumor cells and inhibits angiogenesis
Phase II	Avastin (Bevacizumab)	Humanized antibody against VEGF receptor
Phase II	Campath-IH	Monoclonal antibody (CD 52) in conjunction with stem cell transplant
Phase I/PhaseII	GVAX Myeloma vaccine	Irradiated patient myeloma vaccine that stimulates immune responses in newly diagnosed patients undergoing transplant
PhaseI/PhaseII (Univ. of Arizona)	Imexon	Induces apoptosis, oxidative stress, mitochondrial changes in myeloma cells

12.7 TREATMENT PLAN OF TYPICAL FORM OF MULTIPLE MYELOMA

Although most patients are symptomatic at diagnosis, some remain asymptomatic and should not be treated. Such patients should be evaluated every 2 or 3 months and treatment is delayed till disease progression is evident. An increasing level of monoclonal protein in the serum or urine, an increasing plasma cell labeling index, significant anaemia, hypercalcaemia, renal insufficiency, lytic bone lesion, or development of extramedullary plasmacytoma are some of the indications for starting therapy.

Most physicians initially treat with Vincristine, doxorubicin (adriamycin), and dexamethasone

Chapter 12

(VAD) for 3 to 4 months to reduce the number of plasma cells in the bone marrow and the peripheral blood. Dexamethasone with or without thalidomide is being evaluated as initial therapy. The oral administration of Mephalan (Alkeran) (0.15 mg/ kg daily for 7 days) and prednisone (20 mg thrice daily for the same 7 days) every 6 weeks is a satisfactory regimen and produces objective response in 50–60% of cases. Leukocyte and platelet count should be done at 3 weekly interval and dose of Mephalan should be adjusted accordingly in the mid-cycle as absorption of the drug is variable Multivariate analysis shows higher response rate with various combination chemotherapy than with Mephalan-prednisone but overall survival rate is similar. [10]

In resistant cases, VAD therapy is preferred. Vincristine and Doxorubicin are given in a continuous 4-day infusion (days 1– 4) along with dexamethasone, 40 mg daily on days 1 through 4, 9 through 12, and 17 through 20. The cycle is repeated every 26 days. A major shortcoming is that vincristine and doxorubicin must be given through a central venous catheter. Significant steroid toxicity is manifested by infections, gastrointestinal bleeding, and steroid myopathy. In addition the median duration of response is less than 1 year.

Methylprednisolone 2 g administered intravenously three times weekly for 4 weeks produces similar response to dexamethasone. If response occurs, frequency may be reduced to twice weekly and then to once weekly for maintenance. There are fewer side effects than dexamethasone. Therapy with VBAP (vincristine 2 mg, carmustine [BCNU] 30 mg, doxorubicin 30 mg administered intravenously on day 1, and prednisone 60 mg daily for 5 days every 3 to 4 weeks has produced some benefit in 30% of refractory cases. Interferon produces objective improvement in approximately 10% of cases with refractory myeloma.

Cyclophosphamide 600 mg/M2 given intravenously daily for 4 days, plus prednisone followed by granulocyte-macrophage colony stimulating factor (GM-CSF) has been useful for refractory, aggressive cases but is quite toxic.[11] In younger patients, autologous peripheral blood stem cells should be collected before the patient is exposed to alkylating agents. Chemotherapy is the preferred initial method of treatment for symptomatic multiple myeloma, in patients older than 70 years or in younger patients in whom transplantation is not possible. Peripheral stem cells are collected after high dose cyclophosphamide and granulocyte-colony-stimulating- factor (G-CSF). One then can proceed to transplantation, for which the patient is given high dose chemotherapy or total body irradiation or both followed by infusion. The other choice is to treat the patient with alkylating agents after stem cell collection until a plateau is reached and to treat the patient with α IFN or no therapy until relapse occurs. [12]

12.8 ALLOGENEIC BONE MARROW TRANSPLANTATION IN MULTIPLE MYELOMA

The major advantage is that the graft does not contain any tumor cell. Unfortunately, fewer than 10% of patients with multiple myeloma are eligible for transplantation because of their age, lack of HLA-matched sibling donor or inadequate cardiac, pulmonary, renal function. In addition, the mortality rate is 25$ Depletion of T-cells from infusion of stem cells decreases the incidence of growth-versus-host reaction. If a patient has relapse after transplantation, infusion of donor lymphocytes results in benefit in half of the patients. Currently, the conventional allogeneic transplant is not recommended because of its high mortality rate and lack of cure. [13]

12.9 TREATMENT PLAN OF SOME ATYPICAL FORMS OF THE DISEASE

Solitary Plasmacytoma

Treatment consists of tumorocidal radiation (40–50y). Overt multiple myeloma occurs in 55% of patients during 10 years of follow-up, whereas new solitary bone lesionsor local recurrences occur in 10% of cases. About 50% of patients survive 10 years. There is no evidence that adjuvant chemotherapy influence the incidence of conversion to multiple myeloma. Progression to myeloma occurs within 3 years in two-third of patients who have disease progression. [14]

Extramedullary Plasmacytoma

Here also the mainstay of treatment constitutes tumorocidal irradiation and in this case it is curative most of the time. Progression to overt multiple myeloma occurs in 15% of cases, in contrast to solitary plasmacytoma.

Waldenstrom Macroglobulinaemia

Therapy should be withheld until the patient has constitutional symptoms. Chlorambucil, in an initial dose of 6–8 mg, produces objective benefit in 70% of cases. The dosage must be altered, depending on the leukocyte and platelet count. Chorambucil may be given on an intermittent schedule in combination with prednisone. Cyclophosphamide or combination of alkylating agents such as VBMCP have been beneficial. Chemotherapy should be discontinued when the patient has reached a plateau state. Cladiribine (2-deoxyadenosine) (2CDA) and fludarabine have produced impressive responses. These agents are more effective in previously untreated patients. Rituximab, an anti CD-20 monoclonal antibody is effective in half of refractory patients. Plasmapharesis is used for treating symptomatic hyperviscosity. The use of a cell seperator alleviates the symptoms quickly. The median survival of patients is approximately 5 years after diagnosis. [15]

Non-secretory and IgD Myeloma

Treatment of these two varieties is the same as in case of multiple myeloma. For non-secretory myeloma as less renal involvement is seen, survival is longer than typical multiple myeloma. For IgD myeloma, as the condition is detected late survival is generally shorter than other varieties, though survival as long as 5 years have been reported.

Osteosclerotic Myeloma

Radiation of solitary lesions decreases the neuropathy in most patients. If the patient has widespread osteosclerotic lesions, autologous stem cell transplantation should be considered. Chemotherapy is less effective. Patients can survive for many years. Death is rarely due to multiple myeloma.

Plasma Cell Leukaemia

Treatment is unsatisfactory in this case. VAD is the usual form of treatment. If the patient responds, autologous stem cell transplantation should be considered. Secondary plasma cell leukaemia that occurs in 1–2% of cases of multiple myeloma seldom responds to chemotherapy, because patients already received these agents and are resistant to them. Survival is shorter than any other group. [16]

Heavy Chain Disease

Most often α HCD is progressive and fatal. Remissions, however, have been recorded with mephalan or cyclophosphamide and prednisone and surprisingly, with antibiotics. Patients with superficial lesions limited to bowel and mesenteric lymph nodes should be treated initially with oral antibiotics. Any documented parasite should be eradicated. If patients do not respond or if more advanced disease is present, initially they should be treated with cyclophosphamide, doxorubicin, vincristine, and prednisone. (CHOP)

The complete remission rate is about 50%, with two-thirds of patients surviving at 3 years. [17] μ (chain) HCD Treatment with corticosteroids and alkylating agents is beneficial. The median survival is about 2 years.

12.10 CONCLUSION

Multiple myeloma is a unique type of hematological malignancy regarding its multidimensional pathogenesis and clinical manifestations. The treatment options are also varied attacking almost every aspect of its molecular pathology. Researches are going on and on so that we become more and more acquainted with various aspects of this disease.

In future, probably we become able to control the disease progress with right choice of therapeutic modality.

REFERENCES

1. Berenson JR, et al. *Long term pamidronate treatment of advanced multiple myeloma patients reduce skeletal events: Myeloma Aredia Study Group*. J Clin Oncol (1998); 16:593.
2. Kyle RA.(2000). *The role of bisphosphonates in multiple myeloma [Editorial]*. Ann Intern Med 00; 132: 734.
3. Durie BG, Salmon SE (1975). *A clinical staging system for multiple myeloma: correlation of measured myeloma cell mass with presenting clinical features, response to treatment, survival*. Cancer 36: 842.
4. Griepp PR et al.(1993). *Plasma cell labeling index and beta2- microglobulin predict survival independent of thymidine kinase and C-reactive protein in multiple myeloma*. Blood 81:3382.
5. Kyle RA (1999). *Sequence of testing for monoclonal gammopathies*. Arch Pathol Lab Med 123:114.
6. Myeloma Trialists' collaborative Group (1998). *Combination chemotherapy versus mephalan plus prednisone as treatment for multiple myeloma: an overview of 6,633 patients from 27 randomized trials*. J Clin Oncol 16: 3832.
7. Alexanian R. et al. (1992). *Primary dexamethasone treatment of multiple myeloma*. Blood 80:887.
8. Fermand JP, et al. (1998). *High–dose therapy and autologous peripheral stem cell transplantation in multiple myeloma: up-front or rescue treatment?* Results of a multicenter sequential randomized clinical trial. Blood 92:3131.
9. Singhal S, et al. (1999). *Antitumor activity of thalidomide in refractory multiple myeloma*. N Engl J Med 341: 1565.
10. Kyle RA. (1999). *High–dose therapy in multiple myeloma and primary amyloidosis: an overview*. Semin Oncol 26:74.

11. Comenzo RL, et al. (1999). *Intermediate dose intravenous mephalan and blood stem cells mobilized with sequential GM+G- CSF or G-CSF alone to treat AL amyloidosis.* Brit J Haematol 104: 553.
12. Gahrton G, Bjorkstrand B. *High dose treatment of multiple myeloma.* Crit Rev Oncol Haematol 30:173.
13. Gahrton G, et al. (1995). *Prognostic factors in allogeneic bone marrow transplantation for multiple myeloma.* J Clin Oncol 13:1312.
14. Leiobross RH, et al. (1998). *Solitary bone plasmacytoma: outcome and prognostic factors following radiotherapy.* Int J Radiat Oncol Biol Phys 41: 1063.
15. Dimopoulos MA, et al. (1993). *Treatment of Waldenstrom Macroglobulinaemia with 2—chlorodeoxyadenosine.* Ann Intern Med 118:195.
16. Noel P, Kyle RA (1987). *Plasma cell leukaemia: an evaluation of response to therapy.* Am J Med 83:1000000000062.
17. Ben-Ayed F, et al. (1989). *Treatment of alpha-chain disease: results of a prospective study in 21 Tunisian patients by the Tunisian-French Intestinal lymphoma study group.* Cancer 63:1251.

CHAPTER

13 Malignant Lymphoid Disorder

This is a group of disorders, which are produced by neoplastic proliferation of lymphocytes and plasma cells. Clinically it produces a particular clinical syndrome characterized by variable clinical picture, consisting of hyperviscosity syndrome, Raynaud's syndrome, autoantibody-mediated neuropathy, monoclonal immunoglobulin-mediated abnormal platelet function or abnormal coagulation protein producing impaired hemostasis, renal tubular dysfunction and renal insufficiency. In this category four different diseases are included e.g. chronic lymphocytic leukaemia, acute lymphoblastic leukaemia, Hodgkin lymphoma and non-Hodgkin lymphoma.

13.1 CLASSIFICATION

According to cells of origin:

1. Acute lymphoblastic leukaemia (ALL) arising from primitive stem cells, at a stage prior to T and B lymphocyte differentiation.
2. Chronic lymphogenous leukaemia (CLL) arising from primitive lymphoid stem cells that may give rise to either T-cell or B-cell phenotype.
3. Hairy cell leukaemia, natural killer cell granular lymphocytic leukaemia, plasma-cytoma arising from lymphocyte stem cell with variable expression of B- or T-lymphocyte phenotype.
4. Hodgkin lymphoma arising from neoplastic B-cell that has highly mutated genes, And that are no longer expressed into protein.

International lymphoma study group, revised by European-American lymphoma group, (REAL) classification was modified by W.H.O in 2001. [1]

The REAL/WHO classification recognizes a basic difference between lymphocyte preponderance and classic Hodgkin lymphoma in behavior, morphology, phenotype and clinical feature. Therefore, the original classification of malignant lymphoid disorder has been changed to the new one, which is based on differences of cells of origin. [2]

13.2 ASSOCIATED CLINICAL SYNDROME

1. When B-lymphocytes undergo malignant transformation, and clonal proliferation, they can secrete monoclonal proteins inappropriately. If monoclonal protein is IgG or IgM or any of the subclasses

IgA, its presence may increase viscosity of blood, impairing blood flow through microcirculation. This process may be impeded by erythrocytes further in the process of aggregation, the condition being known as **hyperviscosity syndrome.** The syndrome is characterized by headache, dizziness, diplopia, stupor, retinal vein engorgement or frank coma.

2. Monoclonal immunoglobulin can interact with cell surfaces, producing abnormal granulocyte function and susceptibility to bacterial infection, on one hand or abnormal platelet function and impaired hemostasis.
3. Excessive production of immunoglobulin light chains can lead to several types of renal tubular dysfunction and renal insufficiency. IgM deposited on glomerular tufts may give rise to renal disease.
4. Cryoglobulins (immunoglobulins that precipitated at temperature below 37° C) can result in Raynaud's syndrome (skin ulceration, purpura, digital infarction, gangrene). Finally excessive production of monoclonal immunoglobulins, immunoglobulin fragments, myeloma proteins or heavy chains in heavy chain disease may result in amyloidosis. [3]
5. Production of autoreactive antibodies spontaneously or in relationship to B lymphocyte neoplasia may lead to autoimmune haemolytic anaemia, autoimmune thyroid disorder or rarely autoimmune neutropenia. Autoantibodies directed against tissues are implicated in the aetiopathogenesis of thyroiditis, encephalitis, peripheral neuropathies (as a result of demyelination). Neuronal injury is often related to antibody activity against myelin-associated glycoproteins or absorption by nerve tissue. Rarely polyneuropathy is associated with organomegaly, endocrinopathy, monoclonal gammopathy and skin changes. (POEMS syndrome).
6. Symptoms due to marrow infiltration- Well differentiated malignant B lymphocytes such as those found in early stages of CLL may infiltrate marrow. This can suppress normal haemopoiesis, resulting in varying combinations of anaemia, granulocytopenia, thrombocytopenia.
7. Malignant B lymphocyte proliferation may result in any combination of splenomegaly and lymphadenopathy in superficial or deep nodes. Many B cell lymphoma tend to involve isolated lymph node groups. B cell CLL and low grade lymphoma tend to involve many superficial and deep nodes bearing areas and spleen. Prolymphocytic and hairy cell leukaemia are prone to involve marrow and spleen producing massive enlargement.
8. Lymphokine-induced symptoms- Patients with cutaneous T-cell lymphoma have elevated plasma levels of Th-2 associated cytokines, which may account for high incidence of eosinophilia and eosinophilic pneumonia. [4] Myeloma, secretes IL-1cytokines that stimulate osteoclast proliferation and activity, producing osteolytic bone lesions. In addition IL-1 may stimulate production of ADH and contribute to inappropriate ADH syndrome. [5]
9. Dysregulation of extrarenal production of calcitrol, the active metabolite of vitamin D, appears to underlie hyperkalaemia associated with hypercalcaemia.
10. Systemic symptoms- Fever, night sweat, weight loss, anorexia, local or disseminated herpes zoster may occur in 10% or more. Pruritus runs in parallel with disease activity. Fever in CLL or macroglobulinaemia is secondary to infection.

11. Metabolic signs- Some lymphomas and CLL are associated with high proliferation rate, high death fractions of cells, enormous turn over rate of nucleoprotein and extreme hyperuricaemia. Burkitt lymphoma or ALL is particularly likely to cause extreme degree of hyperuricaemia. Cytolytic action of drugs may cause hyperuricaemia, hyperkalaemia, hyperphosphataemia, preciptation of uric acid in renal tubules, collecting ducts (tumor lysis syndrome).Hypercalcaemia, calciuria may occur during osteolysis, tumor cell production of IL-1, ectopic parathyroid hormone elaboration, excessive bone resorption, impaired bone formation. [6]
12. Organ infiltration (Extranodal)- T-cell leukaemias and lymphomas, in addition to causing lymph node and spleen enlargement, also may involve the skin, the mediastinum or CNS. Cutaneous T-cell lymphomas have malignant cells that home to skin, producing a desqumating erythroderma in Seizary syndrome, small (>2cm) subcutaneous nodules or primary cutaneous nodules in CD30+ve lymphoma or a variety of nodular infiltrative skin lesions in mycosis fungoides. T-cell ALL and lymphoblastic lymphoma can cause mediastinal enlargement. These diseases frequently involve the leptomeninges and other structures that are transverse to subarachnoid space. B-cell lymphoma usually involves the salivary glands, endocrine glands, joints, heart, lungs, kidney, bowel, bone, and less frequently often extranodal sites. These diseases may begin as an extranodal tumor or the tumor may develop in the course of the disease. Marginal zone B-cell lymphoma of mucosa-associated lymphoid tissue, frequently involves stomach and salivary glands, although the disease may be encountered in any extranodal site distinguished by the presence of columnar or cuboidal epithelium.

REFERENCES

1. Harris NL Jaffe ES, Stein H et al: *A revised European_American classification of lymphoid neoplasm. A proposal from lymphoma study group.* Blood 84:1361,(1994).
2. Strauchen JA: *Immunohemotype and molecular studies in the diagnosis and classification of malignant lymphoma.* Cancer Invest 22:138, (2004).
3. Kyle RA: *Clinical aspects of multiple myeloma and related disorders including amyloidosis.* Pathol (Biol) Paris 47:148, (1999).
4. Hirschberg B, Kramer MR, Lortem M et al: *Chronic eosinophilic pneumonia associated with cutaneous T-cell lymphoma.* Am J Haematol 60:143, (1999).
5. Chaubachi A, Miura I, Hatano Y et al : *Syndrome of inappropriate secretion of antidiuretic hormone in patients with lymphoma-associated haematophagocytic syndrome.* Ann Haematol 70: 53, (1995).
6. Scymour JF, Gagel RF: *The major humoral mediator of hypercalcaemia in Hodgkin and non-Hodgkin lymphoma.* Blood 82:1383, (1993).
7. Roodman GR: *Mechanism of bone formation in multiple myeloma and lymphoma.* Ann Haematol 70:53, (1995).

Part IV

Coagulation Disorder

CHAPTER 14

Coagulopathy: Bleeding Disorder and Thrombophilia

14.1 NORMAL COAGULATION

The coagulation process is the result of interaction of several coagulation proteins, platelets and tissue factors, derived from damaged tissues. The process begins with contact activation, starting with factor XII, proceeding to factor XI, and activation of factor IX. Resulting factor IX a (a = activated) activates factor VIII, which binds to Von Willebrand Factor (vWF), (an adhesion molecule also for promoting platelet plug). **Factor VIIIa** acts as a template having a negatively charged surface with two binding sites, each for factors IX and X. **Factor Xa,** with its cofactor VIIIa, on phospholipid membrane, activates **factor VII,** which is also activated by tissue factor released by damaged endothelium.

By **mitogenic activity,** Factor Xa induces smooth muscle proliferation and proinflammatory cytokines, thereby promoting healing. Factor Xa forms a complex with factor Va, which activates prothrombin **(Factor II)** to **thrombin**. **Factor XI**, activated by thrombin, on negatively charged surface of activated platelets, activates **Factor IX and factor XII**. **Factor XIII**. With complement Ciq, they help in generation of inflammatory response, to promote healing of damaged endothelium, and liberation of kinins to promote vasoconstriction and haemostasis.

TABLE 14.1: Key Role of Factor X in Coagulation

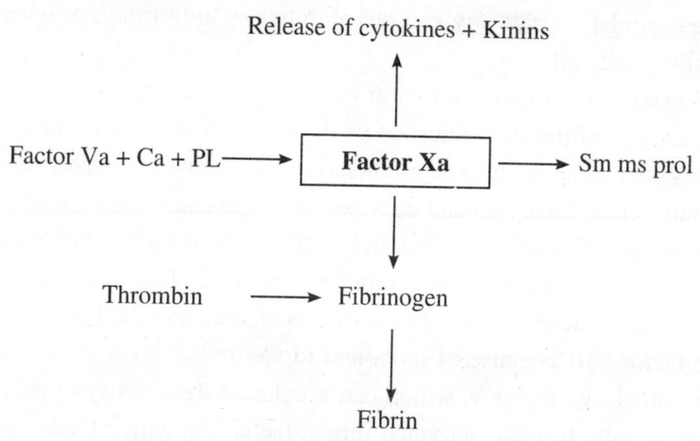

14.2 ROLE OF PLATELETS IN COAGULATION

Activation of platelets on exposure to damaged endothelium induces **release** of cytoplasmic granules, which **bind to receptors** on other platelet surfaces.

Adherence of platelets to collagen occurs **through mediation by von Willebrand factor (VWF). Conglomeration** of platelets takes place by **bridging** and **binding** of **fibrinogen** to **GP IIb/IIIa** receptors on platelet surface.

Steps of Haemostasis

1. Formation of platelet plug, which involves interaction of platelets, vessel wall, and VWF-primary haemostasis.
2. Formation of fibrin clot through humoral coagulation cascade-secondary haemostasis.
3. Bridging and binding of platelets with fibrin-formation of firm clot.

Abnormalities of Haemostasis

Abnormalities in platelet number, morphology, aggregation, adhesion

Abnormalities in coagulation proteins including deficiencies or defective molecule

Abnormalities of contact factors *e.g.*, fibrinogen or connective tissue disease

For hereditary deficiencies, mutation of controlling gene, is usually autosomal recessive, or X-linked, may be dominant in some cases.

Control of Coagulation Reactions

The blood coagulation system, like a powerful engine in idling mode, is always active in generation of thrombin at very low level and is poised for explosive generation of thrombin. In positive feedback reactions pro-coagulant thrombin activates platelets, factor V, VIII and XI. Small amount of thrombin can be generated by trace amount of tissue factor via the extrinsic pathway. Subsequently thrombin can activate factors XI, VIII and V, thereby stimulating each of the steps of the intrinsic pathway and thus amplifying thrombin generation.

The limiting of the clot is accomplished by **two systems** that depend on an intact endothelial surface. The **antithrombin system** requires the presence of endogenous heparins on endothelial surface. Antithrombin inhibits the coagulation mechanism by binding activated proteases in 1:1 proportion. Most enzymes in the coagulation pathway can be inhibited by antithrombin, whereas enzymes in the complexes are partially protected.

The **protein C system** inhibits coagulation by cleaving the large template coenzyme proteins factors V and VIII. Cleavage of these proteins slows the rate of thrombin activation sufficiently to shut down the process. The system requires intact endothelial cells that have a receptor called thrombomodulin. In turn, thrombomodulin binds thrombin and changes its conformation and thereby its specificity from fibrinogen to cleaving protein C. Activated protein C (APC)., in complex with protein S on the plasma of intact endothelial cells, then can cleave factors V and VIII. The inactivation of factor VIIIa is accelerated by protein S and factor C, the latter acting as an anticoagulant protein in this context. APC can't cleave inactive factor VIII because of its bound to vWF.

APC, however, can cleave factor V, which can accelerate the activity of APC along with protein S. Factor V therefore, actually has two activated forms, factor Va, which forms the template complex, and the active form after cleavage by APC, which accelerates the anticoagulant activity of the same enzyme. The common aspects of these systems are that intact endothelial surfaces are required and that the rate of the coagulation reaction is slowed to the point that new clots are not formed.

Negative feedback reactions involve the expression of activated protein C (APC). Anticoagulant activity that is generated by APC cellular pathway involves reactions, mediated by direct effects of APC on cells, which are entirely independent of action of APC on factor V and VIII. These are manifested as anti-inflammatory and anti-apoptotic activities. The direct effect of APC on cells indirectly down regulates thrombin generation as inflammation and apoptosis promote thrombin generation.

Binding of thrombin to thrombomodulin (endothelial cell receptor) converts the thrombin from a pro-coagulant enzyme to an anticoagulant. The surface dependent reaction is enhanced by endothelial cell protein C receptor (EPCR) that binds protein C. In a subsequent negative feedback loop, APC with the aid of non-enzymatic cofactor inactivates factors V and factor VIII. Protein S can also directly inhibit factors VIIIa, Xa, Va. Thus protein S inhibits multiple steps in the intrinsic coagulation pathway.

Table 2: Coagulation Control

Thrombin + Fibrinogen = Fibrin + Aggregated platelets = Clot

Thrombomodulin (Endo cell receptor) + Protein C = APC

APC + Protein S → inhibition → Thrombin + Factor Va + Factor VIIIa

Protein S → Inhibits factors Va VIIIa Xa

14.3 FIBRINOLYSIS

The control and remodeling of thrombus are accomplished by cleavage of fibrin by **plasmin,** the precursor of which is contained within the fibrin clot. Plasmin is activated from its **precursor plasminogen** through a number of pathways. Urokinase, located primarily in the urinary tract, has several active forms and cleaves plasminogen into plasmin. **Tissue plasminogen activator (t-PA),** present in several tissues, also bind to plasminogen to activate it, and causes local fibrinolysis and removes fibrin, when it is no longer necessary, **Plasminogen activator inhibitors** prevent premature activation. Deficiency of these inhibitors can cause a clinical bleeding disorder similar to haemophilia. Plasmin, is inhibited by several inhibitors, one of which is α_1 antiplasmin. The fibrinolytic products produce an inhibitory effect in the coagulation assays by interfering with the protease activity of multiple clotting factors that play important role in the generation of clot.

TABLE 14.2: Control of Thrombus Formation

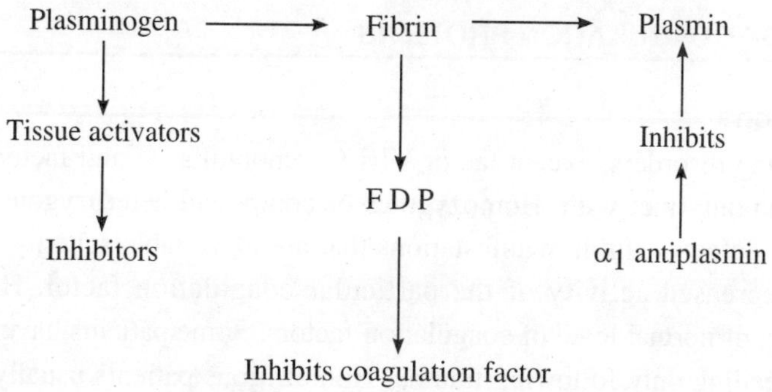

14.4 VASCULAR FUNCTION IN HAEMOSTASIS

The physiologic defense systems render endothelium thrombo-resistant and anti-fibrinolytic, which is also atherogenic and up-regulates expression of leukocytes, adhesion molecules, tissue factor and eisocanoids. Discovery of endoperoxides and thromboxane A_2 in early 1970s show that activated platelets release serotonin and thromboxane A_2. The latter also causes platelet aggregation that operates via ADP release. Subsequently, an endothelium-derived eisacinoids causes vasodilatation and inhibits platelet aggregation. This was named as prostacyclin $PGI_{2,}$ which subsequently inhibits platelet adhesion to vascular endothelium and results in increased intraplatelet concentration of CAMP. This process leads to abolition of platelet secretion and impaired binding of vWF and fibrinogen to platelet surface.

Prothrombin: Its central Role in Coagulation

Prothrombin is a member of vitamin K dependent coagulation proteins, other proteins being factors VII, IX, X. It plays a central role in coagulation, functioning in both tissue factor and surface activation pathways. It is synthesized in the liver as a peptide of 622 amino acids, the active domain consisting of glutamic acid residue, responsible for protein-protein interaction, and the catalytic domain responsible for cleavage of fibrinogen. [1]

Multiple Functions of Thrombin in Coagulation

In addition to converting fibrinogen to fibrin thrombin also acts at multiple sites of coagulation pathway

Thrombin is a serine protease, which:

1. activates platelets by cleavage of protease-activated receptor leading to adhesion and aggregation, as well as factors V, VIII, XIII which lead to cross-linking of fibrin
2. converts plasminogen to plasmin, thereby activating fibrinolytic system
3. activates fibrinolysis inhibitors
4. activates protein C after binding to thrombomodulin in the presence of endothelial protein C receptor
5. stimulates wound healing through its action as growth factor and for pro-angiogenic activity

Site of Synthesis of Coagulation Proteins

The coagulation proteins are synthesized in the liver except factor VIII and von Willebrand factor, the former is synthesized in the hepatic as well as non-hepatic sinusoidal cells, and the latter is synthesized in all endothelial cells.

14.5 DISORDER OF COAGULATION PROTEINS

Clinical Manifestations

These are rare bleeding disorders, except factor VIII (haemophilia A) and factor IX (haemophilia B), which are more commonly met with. Homozygotes or compound heterozygotes for the mutant gene responsible for these defects exhibit manifestations that are of variable severity and usually related to the extent of the decreased activity of the particular coagulation factor. Heterozygotes exhibit approximately 50 p.c. of normal level of coagulation factors. Some patients have only mild bruising or display excessive bleeding only following trauma. Homozygous patients usually with less than 1 p.c.

of normal factor VII, XIII or X activity exhibit intracranial haemorrhage and haemarthrosis, similar to patients of haemophilia A or B.

Genetics

The inherited combined deficiency of factor V and VIII is caused by mutations in two genes encoding for transporter proteins carrying factor V and VIII from the endoplasmic reticulum to the Golgi apparatus. The combined deficiency of all vitamin K dependent factors (factor VII, IX, X, protein C, protein S), has been shown to be result of mutations in two genes, one encoding for carboxylase that introduces γ carboxyl group at the glutamic acid residues of the molecule, into the coagulation factors, and the other, for vitamin K epioxide reductase (VKOR), that replenishes the resources of active vitamin K respectively. Carboxylation is essential for functional activity of these proteins, which yield vitamin K epioxide. These changes enable these proteins to bind calcium ions and become associated with membranes containing negatively charged phospholipids, VKOR, the target for inhibition of coagulaion is blocked by warfarin. [2]

Numerous mutations have been identified in genes encoding coagulation factors II, VII, X, XI and XIII. For some factors, such as factor II, VII and X, mutations giving rise to dysfunctional proteins predominate, whereas factors V, XI, XIII deficiency or true combined deficiency of factor V and VIII, an inherited autosomal recessive trait, results from mutation in genes encoding for carboxylase that carboxylates glutamic acid residue of these proteins or in the gene encoding for vitamin K epioxide reductase.

Therapy

Treatment of patients with varying coagulation deficiencies, plasma replacement has been used. Methods for measurement of specific concentrations of all vitamin K dependent factors and of factors VII, XI, XIII are not available. Replacement therapy with concentrated factor has been practiced in cases of factor VII, VIII or factor IX (haemophilia B) deficiency. In cases of inherited prothrombin deficiency, administration of prothrombin complex containing factor II, VII, IX and X is used.

These complexes are prepared by treating with detergent-solvent and exposure to ultraviolet rays to remove viruses like hepatitis B or C, HIV, but these processes may not remove Parvo viruses or risk of transmission of diseases like Cruetzfeldt disease or its new variant.

Fresh frozen plasma is less expensive and effective in these deficiencies, but it confers a very low level of the factor concerned and carries a measurable risk of transmission of HIV, hepatitis B and C, even if treated with solvent-detergent as the product is prepared from large pools of plasma.

In most cases, the question is whether to treat or not. Bruises and mild superficial bleeding may not require therapy. In case of prothrombin deficiency, as biological half- life of the factor is approximately 3 days, in many occasions, only single treatment is necessary.

Diagnosis

The activated partial thromboplastin time (aPTT) and prothrombin time are variably prolonged in hypo- and dys-prothrobinaemia, but thrombin time is normal. The diagnosis of prothrombin abnormality is established by demonstrating decreased functional level of prothrombin.

Hereditary and acquired deficiency of prothrombin must be distinguished. Acquired deficiency of prothrombin is infrequent but seen in patients with antiphospholipid syndrome, presenting with bleeding tendency.

Prolonged APTT and PT with normal thrombin time has been found in acquired conditions like liver disease, patients with lupus anticoagulant, therapeutic use of warfarin, vitamin K deficiency, as well as inherited conditions like factor V and X deficiency.

Factor VIII or von Willebrand factors are elevated in acute phase response and may show elevated values in hepatic disease as the sites of synthesis of these two factors lie also in cells other than liver cells. Acquired deficiency of vWF occurs (due to formation of antibodies) in collagen vascular disease, para-proteinaemia, Bcell lymphoma, myeloproliferative disorder like congenital deficiency. The condition does not respond pooled plasma and level of factor VIII is also subnormal. [3]

Factor VII Deficiency

Hereditary deficiency is a rare autosomal recessive chromosomal disorder, first described by Alexander and colleagues in 1951. The disorder is symptomatic only in Homozygotes and symptoms vary greatly from mild to severe. A presumptive diagnosis can easily be made as it is the only coagulation disorder that produces a prolonged PT and a normal APTT. Venous and arterial thromboses have been described in several patients. A survey of 514 patients with severe or mild partial factor VII deficiency recorded seven patients with venous thrombosis and one patient with arterial thrombosis. In 6 of 8 patients with venous thrombotic event occurred after surgery or labour. The common causes of acquired factor VII deficiency (the causes being almost similar to factor V deficiency as stated earlier) must be differentiated from the hereditary ones, careful history taking, physical examinations and relevant laboratory tests. Detection of heterozygotes can be facilitated by concomitant measurement of factor VII activity, antigen levels by ELISA method or factor VIIa can be measured by a soluble tissue factor, which is insensitive to native factor VII or by using an antibody in ELISA, which shows 3000 greater reactivity with factor VIIa. Hereditary deficiency must be distinguished from deficiency of all vitamin K dependent factors and combined deficiency of factors VII and X or VII and IX.

When surgery is required, the following factors should be considered

1. The site of surgery, as dental extraction, tonsillectomy, nasal surgery, urologic interventions may produce serious bleeding.
2. H/O bleeding like haemarthrosis, intracerebral haemorrhage.
3. Basic level of factor VII with very low activity (<3% normal).
4. Factor VII level 20 to 25 p.c of normal usually bleed after extensive trauma.
5. Volume overload is expected when plasma replacement is done.
6. Short half life of factor VII *i.e.*, 5 hours may need repeated administration.
7. Safety of blood components should be considered in cases of subsequent procedure like liver transplantation.

When plasma is used for major surgery, a loading dose of 15 ml/kg should be administered by 4 ml/kg every 6 hours for 7 to 10 days. Specific factor VII concentrate have been successfully used, the dose ranging 8–40 ml/kg in 4–6 hours intervals. Another option is to use recombinant factor VIIa in doses of 20 to 25 μg/kg at intervals of 2–3 hours. In children and in females, the half life of factor VIIa is even shorter than usual *i.e.*, 2.5 hours, so treating such cases is more difficult.

TABLE 14.3: Inherited Deficiencies of Coagulation Factors Compared

Type of Deficiency	Inheritance	Clinical Picture	Therapy	Activity Required
Factor XII	————	Not assoc. with bleeding, APTT > 65 sec	Does not require replacement	Activator of factor XI
Factor XI (Haemophilia C)	Autosomal recessive	Intraartcular and muscle bleeding, variable for a given level	FFP replacement, chance of thrombosis with concentrate	Haemostasis with level > 30%
Factor IX (Haemophilia B or Christmas disease)	X-linked recessive (1:10 as common as factor VIII def)	Intraarticular and muscle bleeding, spontaneous in severe disease	Recombinant factor, 75 U/kg, initially every 24 hours	Critical for normal in vivo regulation
Factor VIII	X-linked recessive (Haemophilia A)	Intraarticular, muscle bleeding, (6–35% Mild, 1–5% Moderate, <1% severe)	Recombinant factor VIII, in a dose of 50 U/kg as a bolus, then 4U/kg/hr for 100 % activity	75% – 100% activity for surgical haemostasis
Factor X	Rare congenital, acquired in primary amyloidosis	Bleeding on trauma	Replacement with FFP	Requires 30% level for haemostasis
Factor V	Rare congenital, Acquired in liver disease, myeloprol, Dis.	Mucosal bleeding-gingivial, epistaxis, easy bruising, menorrhagia	Contained in platelets, platelet transfusion for therapy	————
Factor II	Very rare congenital, acquired in cases of nutritional def or warfarin therapy		FFP is the best therapy	Requires about 30% activity
Factor VII	Congenital not rare but unusual	Most do not bleed, level varies, spontaneous thromboses may occur	FFP is the best replacement	
Combined deficiency of vit K dependent factors	Rare autosomal recessive-first reported in1966 mutation in the gene for carboxylase		Large dose of vit K, FFP or prothrombin complex concentrate	

Gene Therapy for Bleeding Disorder

Transduction of muscle cells by an adeno-associated virus (AAV) containing a factor IX construct resulted in phenotypic correction in haemophilic B mice for more than 17 months. Likewise transduction of hepatocytes with an AAV vector containing factor IX DNA reportedly corrected the haemophilic defect in haemophilia B-mice and dogs for approximately 7 to 8 months.

One of the interesting approach is the introduction of AAV vector containing cDNA of factor VII, which when secreted, becomes activated. This produces fewer bleeding episodes and no thromboembolic side effects are seen. [4]

14.6 SCREENING TESTS FOR BLEEDING DISORDERS

1. **Bleeding time** has been criticized extensively and is vulnerable to many variables *e.g.*, age, skin elasticity, condition of capillary wall, thickness of subcutaneous tissue. It remains, however, the only broadly available screening test for platelet function and platelet adhesion molecule abnormalities such as von Willebrand disease. The bleeding time is sufficiently variable that it is unusual to obtain meaningful serial measurements in response to various interventions.
2. (i) **History regarding previous bleeding** is most important in evaluation of a bleeding disorder. Specific questioning about prolonged bleeding after dental extraction, tonsillectomy, frequent epistaxis, may reveal thrombocytopenia.
   - (ii) **Type of bleeding:** Bruising > 3 at a time, bruising on the trunk, pain and swelling persistent on the site of bruising, without severe trauma, indicates presence of coagulation disorder. Circumcisional bleeding may be the firs indication of factor VIII deficiency. Very prolonged wound bleeding or prolonged bleeding from an umbilical stump may be due to factor XIII deficiency inhibiting cross-linking and stabilization of fibrin clot. Bleeding in joints or deep muscle is indicative of deficiency of coagulation proteins, whereas, mucosal bleeding or extended bleeding from superficial clot indicates platelet related disorder.
   - (iii) **Timing of bleeding** after trauma is very much important. Bleeding immediate after trauma, suggests severe deficiency of coagulation protein or platelet disorder. Initial good haemostasis with bleeding 2–5 days later, suggests a plasma protein disorder.
3. **Family history** of at least two prior generations is important to confirm he presence of a familial pattern to the disorder. Disorder may be autosomal or sec-linked recessive. When there is a positive family history, careful documentation of entire pedigree is essential. Death due to bleeding or surgery in the family carries additional information. Analysis of pattern of age and sex prevalence allows the probability of various disorders to be detected.
4. Acquired coagulopathy is more common in practice. Hence, following histories are important.
   - (a) **History of medication** such as aspirin, clopidrogel (which interfere with Gp IIb/IIIa receptors of platelets), heparin or warfarin.
   - (b) **Medical problems** like hepatic disease, renal failure, malabsorption.
5. **Physical examination** must include examination of skin for evidences of connective tissue disorder, telengiectasis for evidence of vascular disorder, examination of abdomen for splenomegaly (which indicates some systemic disease), examination of joints for secondary changes due to haemarthrosis.

6. **Prothrombin time (PT), Activated partial thromboplastin time (APTT)** have sensitiveness that cannot exclude clinically important deficiencies *e.g.*, most APTT reagents will have a normal clotting time with a 35% factor VIII level.
7. **Coagulation protein abnormality approach:** Preliminary testing with PT and APTT may detect a prolonged clotting time. If it is found, the next step is to perform a 1:1 mixture of normal plasma and patient's plasma, if the repeat test with this mixture becomes normal, a protein deficiency is suggested. A 50% level of any single coagulation protein will support a normal clotting time. If the test time of the mixture remains prolonged, an inhibitor is suggested. Mild or moderate deficiencies of coagulation proteins may have normal or minimal coagulation time. If the test is normal but the history is suggestive of a bleeding disorder, additional testing should be performed, including individual coagulation factor assays and platelet function testing.

   PT = Prothrombin Time, which measures the clotting time of plasma in the presence of an optimal concentration of tissue extract (thromboplastin) and indicates the overall efficiency of the extrinsic clotting system. Although originally thought to measure prothrombin, the test is now known to depend also on reactions with factors V, VII and X, and on the fibrinogen concentration of the plasma. The test result is compared with that obtained from normal healthy persons. The result is expressed in International standard unit (INR). Normal value depends on thromboplastin used. With most rabbit thromboplastin, normal range of PT is 11 to 16 sec withan INR of 1.0 to 1.3.

   APTT = Activated Partial Thromboplastin Time, which measures the clotting time of plasma after activation of contact factors, but without added tissue thromboplastin. It indicates overall efficacy of the intrinsic pathway. To standardize the test, the plasma is first preincubated with kaolin, and a standardized phospholipid is provided to perform the test on platelet-poor plasma. The test measures the contact factors, factors VIII, IX and depends also on factors X, V prothrombin and fibrinogen. It is also sensitive to inhibitors and heparin. Normal range is 30–40 sec, when pooled normal plasma is used as a control. In case of prolonged APTT, a 50 : 50 mixture of normal and test plasma is used. If APTT is corrected, there is probably a deficiency of one or more clotting factors.

   TT = Thrombin Time is measured by adding thrombin to test plasma and clotting time is noted. The time is affected by concentration and reaction of fibrinogen, and the presence of inhibitors, including fibrinogen and fibrin degradation product (FDP) as well as heparin. Times of 20 s and over are definitely abnormal.

   If all of these first line tests, PT, APTT, TT, platelet count, are normal, in a case of bleeding disorder, patient may have

   1. Disorder of platelet function
   2. Factor VIII deficiency
   3. Disorder of vascular haemostasis
8. **Examination of platelets—** Platelet count less than 100,000/c mm will prolong bleeding time.

   Morphology of platelets in PBS

Giant megakaryocytes may indicate thrombocytosis or malignant disorder, or rare hereditary disorder like Bernard Soulier disease.

Chapter 14

Platelet Function Test

(i) **Platelet aggregability test:** The platelet studies are performed using a platelet-rich plasma harvested from anticoagulated blood, and responses are monitored to various agonists including ADP, epinephrine, collagen, Thromboxane A_2, thrombin receptor peptides and ristocetin.

Abnormalities in platelet aggregaion may be due to **severe deficiency of fibrinogen,** quantative or **qualitative abnormality** of the platelet membrane **GP Iib-IIIa complex** (Glanzman thromboasthenia) or defect in vWF, which is an adhesion molecule.

(ii) **Impaired response to Ristocetin but normal response to other agonists suggests von Willebrand disease or the Bernard Soulier syndrome.** In the latter, platelet count is decreased, platelet size is increased, but plasma levels of vWF and factor VIII are normal. [5]

(iii) **Platelet secretion and signal transduction defects are** a heterogenous group of disorders. The major characteristic of this group is an inability to release intracellular granule contents on activation of platelet-rich plasma with agonists such as ADP, epinephrine and collagen. A group of patients show **deficiency of platelet or granules (factor V binding protein), deficiency of dense platelet granules (storage pool deficiency).** This group of disorder shows muco-cutaneous bleeding, impaired response to epinephrine and the second wave of aggregation is blunted.

Deficiency or defect of von Willebrand factor may be of various types.

The clinical feature includes mucosal bleeding, especially epistaxis, many have normal APTT values. Patients with severe vWF deficiency (type 3) have similar feature as haemophilia, as a result of concomitant decrease of Factor VIII level, the cause is not understood. In type 2 deficiency, the protein structure is abnormal, in type 1, there is normal protein with decreased but detectable von Willebrand factor.

14.7 ACQUIRED COAGULOPATHY

I. Vitamin K Deficiency

Vitamin K is essential for the carboxylation of factors I, VII, IX and X as well as proteins C and S in the natural anticoagulant system. In the absence or deficiency of vitamin K abnormal coagulation molecules called PIVKA (proteins induced by vitamin K absence) are produced, which have minimal coagulation activity because they cannot bind calcium and participate in the coagulation reaction.

Causes of vitamin K deficiency are inadequate die, alcohol dependency, or hospitalized patients receiving (total parenteral) nutrition without vitamin K supplementation. Impaired absorption of vitamin K is caused by deficiency of bile salt resulting from bile duct obstruction, inflammatory bowel disease due to tropical sprue or inflammatory bowel disease. It is common in postoperative patients who are not taking nothing orally and taking antibiotics for extended period. Vitamin K antagonists such as warfarin or its newer analog *e.g.*, brodifacum may also produce this deficiency.

Diagnosis is done by measuring PT: Sometimes specific factor assays will uncover the condition. There is normal factor VII and depressed levels of longer surviving factors II and X.

Therapy

Moderate prolongation of PT may be treated with small doses of vitamin K (1 mg) if continued anticoagulation is desired. 5 mg of vitamin K is administered S.C. daily for 3 days and that will differentiate the condition from liver failure.

II. Haemostatic Dysfunction in Liver Disease

Chronic or acute liver failure initiated by viral hepatitis, alcohol abuse or acetaminophen intoxication results in substantial changes in the haemostatic system. If synthetic function of the liver is compromised, haemostatic proteins are reduced in amount. Furthermore, a diseased liver has reduced ability of clearing activated haemostatic proteins, activators of fibrinolysis or protein inhibitor complexes from the circulation. These alterations lead to a bleeding tendency. On the other hand, thrombosis of portal vein and hepatic artery may occur in patients with liver disease or after liver transplantation. A reduced platelet count and impaired platelet function are commonly observed in patients with liver disease. [6]

The following abnormalities are noted in haemostatic function in liver disease:

Platelet count, 100,000/μl, is frequently present in patients with liver disease. The main causes for **thrombocytopenia** in liver disease are

(i) increased platelet sequestration due to congestive splenomegaly related to portal hypertension.
(ii) reduced platelet half life possibly related to autoantibodies.
(iii) in patients with alcohol-induced liver disease, folic acid deficiency, or consequences of toxic effect of alcohol on platelet production.
(v) Low-grade DIC resulting in further platelet consumption.

Changes in platelet function

(a) Platelet aggregation in response various agents is diminished as well as interaction of platelets with extracellular matrix components.
(b) Defective platelet resulting from impaired signal transduction, due to proteolysis of platelet membrane.
(c) Increased production of endothelial-derived platelet inhibitors, nitric oxide and prostacycline.
(d) Reduced haematocrit may contribute to reduced platelet vessel wall interaction.

von Willebrand factor

Profoundly elevated level of vWF is frequently observed in liver disease and probably results from endothelial damage mediated by bacterial infection. vWF in RNA and protein expression in the liver itself are enhanced in cirrhosis.

Coagulation and anticoagulation

The liver is the site of synthesis of most **procoagulant factors** *e.g.*, factors V, VII, IX, XI and prothrombin. These are found to be **decreased** in liver disease. **Factor VIII level is increased** due to decreased hepatic expression of LDL related receptor and increased level of vWF may be related to elevated level of its clearance protein. Hepatic sinusoidal epithelial cells may maintain the capacity to synthesize factor VII when liver function is severely compromised. Because of vitamin K **deficiency or decreased vitamin K dependent carboxylation factors II, VII, IX and X may be deficient** and their function is impaired. The markedly elevated level of γ carboxy-prothrombin in patients with hepatocellular carcinoma may be used to distinguish between malignant and non-malignant liver disease.

Anticoagulant factors like protein C, protein S, antithrombin, heparin cofactor II and α_2 macroglobulin are **decreased** in patients with liver disease, a consequence of reduced synthesis. Hyperfibrinolysis has been associated with low grade DIC, induced by endotoxinaemia. In acute liver failure there is increased level of D-dimer, which is indicative of augmented fibrinolysis, though there is apparent hypofibrinogenaemia.

Diagnosis: is confirmed by abnormal or elevated hepatic enzymes. APTT is prolonged as well as PT in severe cases, although the elevated factor VIII suggests chronic liver disease.

Therapy of coagulopathy in liver disease: Spontaneous bleeding is uncommon. Preceding or following some surgical procedure, haemostatic defect should be corrected.

Replacement therapy with FFP is the most common therapy as it replaces all plasma components. If fibrinogen level is to be replenished, cryoprecipitate is most appropriate. Anti-fibrinolytic therapy must be used in cases of disseminated coagulation, either transexamic acid 20 mg/kg three times daily or epsilon-amino-caproic acid (EACA) 4 g every 4 hours.

Disseminated intravascular coagulation (DIC)

This is a **condition of coagulation activation** to an abnormal degree resulting in generation of sufficient thrombin **to overwhelm the physiologic thrombin inhibitors,** including antithrombin and thrombomodulin. Thrombin activates the coagulation factors rapidly enough for their levels to fall to levels, that do not allow normal haemostasis to occur. The generation of fibrin also initiates the overproduction of fibrin degradation products (FDP). The presence of fibrin strands can damage red blood cells, producing an abnormal blood smear with fragmented red cells, which are considered diagnostic of a microangiopathic haemolytic anaemia. [7]

Aetiology

Although DIC is not a disease, it is a condition that is produced by some other disease processes, like infection (endotoxin), trauma, cell necrosis. DIC is found in infections *e.g.*, typhoid fever, Gram +ve and Gram –ve septicaemia, viraemia, tuberculosis or parasitic infection *e.g.*, malaria. Tissue injury such as renal allograft rejection, heat stroke, brain injury or crush injury, necrotizing enterocolitis, haemolytic transfusion reaction, may also produce this condition.

Foreign substances (chemicals, and hypotonic solution), foreign enzymes (snake venom), obstetric hazards *e.g.*, amniotic fluid embolism, abruptio placentae, that activate the coagulation process by overproduction of thrombin, may be responsible for DIC. Connective tissue disorder, malignancy like acute promyelocytic leukaemia or mucin producing adenocarcinoma, may produce activation of disseminated coagulation.

TABLE 14.4: Key Role of Thrombin in Pathogenesis of DIC

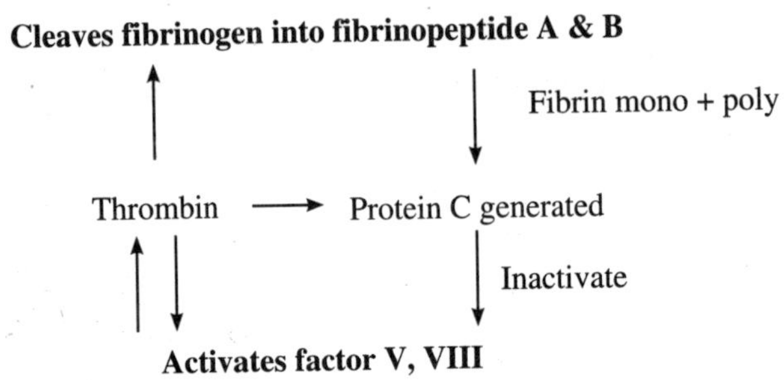

14.8 CLINICAL MANIFESTATIONS

Bleeding is the most commonly recognized clinical sign and usually is in more than one site. Thrombotic events may be more subtle but can manifest as changes in mental state, renal failure, or other localized organ ischaemia caused by small vessel obstruction.

There is no single test that can diagnose the condition. The presence of fibrinolysis products such as D-dimers (plasmin cleaved cross-linked fibrin), detection of soluble fibrin monomer complex (SFMC), decreases of fibrinogen or platelets and the prolongation of PT reflecting reduced levels of circulating coagulation factors, are common abnormalities associated with this condition. Fibrin degradation products (FDP) are indicative of fibrinolysis.

Therapy: If coagulation factors are decreased and the patient is bleeding, factor replacement with FFP (the plasma coagulation proteins), cryoprecipitate concentrate, concentrated fibrinogen and platelets is indicated. The condition should never be treated only for abnormal tests. If thrombosis occurs, anticoagulation usually with heparin is appropriate. Anti-thrombin concentrates may be needed. Heparin in the absence of thrombosis is rarely indicated. Accurate diagnosis and vigorous treatment of underlying cause are necessary for successful outcome.

Fibronolysis: It is very rare, occurring in amyloidosis, sometimes with liver disease, (though decreased clearance of fibrinogen degradation products complicates the picture), and rare malignancies, where a fibrinogen cleaving enzyme may be present. [8]

Diagnosis and differentiation from DIC is difficult, but no decrease in coagulation factors other than fibrinogen, plasminogen, and α_2 antiplasmin should be present. Treatment for fibrinolysis with inhibitors, transexamic acid, (1500 mg three times daily for the average adult), or EACA (4 g every 6 hours or 1 g per hour continuous infusion) may be helpful.

TABLE 14.5: Differences between DIC and Primary Fibrinolysis

	DIC	Primary fibrionlysis
Platelet count	Low	Usually normal
Fibrinogen	Low	Low
Factor V	Low	Low
Factor VIII	Low	Normal to moderately decreased
Protamine sulphate test	Positive	Negative
Euglobulin lysis time	Normal	Short
FDP	Increased	Very large in amount

14.9 CARDIOPULMONARY BYPASS INDUCED BLEEDING DISORDERS

All patients have an acquired platelet defect that reverses in first after stopping bypass. The bleeding tendency can be treated with platelet transfusion. Partial activation can cause part of platelet defect and complex activation of the platelets can cause thrombocytopenia. If transfusion is massive, additional coagulation factors should be replaced with FFP, and cryoprecipitate will replace fibrinogen and improve qualitative platelet defect.

Chapter 14

14.10 COAGULOPATHY IN CONNECTIVE TISSUE DISORDER

Varities of Coagulopathy

1. Prothrombotic state and clinical thrombosis due to antiphospholipid antibodies is common rather than bleeding disorder.
2. Incidence of lupus anticoagulant is high (30–37%) of diagnosed cases, in which, bleeding tendency is present.
3. Antibodies to factor VIII and vWF produce surgical bleeding, or large haematoma, ecchymoses, spontaneous or on trivial trauma. The condition responds to desmopressin but not to factor VIII, unlike hereditary variety.
4. Acquired vWF disease-Antibodies to vWF factor are reported in collagen vascular disease, paraproteinemia, B cell lymphoma, myeloproliferative disease Reduced activity of both vWF and factor VIII distinguish the acquired variety from congenital form Prolonged APTT is not corrected by pooled plasma unlike congenital deficiency.
5. In SLE incidence of immune thrombocytopenia is 25% in lupus anticoagulant negative patients and overall incidence is 54–60%. It may be associated with bleeding. DIC (in lupus anticoagulant +ve cases) may precipitate secondary bleeding.

   Antiphospholipid antibody (APLA) may produce cerebral infarction or digital gangrene.

Pathogenesis of Coagulopathy in Connective Tissue Disorder

1. **Activation of coagulation system:** This has been found in studies (with labeled fibrinogen) of different connective tissue disorder in active or sub-clinical state. In patients with SLE, enhanced fibrinogen consumption was significantly correlated with disease activity, DNA-binding activity test, serum complement level, serum mucoprotein level (which is a specific inflammatory index). These data suggest usefulness of complementary treatment in connective tissue disease to counteract its pathogenetic mechanism. [8]
2. **Antiphospholipid antibody syndrome:** These are natural antibodies to cardiolipin and a B cell clone from a patient with CLL has been first demonstrated producing these antibodies. [9]

Antigens, stimulating these antibodies, are variable. In acute syndrome, antibodies are found in association with infections, after cardiac surgery or infarction, but not always associated with thrombosis. [10] Chronic antibodies are found in connective tissue disorder, and further associated with lupus anticoagulant activity. These antibodies can bind to cardiolipin in association with cofactors, histones or DNA, in connective tissue disorder. [11]

Clinically important antibodies react with anionic rather than zwitteronic phospholipids, as a result there is persistent endothelial cell damage and interaction both with β_2 GP1 and prothrombin. The former cofactor would change and induce lupus anticoagulant activity.

Therapy

For oral anticoagulant, recommended INR is to be kept in the range of 3–3.5.

Patients with arterial thromboembolism or pregnancy should be treated with low dose aspirin and prednisone.

Alternatively full dose heparin therapy (BD, SC) has been shown to be equally effective but less toxic. [12]

14.11 THROMBOPHILIC DISORDER

The majority of thrombophilic disorders involve the anticoagulant protein C pathway, including thrombomodulin, endothelial protein C receptor, protein S, high density lipoprotein and factor V. The substrate for enzymatic action of activated protein C include the plasma clotting factors Va and VIIIa and protease activated receptor-I as a key cell signaling target. Tissue factor pathway inhibitor neutralizes coagulation pathway factors VIIa and Xa. Other plasma protease inhibitors can also neutralize various coagulation proteases, although clinical significance is less apparent. [13]

14.12 INHERITED THROMBOTIC DISORDER

The well defined congenital hyper-coagulable disorders are clinically indistinguishable from one another, all characterized by predominantly venous thrombosis, which may range from peripheral venous events in the extremities to central nervous system thrombosis. Isolated arterial events are less likely to indicate one of these conditions are less likely to occur. [14]

1. The most common inherited disorder is a point mutation in factor V molecule, rendering it resistant to degradation by APC. Variant factor V containing glycine 506 in place of arginine 506 (factor V Leiden) causes hereditary disorder. The condition is associated with recurrent venous thrombosis in 25% to 45% of cases. The mutant factor V has full coagulant activity but prolonged half- life, giving rise to hyper-coagulable state. This form of factor V accelerates APC formation and slows down factor VIII inactivation. This is called factor V Leiden, which shows an ethnic variation, ranging from up to 5% of Northern European to extremely rare in Asian population.
2. The second most common abnormality is an abnormality of the non-coding portion of prothrombin, which results in its slight elevation, but thrombotic risks are multiplied by presence of other prothombotic states.
3. Protein C or S deficiencies are present in about 1 in 300 persons and present in 1% to 3% of persons with venous thrombosis. Protein C deficiency may be homozygous or heterozygous, the homozygous form being associated with neonatal purpura fulminans. Protein S deficiency may be of total amount, its free form or abnormal bioactivity.
4. Antithrombin, the first described deficiency, is rare, occurring in 1 in 2000. Antithrombin neutralizes all proteases of intrinsic pathway, including thrombin, factor IXa, XIa, XIIa in reactions stimulated by physiological or pharmacological heparin The antithrombin activity may be affected by concomitant heparin therapy. Heparin binds to antithrombin, greatly increasing its anticoagulant effect by inhibiting thrombin and factor Xa. The presence of an abnormal form with a normal antigen level makes measurement of activity mandatory.

Acquired Inhibitors of Coagulation

1. Lupus-type anticoagulant— is the most common type of acquired inhibitor in clinical practice. The inhibitor appears to be directed against a combination of a coagulation protein epitope and β_2 microglobulin and is enhanced by phospholipid. There is general inhibition of multiple coagulation factors in vitro. There is prolonged APTT. The condition is associated thromboses, bleeding is extremely rare, except when associated with hypothrombinaemia or severe

Chapter 14

thrombocytopenia. LAC belongs to anticadiolipid antibodies' family, which is also associated with thromboses. [15]

Therapy is with coumarin anticoagulants with minimum target international normalized ratio of 2.5 to 3.0 needed because of in vitro effect of the LAC on the PT. Some investigators argue for LMW heparin, but prolonged therapy is needed which may be problematic.

2. Acquired inhibitor to factor VIII- Antibodies to factor VIII are the most common inhibitors to a specific coagulation factor. This may occur in the following conditions:
   - Elderly people
   - Post-patrum (usually after 3–12 months)
   - Diagnosis
     (i) No correction of APTT with factor VIII (normal citrated plasma).
     (ii) Quantified by Bethesda unit, a less confusing unit that is best thought as the amount inhibitor required to reduce the factor VIII activity in a volume of plasma by 50%.
     (iii) Low levels of inhibitors are fewer than 5 Bethesda units.
     (iv) High levels of inhibitors are more than 5 Bethesda units.

Treatment of acquired factor VIII inhibitors include the use of prednisolone 100 mg to 1 gm daily, with or without other immunosuppressives such as cyclophosphamide. The higher the inhibitor, the less likely a complete response will occur and the greater the risk of fatality. For acute bleeding plasmapharesis may be effective in lowering antibody titre. Antifactor V antibodies are rare, but a number of cases have been reported in late 1980s, with the use of topical bovine thrombin containing a small amount of bovine factor V. Antibodies with varying degree of cross-reactivity with human factor V developed in some cases and may cause fatal bleeding disorder.

Predisposing Factors for Thrombosis

1. Increased Factor VIII may occur in pregnancy, oral contraceptive (OCP) therapy, old age, acute phase response, liver disease, hypothyroidism.
2. Decreased Protein C as found in liver disease, OCP therapy, vitamin K deficiency,in childhood, in presence of autoantibodies.
3. Decreased Protein S found in liver disease, therapy with oral anticoagulants, in pregnancy, as nephrotic syndrome, OCP therapy, in presence of autoantibodies.

Prothrombotic States

1. Hereditary or acquired Pr C or Pr S def, elevated Factor VIII
2. Antiphospholipid syndrome
3. Prothrombin gene polymorphism
4. Increased fibrinogen or dysfibrinogenaemia
5. Homosystinaemia

Added Risk Factors for Thromboses

1. Acquired Anti thrombin deficiency— liver disease,heparinisation, nephrotic syndrome, chemotherapy with asparaginase, pre-eclampsia, DIC.

2. Increased level of fibrnogen-Acute phase reaction, old age, atherosclerosis, smoking, excessive coffee consumption.
3. Dys lipidaemia and lipoproteinaemia.

Homocystinaemia-is the Condition Which Shows:

1. Plasma level of homocysteine > 100 mmol/l.
2. Genetic polymorphism of the enzyme cystathione b synthetase.
3. Suboptimal vit B_6 or vit B_{12} therapy may produce the condition.
4. Renal failure, hypothyroidism, inflammatory bowel disease, Psoriasis, rheumatoid arthritis, may be the other causes.

Clinical Features of Thrombotic Disorders

I Venous thrombosis is more common than arterial

Portal or hepatic vein thrombosis is common, specially in liver disease

Renal vein thrombosis is common in nephrotic syndrome

Pulmonary. thromboembolism is common in septicaemia

Superficial venous thrombosis is common in Protein C or S def

Arterial thromboses, though less frequent than venous, may occur with an onset in 30% of cases below 35 years and in 70% onset is above 50 years, when added risk factors are present. Cerebral or coronary arterial thrombosis is found in APLA positive cases or thrombocytosis, the latter showing also digital arterial thrombosis and gangrene. Hepatic, mesenteric arterial thrombosis is very rare.

14.13 LABORATORY DIAGNOSIS

1. Clot-based testing can identify presence of APC resistance, presence of lupus anticoagulant, protein C and protein S levels and antithrombin deficiencies.
2. The measurement of antigen level as well as activity should be done because abnormal forms of protein may produce apparent deficiency.
3. Free protein S should be measured because the balance between balanced bound and free protein S may cause a prothrombotic state.
4. Concomittant heparin therapy may produce transient decrease of antithrombin level, so, the diagnosis of deficiency may require confirmatory test after recovery.
5. An elevated level of homocysteine arising from numerous enzyme abnormalities and nutritional deficiency increases the thrombotic risk.
6. Elevated level of factor VIII and fibrinogen are additional risk factors, but they are not included in the screening tests.

14.14 THERAPY OF THROMBOTIC STATE

1. Heparin and Low Molecular weight heparin- Low molecular weight heparin has a more predictable pharmacokinetics than standard heparin. It can be administered subcutaneously and can be monitored easily. Standard heparin is associated with more commonly with induced thrombocytopenia, mediated by antibodies against platelet factor 4, complexed with heparin.

Both forms of heparin require the presence of antithrombin for the anticoagulant defect. The high molecular forms have some antiplatelet effect.

2. The family of vitamin K antagonists inhibit the addition of carboxyl group to glutamic acid, which confers calcium binding for localization of the coagulation reaction. In the presence of vitamin K anagonists, there are abnormal forms of coagulation factors II, VII, IX, and X as wellas proteins C and S, both naturally occurring anticoagulants, are also vitamin K dependent, it is also little confusing as to why the overall effect is anticoagulation. In the presence of an inherited deficiency of protein C, however, there is increased risk of warfarin associated skin necrosis, a phenomenon of microvascular thrombosis.

   Most common side effect of therapy is bleeding and monitoring the therapy should be done by measurement of PT and monitoring frequency is determined by stability of INR but should not be less frequent than every 3 to 4 weeks.
3. Duration of treatment should be judged by the clinical set up. More prolonged the therapy, there is less chance of recurrence. The balance in a person with single episode of thrombosis is usually maintained by 6-12 months of therapy.
4. Added risks of thrombosis must be evaluated and properly treated. Elevated homocysteine must be treated with folic acid 1 mg daily.

   Broad investigation in absence of symptoms or previous thromboembolic event is unjustified. History-based evaluation and therapy is most appropriate.

REFERENCES

1. Jagenson M, Cantor A, Furie B, et al., (1987): *Recognition site of Vit K-dependent γ carboxylation resides on the propeptide of factor V.* Cell 48:185.
2. Sten L, Dahlback B (1994): *Factor V and protein S as synergistic cofactors in activated protein S as synergistic cofactors in activated protein C in degradation of factor VIIIa.* J Biol Chem. 269:18735.
3. Tuddenhan EGD (1995): *Factor VIII, in Molecular basis of Thrombosis and Haemostasis, edited by K.A. High, H.R. Rolents* p167, Marce Dekken, New York.
4. Margaretes P, Arruda VR, Aljamali M,et al., (2004): *Novel therapeutic approach for haemophilia using gene delivery of an engineered secreted activated factor VII.* J clin Invest 113:1025.
5. Dale GL, Biese P, Batar P, et al., (2002): *Stimulated platelets are serotonin to enhance their retention of procoagulant proteins on the cell surface.* Nature 415:175.
6. Pareti FL, Capitanio A, Mannuci Li (1976): *Acquired storage pool disease in platelets during disseminated intravascular coagulation.* Blood 48: 511.
7. Kitchens CS (1995): *Disseminated intravascular coagulation*; Curr Opin Haematol 2:402–6.
8. Liebman HA, Carfango MK, Weitz IC, et al., (1992): *Excessive fibrinolysis in amyloidosis associated with elevated plasma single chain urokinase.* Am J Clin Pathol 98:534 – 41.
9. Mariette X, Levy Y, Dulurekil ML, Intrator L, Datton F, Brouet Jc (1993): *Characterisation of a human monoclonal autoantibody directed to cardiolipin (beta 2 glycoprotein 1) produced by chronic lymphocytic leukaemia B cells.* Clin Exp. Immunol 94:385–90.

10. Adelajo AO, Charles P, Maini RS, Hazlleman BL (1994): *Autoantibodies in malaria, tuberculosis, hepatitis B in a West African population*. Clin Exp Immunol 92:73–6.

11. Pereira LF, Marco FM, Boimato R, Caturia A, Bustos K, de la Concha EG, Suliza JL (1994): *Histones interact with anionic phospholipids with high avidity*. Clin Exp Immunol; 97:175–80.

12. Kearon C, Gent M, Hirsh J, et al., (1999) *A comparison of three months of anticoagulation with extended anticoagulation for a first episode of idiopathic venous thromboembolism*. N Engl J Med 340:901–7.

13. Rezende SM, Simmonds RE, Lane DA (2004): *Coagulation, inflammation, and apoptosis: Different roles for protein S and proteins-c4b complex*. Blood 103:1192.

14. Esman CT (2000): *Regulation of blood coagulation*. Biochem Biophys Acta 1477:349.

15. Bevers EM, Galli M, Barbui T, Comifarmis P, Zwal RR, (1991): *Lupus anticoagulant IgG3 are directed to phospholipids not only but also to lipids bound to human prothrombin*. Thrombo Haemost 66:629–32.

CHAPTER

15 Coagulopathy in Chronic Kidney Disease

15.1 INTRODUCTION

Coagulopathy comprises of heightened or suppressed coagulation function of the body. Actually, the hyper- and hypo-activity of the system are interdependent. The process which is initiated as disseminated intravascular coagulation may culminate in torrential haemorrhage. In chronic kidney disease, both of the varieties of coagulopathy e.g., haemorrhagic and thrombotic complications may occur.

15.2 NORMAL COAGULATION PROCESS

Normal coagulation is a complex physicochemical process. The reactions occur in cascade fashion. There are two arms of the system. On one side, there is a number of coagulation factors present in the streaming blood, on the other side, there are platelets and leukocytes.

The process is initiated by **platelets** following tissue injury or breach in continuity of the inner endothelial lining of the vessel wall, so that platelets are activated on exposure to subendothelial tissue. Being activated, they release the content of cytoplasmic granules, including ADP, which binds to receptors on nearby platelet surfaces. Adherence of platelets to collagen occurs through von Willebrand factor, a coagulation factor present in the blood. Conglomeration of activated platelets occurs through bridging by fibrinogen, which binds to GP IIb/ IIIa receptors on platelet surfaces. Further activation occurs through Thromboxane A2, generated from Arachidonic acid in the platelet. This is strongly opposed by prostacyclin released from endothelial cells and a balance is maintained in health between the two to preserve the fluidity of the blood. Platelets also release growth factors which induce vascular endothelial cell proliferation and thereby promote healing. Thus, the platelets form the primary haemostatic plug.

Sequence of events may be represented as follows:

- **Activation** of platelets on exposure
- **Release** of cytoplasmic granules
- Granules **bind to receptors** on other platelet surfaces
- **Adherence** of platelets to collagen **through VWF**
- **Conglomeration** of platelets by **bridging** and binding of **fibrinogen** to **GP IIb/IIIa** receptors
- Further activation through **Thromboxane A2** generated from Arachidonic acid

The coagulation factors cascade is initiated by contact activation of receptors on an uneven surface, serially, starting from factor XII, to factor XI, factor IX, factor VIII in that order, the activated factor being designated by fixing -a at the end of the number of corresponding factor. Factor IXa can activate factor VIII, which circulates to von Willebrand factor, an adhesion molecule key in the formation of the platelet plug. Factor VIIIa acts as template for binding site of factor IXa and X. This juxtaposition of factor IXa and X increases the rate of activation of X to Xa. Factor X then migrates over membrane surface of factor Va, which has homology with the factor VIII, bridging together factor Xa and its substrate factor II. Factor Va, Xa, calcium, phosphate lipid complex together, is referred to as, **prothrombin complex**. The complex then cleaves factor II to IIa and factor IIa cleaves fibrinogen to fibrin, when the firm clot is ultimately formed.

Coagulation Cascade may be represented as follows:

- **Contact activation** of factor XII
- **Sequential activation** of XI, IX, VIII
- **Activated factor VIII** circulates to VWF to form the **template for factor IXa, X**
- Formation of **prothrombin complex** with factor Va, Xa, calcium, phosphate, lipid
- The complex **cleaves factor II to IIa**
- **Factor IIa cleaves fibrinogen to fibrin = Clot**

15.3 CLINICAL MANIFESTATIONS OF ABNORMAL HAEMOSTASIS

Haemostatic problems are frequently observed in chronic renal failure patients. This may be manifested as spontaneous bleeding e.g.,

1. Purpura and ecchymoses.
2. Epistaxis
3. Menorrhagia-surprisingly uterine bleeding often occurs when kidney function returns after haemodialysis.
4. Gastrointestinal bleeding e.g., blood vomiting or bloody diarrhoea-usually terminal event.
5. Haemopericardium and subdural haematoma are usually rare.
6. Intraocular haemorrhage.

Bleeding may also occur in the following forms.

1. Bleeding from kidney biopsy site in the form of haematuria.
2. Prolonged bleeding after dental surgery, which should be done more safely on the day following dialysis.
3. Bleeding complication of regional anaesthesia.
4. Bleeding from vascular access site in patients on haemodialysis.

It is a fortunate event that the anticoagulant effect of heparin, used during dialysis, does not cause residual bleeding abnormalities because the effects last only 3–4 hours post-infusion.

Standard Laboratory tests to establish the diagnosis of coagulopathy are usually normal in cases of uraemia. e.g.:

1. Clotting time is normal.
2. Prothrombin time is normal.
3. Partial thromboplastin time and INR are normal.
4. Platelet count is usually within normal limit.

Abnormal Laboratory tests revealing abnormality of haemostasis in uraemia:

1. The skin bleeding time is the best indicator of uraemic bleeding. [1]
2. Platelet activity is however abnormal. There is decreased adhesiveness and aggregation of the platelets. [2]

15.4 PATHOGENESIS OF URAEMIC HAEMOSTATIC PROBLEM

From the laboratory tests, it is evident that the main defects involve ***platelet-vessel wall and platelet-platelet interaction.*** The skin bleeding time depends on platelet number and function, vascular integrity, and haematocrit and thus gives an excellent assessment of primary haemostasis.

Different experimental evidences show different structural abnormality in platelets in uraemia:

1. Dense granule content of platelet is reduced.
2. A storage pool defect of platelet develops with reduction of platelet adenosine diphosphates (ADP) and serotonin. Decreased subnormal platelet adenosine triphosphate release in response to stimuli indicates a defect in granule secretion. [3]
3. Calcium content of platelets is increased.

Several platelet functional abnormality are found in uraemia, these are:

1. Subnormal ATP release in response to stimuli. [3]
2. Abnormal calcium mobilization in response to stimuli. [4]
3. Defective platelet Thromboxane A2 production in response to exogenous and endogenous stimuli. [5]
4. Deficiency of platelet activating factor exists in plasma that promotes irreversible platelet aggregation. [6]

Elevation of cyclic adenosine monophosphate (c AMP) in platelet and abnormal calcium mobilization point to the fact that raised Parathyroid Hormone (PTH) may be responsible for platelet dysfunction in uraemia. However, the bleeding time does not correlate with the serum concentration of intact PTH or PTH fragments, suggesting that elevated PTH is not solely responsible for defect in the platelet in chronic kidney disease. [7]

15.5 ABNORMALITIES OF VESSEL-PLATELET INTERACTION

1. There is inadequate vascular endothelial release of von Willebrand factor/factor VIII complex, which binds to and activates platelets. [8]
2. Increased platelet release of beta thromboglobulin and vascular production of PGI_2 also contribute to this defect.

15.6 ABNORMALITIES IN PLATELET-PLATELET INTERACTION

1. Defective platelet aggregation and defective thromboxane A2 production in response to various exogenous and endogenous stimuli have been demonstrated in vitro. The latter is not correctable by fibrin.
2. In some uraemic patients, irreversible platelet aggregation does not occur in response to platelet activating factor (PAF). This abnormality is probably independent of a plasma factor and is possibly due to platelets' reduced capacity to produce thromboxane A2 in response to PAF.

15.7 BASIC AETIOLOGY OF PLATELET DYSFUNCTION

Evidences

1. The plasma obtained from patients of chronic renal failure has been shown to be a potent inducer of vascular endothelial nitric oxide (NO) production. Plasma concentration of NO metabolites, nitrites and nitrates, is found to be higher than normal in uraemic rats. [9]
2. Excess formation of NO at systemic levels is derived from vessels, as shown by increased NO synthetase activity and by higher expression of both inducible NO (iNO) and endothelial NO (eNO) in the aorta of uraemic animals. Besides its vasoactive properties, NOs inhibit platelet aggregation in vitro and platelet adhesion of cultured endothelial cells. The in vivo counterpart of this activity is the prolongation of skin bleeding time observed in healthy volunteers given NO by inhalation. [10]
3. The possibility that high systemic NO may play a role in the abnormal primary haemostasis in uraemia is supported by the observation that N-monomethyl-L-arginine, a competitive inhibitor of NO synthesis, normalized the prolonged bleeding time in uraemic rats. The shortening effect of conjugated oestrogen on bleeding time, in uraemia, is abolished by L-arginine administration, and is also found to be associated with complete normalization of NO metabolites in the plasma, and vascular expression of NOs isoenzyme. [11]
4. Cultured human micro-vascular cells show potently induced NO synthesis when exposed to uraemic plasma.
5. Plasma from chronic renal failure patients on haemodialysis, unlike normal plasma, potently induced NO synthesis in human umbilical vein endothelial cells. [12]

Thus, all the available evidences suggest that substances which accumulate in plasma of uraemic patients, are capable of up regulating vascular NO synthesis. The stimulatory activity is attributed to cytokines such as TNF alpha and IL-1 beta which are potent inducers of the inducible isoform of NOs and circulate in increased amounts in the plasma of patients of chronic renal failure who either do not receive dialysis or are on maintenance haemodialysis. [13]

15.8 PLATELET DYSFUNCTION AT RECEPTOR LEVEL

Two adhesive proteins, fibrinogen and von Willebrand Factor (vWF), and two adhesion receptors, glycoprotein (gp) Ib and the gpIIb-IIIa complex, play a vital role in the ***formation*** of platelet thrombi at the sites of injury. Binding of gpIb to vWF is normal in uraemia as is the surface expression of receptors. In patients with chronic renal failure, **a decrease in total content of platelet gpIb** has been documented, accompanied by an increase in soluble glycocalcin (a soluble proteolytic fragment of gpIb) and this is probably due to proteolytic damage to membrane gpIb. The normal surface expression of this receptor on the surface of the platelets coupled with total decrease in its content point out **a redistribution of the molecules from the intraplatelet pool to the surface pool. The activation-dependent receptor function of gp IIb- IIIa complex is defective** in uraemia, as shown by decreased binding of both vWF and fibrinogen to stimulated platelets. [14] The number of gpIIb-IIIa complex expressed on platelet surface is normal. Removal of **substances accumulated in uraemic plasma** markedly improves the defect. However, no correlation has been found between bleeding time or platelet adhesion and the serum level of metabolic toxin. Activation dependent receptor function may be also defective due to **receptor occupancy by fibrinogen fragments** present in uraemic plasma. The impaired gpIIb-IIa activation in uraemia may explain aggregation defects as well as reduced vWF-dependent adhesion and thrombus formation. [15]

15.9 POSSIBLE CAUSES OF PLATELET DEFECT AT MACROMOLECULAR LEVEL

(1) "Metabolic" Toxins

Several dialyzable "toxins" (e.g., urea, creatinine, phenol, phenolic acids or guanidosuccinic acid) may possibly be involved in the genesis of uraemic platelet dysfunction. Guanidosuccinic acid which accumulates in uraemic plasma, inhibits the second wave of platelet aggregation to ADP, when added to normal platelet rich plasma.[16] The phenolic acid, concentration found in the uraemic plasma, also impairs primary aggregation to ADP. [17]

(2) von Willebrand Factor

Quantitative and functional abnormalities of the vWF molecules which promote platelet adhesion and aggregation to sub-endothelial collagen, have been reported in uraemia. They may alter platelet-vessel wall interaction and contribute to the haemorrhagic tendency of uraemia. A cryoprecipitate, a plasma derivative rich in factor VIII and vWF, and Desmopressin, a synthetic derivative of antidiuretic hormone, which releases autologous vWF from storage sites, significantly shorten the bleeding time of uraemic patients. This suggests that a functional defect in the vWF-platelet interaction may indeed play a role in the abnormal haemostasis of uraemic patients. Some authors reported elevated vWF antigen levels and others reported elevated vWF antigen levels but reduced ristocetin cofactor activity in uraemic plasma. [18]

(3) Erythrocytes

Platelet adhesion has been found to be potentiated by Erythrocytes. Erythrocytes enhance platelet function by releasing ADP, by inactivating prostacyclin, and by increasing platelet-vessel wall contact by displaying platelets from axial flow toward the vessel wall. A significant negative correlation was found between bleeding time and packed cell volume (PCV) in uraemic patients on haemodialysis. A significant shorter bleeding time was demonstrable in uraemic bleeding when haemostatic improvement was achieved by treatment with recombinant Erythropoietin in uraemic anaemic patients. Thus, partial correction of anaemia was sufficient to correct defective primary haemostasis in uraemia. [19]

15.10 DREADED CONSEQUENCES OF HAEMOSTATIC DEFECT IN URAEMIA

(1) **Gastrointestinal Bleeding:** Upper gastrointestinal bleeding is the second leading cause of death in renal failure. The most common pathologies are peptic ulcers, haemorrhagic oesophagitis, gastritis, duodenitis and gastric telegiectasia. Angiodysplasia with gastrointestinal bleeding has been observed in stomach, duodenum, jejunum, colon. This abnormality affecting the microcirculation, occurs most often in haemodialysis patients. Finally, dialysis patients suffering from Human Immuno-deficiency Virus nephropathy may have specific lesions, such as Kaposi's sarcoma, cytomegalovirus colitis, and non-Hodgkin lymphoma that contribute to gastrointestinal bleeding. G.I. bleeding produces higher mortality among dialysis patients than in general population. [20]

(2) **Haemorrhagic Pericarditis and Cardiac Tamponade**, though rare, can occur in uraemia. The clinical features of this condition include normal cardiac shadow, increased jugular venous distension with hypotension, shortness of breath, and a pericardial friction rub. Deaths due to haemorrhagic pericarditis has been reported as high as 3% to 5% among dialysis patients. [21]

(3) **Subdural Haematoma** has been reported in 5% to 15% of patients on haemodialysis. It usually occurs in frontal or parietal lobe and is bilateral in 15% of cases. Headache, vomiting, drowsiness, confusion, coma, are the usual symptoms. Head trauma, hypertension and systemic anticoagulation are risk factors. The prognosis is at least, partly related to the stage of diagnosis and mortality rate may be as high as 90% in patients requiring emergency surgery. [22]

(4) **Haemorrhage into the Pleural Cavity** may occur as a rare complication in patients having fibrinous pleurisy, when put on anticoagulation therapy. [23]

(5) **Spontaneous Retroperitoneal Bleeding** is a rare complication inpatients receiving haemodialysis. Trauma, anticoagulation, and the presence of polycystic kidneys are predisposing factors. The symptoms and signs include sudden onset of pain in the abdomen, flank, back and hip, with an associated drop of blood pressure. The haematocrit drops in absence of any obvious blood loss. Computed tomography is useful in the diagnosis of retroperitoneal bleeding. [24]

(6) **Spontaneous Subcapsular Haematoma in Liver** is a newly recognised complication of uraemia. Typically patients have right upper quadrant abdominal pain, fever, sometimes elevated serum bilirubin level and alkaline phosphatase levels accompanied by a falling haematocrit. [25]

(7) **Intraocular Haemorrhage** can also occur in uraemia, and spontaneous hyphaema has been reported during dialysis. There is no visual loss and the haemorrhage generally resolves during therapy. Intraocular bleeding with temporary visual loss has also been reported in large percentage of dialysis and transplant patients. [26]

15.11 USE OF ASPIRIN IN CHRONIC KIDNEY DISEASE

In patients of chronic renal failure, when on maintenance haemodialysis, aspirin is usually given to prevent vascular access thrombosis or platelet activation on dialyzer membrane. Aspirin is also given to prevent thrombotic complications in uraemic patients treated with rh EPO, when the haematocrit value is rising. The beneficial effect of aspirin can be achieved with a moderate dose (160 mg/day), which inhibits platelet thromboxane A_2 generation without affecting vascular prostacyclin formation. However, even a moderate dose of aspirin prolongs the bleeding time. [27]

15.12 ABNORMALITIES OF COAGULATION FACTORS IN URAEMIA

As stated earlier, activated partial thromboplastin time, prothrombin time, and thrombin time are generally normal in uraemia. ***Fibrinogen and factor VIII:C*** are usually ***increased.*** Changes in major inhibitors of coagulation have been found. Previous reports demonstrated increased levels of this natural anticoagulant. ***Reduced levels of Antithrombin II*** have been found in uraemic patients. This evidence, together with the observed ***decrease in Protein C anticoagulant activity with normal Protein C amidolytic activity*** and antigen and ***decreased Protein S*** may further contribute to thrombotic tendency. ***Thrombin is continuously formed,*** *as evidenced by increased levels of thrombin-antithrombin III, D dimer, and fibrinopeptide A. These suggest that a* ***hypercoagulable state*** *exists in uraemia.* [28]

Contrasting results regarding ***fibrinolytic system*** have been obtained. Previous reports demonstrated decreased fibrinolytic activity either absolute or relative (to the extent of activation of platelets) exists in uraemia. ***Activation of fibrinolytic system*** has been found in uraemia with an increase of plasmin-plasminogen complexes, fibrinogen and fibrin degradation product as well as a decrease in the activity of plasminogen activator inhibitor. These findings suggest a fibrinolytic response secondary to fibrin deposition. These abnormalitics arc partially corrected by dialysis. [29]

15.13 CONSEQUENCES OF ABNORMALITIES IN COAGULATION FACTORS

The abnormalities of coagulation or fibrinolysis predispose more to thrombosis rather than bleeding. One interesting finding is that levels of protein C and its cofactor protein S are significantly decreased in association with Erythopoietin therapy, a finding that may contribute to increased risk of **thrombosis of vascular access** in patients receiving chronic haemodialysis as well as Erythropoietin therapy.

Atherosclerotic cardiovascular disease is more prone to occur in patients on haemodialysis as lipoprotein (a) is found to be markedly elevated in such patients.

Disseminated intravascular coagulaton (DIC)

This condition usually results from sepsis, which is very much common in immunocompromised state of uraemia. There is increased production of proinflammatory cytokines suggesting activation of monocytes play a role in uraemic immune dysfunction. Various factors may activate coagulation system in sepsis, but the end result is formation of fibrin, a mesh like protein, the fibrin deposition may block microcapillaries, leading to ischaemic damage to vital tissues Red blood cells are damaged and shredded by fibrin leading to microangiopathic haemolytic anaemia. Platelets are consumed in the formation of clots leading to thrombocytopenia. And the whole process culminates in haemorrhage.

Fibrinolytic agents e.g., streptokinase, or urokinase, produce contrasting results in such condition. A new development in treatment of DIC is, Drotrecogin alfa (Xiris @), a recombinant activated protein C product. It deactivates clotting factors V and VIII. Due to high cost, it is used only in ICCU. [30]

15.14 EFFECT OF HAEMODIALYSIS (HD) AND PERITONEAL DIALYSIS (PD) ON HAEMOSTATIC PROBLEM

HD is accompanied by a transient form of platelet activation related to interaction of platelets with artificial membranes and vascular access itself. Dialysis patients have an accelerated platelet turnover. Repeated platelet activation on dialysis membrane may induce refractionariness to further platelet stimulation, contributing to clinical bleeding that can occur at the termination of dialysis process. Thrombosis of the arteriovenous shunt is a frequent complication in uraemic patients undergoing haemodialysis. [30]

PD has been reported to cause platelet hyperactivity which in some cases may be related to hypoalbuminaemia. [31]

Il-1 and TNF alpha, the two inducers of NO, are generated by circulating monocytes, during dialysis. Production of cytokines is enhanced by bacterial endotoxin intact or fragments, that cross dialysis membrane, and also by acetate containing dialysis fluid. Thus, the capacity of the dialysis procedure to remove uraemic toxin is negated by its effects on platelet activation and NO synthesis. [32]

Plasma levels of lipoprotein (a), an independent risk factor for atherosclerotic cardiovascular disease, are markedly increased in uraemic patients either on haemodialysis or peritoneal dialysis. [33]

15.15 THERAPEUTIC MODALITIES IN URAEMIC COAGULOPATHY

Frequent low dose heparin rather than constant infusion along with protamine or low molecular weight heparin has been proposed as therapy for thrombosis of vascular access. Dermatan sulfate has been also proposed as an alternative to heparin as it causes less bleeding in animal models. This may be due to its reduced effect on platelets. Effective doses range from 6–10 mg/kg body weight per dialysis session. Dermatan sulphate can be given as a pre-dialysis bolus dose when the dialysis is of short duration (4 hours), and combination of bolus dose plus infusion, when dialysis lasts for a longer period. [34]

Aspirin and dipyridamole analogue reduce deposition of fibrin and cellular deposit on filter membrane, but increase the risk of gastrointestinal bleeding.

Prostacyclin, given in a continuous infusion, of 5 ng/kg/min, completely inhibits platelet aggregation without causing bleeding. However, it causes headache, flushing, tachycardia, chest and abdominal pain, which require careful monitoring by a physician. The use of prostacyclin should be thus restricted to patients with high risk of haemorrhage. [35]

Fibrinolytic agents such as urokinase or streptokinase have produced contrasting results. [36(a) and (b)]. Usually heparin is given by constant infusion through the inlet line of the dialyzer. Simultaneously protamine sulphate is infused into outlet part before the blood returns to the patient. Even this schedule may be associated with high incidence of bleeding. Usually 40–50 IU/kg of heparin is given at the beginning of haemodialysis, followed by 60% of the initial dose after 1 hour and 2 hours and 30% of initial dose after 3 hours. The activated partial thromboplastin time (APTT) is measured hourly and should be maintained at 1.5 to 2.0 times the basal value. [37]

Patients with high risk of bleeding may use an ethylene vinyl alcohol copolymer **hollow-fibre dialysis membrane** that does not require systemic anticoagulation, provided that blood flow is maintained at more than 200 ml/minute. [38]

The progressive increase in haematocrit associated with **rhEPO therapy** is seen to be decreased with shortening of bleeding time. No consistent changes are found in platelet number, platelet aggregation, platelet TXA2 formation. Several studies reported a significant increase in vWF and ristocetin cofactor activity. In a study, EPO was given in a dose of 50 IU/kg thrice a week; every 4 weeks the dose is increased by 25 IU/kg until bleeding time became normal. An EPO dosage of 150–300 IU/kg/week increased PCV to a range of 27% to 32% and normalized bleeding times in all patients. A significant negative correlation was found between PCV and bleeding time. Thus rh EPO therapy may significantly prevent and control the bleeding in uraemia. [39]

Low molecular weight heparin has been proposed as an alternative to unfractionated heparin in patients receiving chronic haemodialysis who are at high risk of bleeding. [40]

Cryoprecipitate, a plasma derivative rich in vWF, fibrinogen, fibronectin, that has been traditionally used in haemophilia, von Willebrand disease, hypofibrinogenaemia, dysfibrinogenaemia is found to correct prolonged bleeding time in uraemic patients within 4–12 hours, and the effect lasts for 24 to 36 hours. The mechanism of action of cryoprecipitate is not known. A small rise of platelet level of fibrinogen and vWF related proteins were the only changes noted after cryoprecipitate infusion. Different preparations of cryoprecipitates, however, have different effects on bleeding time. The poor reproducibility of results and risk of disease transmission prompted the search for alternatives to cryoprecipitate. [41]

Desmopressin (i-deamino-8-D-arginine-vasopressin)-a synthetic derivative of antidiuretic hormone-induces release of autologous vWF from storage sites. In a randomized, double blind, cross-over trial, desmopressin given intravenously at a dose of 0.3 mg/kg body weight in 50 ml of physiologic saline over a period of 30 minutes temporarily corrected prolonged bleeding in chronic renal failure. [42] Shortening of bleeding time was significant one hour after the end of infusion, and the effect lasts for 6 to 8 hours. Desmopressin looses its efficacy after repeated administration. Desmopressin also can be given by the intranasal route which is well tolerated and safe. At 10 to 20 times the intravenous dose (3 mg/kg), intranasal desmopressin shortens the bleeding time and decreases clinical bleeding. Desmopressin has also been given subcutaneously, with the dose same as that used for intravenous administration. Peak responses are achieved after 30 to 90 minute of delay.

Adverse effects include facial flushing, headache, nausea, abdominal cramp, and mild tachycardia. Protein C anticoagulant decreases after desmopressin infusion.

However, desmopressin is found to be useful in the treatment of bleeding and in the prevention of bleeding during surgery or invasive procedure.

The observation that there is diminished gastrointestinal bleeding with conjugated oestrogen in uraemia and the improved haemostasis in von Willebrand disease in pregnancy led to the therapeutic trial of conjugated oestrogen in uraemic bleeding. One oral dose of 25 mg normalizes bleeding time for 3 to 10 days with no apparent ill effect. A controlled study shows that conjugated oestrogen given intravenously at a cumulative dose of 3 mg/kg divided over 5 consecutive days has got long lasting effect. [43] At least 0.6 mg/kg is needed to reduce the bleeding time and four to five infusions, spaced 24 hours apart, is needed to reduce bleeding time by 50%. The effect of oestrogen on bleeding time in an animal model of chronic uraemia is completely reversed by the NO precursor L-arginine, suggesting that the effect of oestrogen might be mediated by changes in NO synthesis. Thus, oestrogen may be a useful alternative to cryoprecipitate or desmopressin in the treatment of uraemic bleeding especially when long lasting effect is required.

15.16 THERAPEUTIC GUIDELINES IN URAEMIC COAGULOPATHY

(1) For all patients with haemorrhagic complications or undergoing major surgery, the adequacy of dialysis should be checked. It is also advisable to change the dialysis schedule for 1 or 2 months in patients who have experienced severe bleeding or who have undergone recent cardiovascular surgery so that heparin can be avoided.

(2) Acute bleeding episode may be treated with Desmopressin at a dose of 0.3 microgram/kg IV (added to 50 ml of saline over 30 minutes) or subcutaneously. Intranasal administration of this drug at a dose of 3 micro gm/kg is also effective and is well tolerated. The effect of desmopressin lasts only a few hours, a major limitation to its use in treating severe haemorrhage. This is also so due to loss of its efficacy with its repeated use.

(3) The ideal treatment of persistent chronic bleeding should have a long-lasting effect. Conjugated estrogen treatment given by IV infusion in a cumulative dose of 3 mg/kg as daily divided doses (e.g., 0.6 mg/kg for 5 consecutive days) is the most appropriate way of achieving long-lasting haemostatic competence.

(4) Severely anaemic patients should receive blood or RBC transfusion to improve haematocrit values. RBC transfusions are effective only when the haematocrit rises above 30%. As an alternative, bleeding in renal failure and haematocrit less than 30% can be treated successfully with erythropoietin.

(5) Cryoprecipitate has got very limited use in chronic renal failure patients due to high risk of disease transmission.

15.17 CONCLUSION

With improved knowledge about coagulopathy and with the invention of newer and newer modalities of treatment coagulopathy in chronic kidney disease is now more amenable to treatment. However, it is very difficult to maintain a balance between tendency to bleed and the propensity to form thrombus and each case should be judged on its own merit.

REFERENCES

1. Steiner RW, Coggins C, Carvahilo ACA(1979): *Bleeding time in uraemia: A useful test to assess clinical bleeding*. Am J Haematol 7:107–117.
2. Ekonoyan G, Wacksman SJ, Glueck HI, et al. (1969): *Platelet function in renal failure*. N Engl J Med 280:677–681.
3. Di Minno G, Martinez A, Mackien M, et al. (1985): *Platelet dysfunction in uraemia: Multifaceted defectpartially corrected by dialysis*. Am J Med 1:17–23.
4. Gura V, Crater D, Levi J (1992): *Elevated thrombocyte calcium content in uraemia and its correction by alpha (OH) vitamin D treatment*. Nephron: 237–239.

5. Remuzzi G, Bengini A, Dodesini P et al. (1983). *Reduced platelet thromboxane formation in uraemia: Evidence for a functional cyclooxygenase defect.* J clin Invest 71: 762–768.

6. Macconi D, Vigano G, Bisogno G, et al. (1992): *Defective platelet aggregation in response to platelet-activating factor in uraemia associated withlow platelet thromboxane A2 generation.* Am J kidney Dis. 19: 318–325.

7. Remuzzi G, Benigini A, Dodesini P, et al. (1981): *Parathyroid hormone inhibits human platelet function.* Lancet 2: 1321–1323.

8. Remuzzi G, Livio M, Roncaglioni MC, et al. (1977): *Bleeding in renal failure: Is von Willebrand Factor implicated?* BMJ 2: 359–361.

9. Aeillo S, Noris M, Todeschini M et al. (1997): *Renal and systemic nitric oxide synthesis in rats with renal mass reduction.* Kidney Int 52: 171–181.

10. Marletta MA (1989): *Biosynthesis and biological significance trends.* Biochem Sci 14: 488–492.

11. Zoja C, Noris M, Corna D et al. (1991): *L-arginine, the precursor of nitric oxide, abolishes the effect of oestrogens on bleeding time in uraemia.* Lab Invest 65: 479–483.

12. Noris M, Benigini A, Boccardo P et al. (1993): *Enhanced nitric acid synthesis in uraemia: Implication for platelet dysfunction and dialysis hypotension.* Kidney Int 44: 445–450.

13. Herbelin A, Nguyen AT, Zingraff J J et al. (1990): *Influence of uraemia and haemodialysis on circulating Interleukin-1 and tumour necrosis factor alpha.* Kidney Int 37: 116–37:116–125.

14. Bengini A, Boccardo P, Galbusera M, et al. (1993): *Reversible activation defect of the platelet glycoprotein IIb-IIIa complexin patients with uraemia.* AM J Kidney Dis. 22: 668–676.

15. Gawaz M P, Dobos G, Spath M et al.(1994): *Impaired function of platelet membrane glycoprotein IIb-IIIa in end stage renal disease.* J Am Soc Nephrol 5: 36–46.

16. Horowitz HI, Stein IM, Cohen BD et al. ((1970): *Further studies on platelet inhibitory effect of guanidosuccinic acid and its role in uraemic bleeding.* Am J Med 49: 336–345.

17. Robiner SF, Molinas F (1970): *The role of phenol and phenolic acids on thrombocytopathy and defective platelet aggregation of patients with renal failure.* Am J Med 346–351.

18. Escolar G, Cases A, Bastida et al. (1990): *Uraemic platelets have a functional defect affecting the interaction of von Willebrand Factor with glycoprotein IIb-IIIa.* Blood 76: 1336–1340.

19. Gordge MP, Leaker B, Patel A et al. (1990): *Recombinant human erythopoietin shortens the uraemic bleeding without causing intravascular haemostatic activation.* Thromb Res 57: 171–182.

20. Zuckerman GR, Cornette GL, Clouse RE, et al. (1985): *Upper gastrointestinal bleeding in patients with chronic renal failure.* Ann Intern Med 102: 588–592.

21. Kumar S, Lesch M ((1980): *Pericarditis in renal disease.* Prog Cardiovasc dis 22: 357–369.

22. Bechr M, Lakke JP, van derHem GK, et al. (1972): *Subdural Haematoma diring long term Haemodialysis.* Arch Neurol 26: 513–516.

23. Galen MA, Steinberg SM, Lowrie FG, et al. (1975): *Haemorrhagic pleural effusion in patients undergoing chronic dialysis.* Ann Intern Med 82: 359–361.

24. Vasin HK, Dana CL, (1978): *Spontaneous retroperitoneal haemorrhage in patients on chronic haemodialysis.* Nephron 32: 322–327.

25. Borra S, Kleinfeld M (1980): *Subcapsular liver haematoma in patients on haemodialysis.* Ann Intern Med 93: 574–575.

26. Slusher MN, Hamilton RW, (1975): *Spontaneous hyphema during haemodialysis.* N Engl J Med 293: 561.

27. Livio M, Benigini A, Vigano G et al. (1983): *Moderate dose of aspirin and risk of bleeding in renal failure.* Lancet 1: 414–416.

28. Pancucci F, Sagripanti A, Pinori E et al. (1983): *Comprehensive study of haemostasis in chronic uraemia.* Nephron 33: 5–8.

29. Nakamura Y, Tomura S, Tachibana K et al. (1992): *Enhanced fibrinolytic activity during the course of haemodialysis.* Clin Nephrol 38:90–96.

30. Homma T, Ichikawa T. (1979): *Studies on fibrinolytic activity of uraemic and long term haemodialysis patients with special reference to fibrinolysis inhibitor.* Biocheem Exp Biol15:229–236.

31. Sloand EM, Bern MM, Kaidany A (1986): *Effect on platelet function of hypoalbuminaemia in peritoneal dialysis.* Thromb Res 44: 415–419.

32. Lande-Sharp M, Caroff M, Simard L et al. (1990): *Induction of IL-1 during haemodialysis: Transmembrane passage of intact endotoxin (LPS)> Kidney* Int 38:1089–1094.

33. Cressman MD, Heyka RJ, Paganini EP et al. (1992): *Lipoprotein (a) is an independent risk factor for cardiovascular disease in haemodialysis patients.* Circulation 86: 475–482.

34. Boccardo P, Melacini D, Rota S et al. (1997): *Individualized anticoagulation with dermatan sulphate for haemodialysis in chronic renal failure.* Nephrol Dial Transplant 12: 2349–2354.

35. Zusman RM, Rubin RH, CatoAE et al. (1981): *Haemodialysis using prostacyclin instead of heparin as the sole antithrombotic agent.* N Engl J Med 304: 934–939.

36. (a) Rodkin RS, Bookstein JJ, Heeney DJ et al. (1983): *Streptokinase and transluminal angioplasty in the treatment of acutely thrombosed haemodialysis access fistula.* Radiology149: 425–428.

    (b) Mangiarotti G, Canavase C, Thea et al. (1984): *Urokinase treatment for arteriovenous fistulae declotting in dialyzed patients.* Nephron 36: 60–64.

37. Lindholm DD, Murray SA (1964): *A simplified method of regional heparinization during haemodialysis according to a predetermined dosage formula.* Trans Am Soc Artif Intern Organs12: 207–209.

38. Matsuda T, Takemoto Y, Kishimoto T et al. (1990): *Mechanistic aspect of cellular interaction with artificial dialyzer membrane surfaces.* Biomatter Artif Cells Artf Organs 18: 574–584.

39. Taylor JE, Belch JJF, Mc Laren M et al. (1993): *Effect of Erythopoietin therapy and withdrawal on blood coagulation and fibrinolysis in haemodialysis patients.* Kidney Int 44: 182–190.

40. Ljungberg B.(1985): *A low molecular heparin fraction as an anticoagulant during haemodialysis.* Clin Nephrol 25:15–20.

41. Triulzi DJ, Blumberg N. (1990): *Variability in response to cryoprecipitate treatment for haemostatic defects in uraemia.* Yale J Biol Med 63:1–7.

42. Akpolat T, Ozdemir O, Anik N, et al. (1993): *Effect of Desmopressin (DDAVP) on protein C and protein C inhibitors in uraemia.* Nephron 64:232–234.

43. Vigano G, Gaspari F, Locatelli M, et al. (1988): *Dose-effect and pharmacokinetics of oestrogens given to correct bleeding time in uraemia.* Kidney Int 34: 853–858.

Part V

Platelet Disorder

CHAPTER

16

Thrombocytopenia

16.1 DEFINITION

Thrombocytopenia is defined as the clinical condition in which platelet count in the peripheral blood is reduced to below 150×10^9/l. The condition may result from (1) peripheral destruction by immune or non-immune mechanism (2) decreased production due to inherited or acquired marrow disease (3) splenic poling or in vitro pooling of platelets due to massive splenomealy and cosequent hyperfunction or disseminated intravascular coagulation (5) in asymptomatic patients this may occur after blood collection.

Thrombocytopenia may occur in the neonates in the following ways (*a*) neonatal alloimmunization (*b*) passive transfer of antibodies from mother suffering from idiopathic thrombocytopenic purpura (*c*) acute viral infection (*d*) inherited thrombocytopenia.

Congenital or inherited thrombocytopenia [1] may have recognizable changes in platelet morphology, such as giant or small platelets, abnormal platelet granules, or associated leukocyte or erythrocyte changes.

16.2 PATHOPHYSIOLOGY

The basis of thrombocytopenia is the loss of balance between platelet production and destruction. Platelet turnover is a measure of net effect of platelet production and platelet destruction under steady state conditions. Although high platelet turn-over is expected in patients with idiopathic thrombocytopenic purpura (ITP), platelet production measured by using ^{iii}I oxime, is not increased. [2] Low production may result from binding of antibodies to megakaryocytes that inhibit their development or lead to their destruction. The normal rate of platelet production varies from 160×10^9 to 280×10^9 per day. [3]

In late 1980s two specific assays of target antigens were described: (*a*) immune-absorbent assay (*b*) monoclonal antibody specific immobilization of platelet antigen assay. These assays showed that majority of anti-platelet antibodies in patients with idiopathic thrombocytopenic purpura (ITP) are directed against GpIIb-IIIa (approximately 80%) and the remainder against GpIb-Ixa complex and the other platelet glycoproteins such as GpIV and GpIa-IIa. [4]

Antibody coated platelets and antigen-presenting cells through FcY receptors are pooled primarily in the spleen and also in other organs of mononuclear-phagocytic system. [5] The mechanism involves presentation of platelet antigens by activated antigen-presenting cells, which thereby activate both CD_4+ cell clones and antigen-specific T cell clones. These T cell clones induce different B cell clones to produce antibodies against distinct platelet antigens. At least some ITP patients had clonal B cell proliferation, as determined by DNA analysis for immunoglobulin heavy and light chain rearrangements and by flow-cytometry of B cells.

Though ITP is antibody-mediated, autoantibodies are under control of T helper cells and their cytokines. [6] Complement activation also plays a role in some patients with ITP.

The large size and increased function of platelets in ITP is attributed to thrombopoietin (TPO), the major regulator of megakaryopoiesis and thrombocytopoiesis. TPO level is markedly elevated in patients with megakaryocytic hypoplasia such as aplasic anaemia or acute leukaemia. In most reports patients, suffering from ITP, have normal or slightly elevated levels of TPO in serum or plasma, but level is lower than in thrombocytopenia resulting from megakaryocytic hypoplasia. Most authorities believe that this finding results from active TPO uptake and destruction by expanded megakaryocytic mass in ITP.

16.3 GENETIC BASIS OF THE DISEASE

Idiopathic thrombocytopenic purpura has been documented in monozygotic twins and in some families. As in other autoimmune disorders, heredity may contribute to development of ITP and may affect response to therapy. Genetic polymorphism of loci for CTLA-4, tumor necrosis factor, and Fc receptor have been suggested to influence the development of ITP and its response to therapy.

16.4 CLINICAL PRESENTATION

Clinical presentation of ITP is entirely different in adults and in children. Chronic ITP is traditionally described in adults as ITP with platelet count less than 150×10^9 /*l* for more than 6 months. A significant number of patients are diagnosed incidentally in routine complete blood counts. Approximately one-third of patients have platelet counts greater than 30×10^9 /*l*, although bleeding symptoms are generally seen on patients with counts below this level. Purpura, epistaxis, menorrhagia gingivial bleeding, ecchymoses, petechiae are common. Haematuria, haemoptysis, G.I. bleeding are less common. Intracerebral haemorrhage is rare and generally occurs in counts less than 10×10^9 /*l* and usually associated with trauma or vascular lesions. The incidence of life threatening complications is highest in patients older than 60 years of age, however, mortality rates are low in patients with ITP, even in those with severe thrombocytopenia.

Purpuric lesions seen in ITP are not palpable, do not blanch with pressure, and often develop on distal regions of extremities and on skin exposed to pressure e.g., around high belts and stockings, anterior to tourniquet sites, Haemorrhagic bullae usually develop on buccal mucosa and generally reflect acute, severe thrombocytopenia. Bleeding after trauma, surgery and tooth extraction are common.

Family history is especially important to discriminate familial thrombocytopenia. Spleen is usually not enlarged, but may be palpable in some. Constitutional symptoms e.g., fever, weight loss, marked splenomegaly, hepatomegaly, lymphadenopathy provide evidence against the possibility of thrombocytopenia resulting from ITP.

TABLE 16.1: Distinguishing features of ITP in children and in adults

Occurrences	Children	Adults
Peak age (years)	2–4 yrs	15–40 yrs
Sex (F : M)	1 : 1	1.2 : 1.7
Onset	Acute (< 1 wk)	Gradual (> 2 m)
Symptoms	Purpura (10% severe)	Purpura (less)
Platelet count	< 20,000/micro L	> 20,000/micro L
Spontaneous Remission	83%	2%
Chronic State	24%	43%
Splenectomy	11%	66%
Complete Remission	64%	89%
Cerebral Haemorrhage	< 1%	> 3%
Haemorrhagic Death	< 1%	> 4%
Chronic refractory state	2%	5%

16.5 LABORATORY INVESTIGATIONS

1. Platelet count and consequent changes in peripheral blood. Platelet count less than 150×10^9/L is the characteristic feature. Platelet anisocytosis is an associated common finding. Mean platelet volume and platelet distribution width are increased. Platelets may be abnormally large or small. The former is associated with accelerated platelet destruction. The latter accompanied by platelet microparticles reflect platelet destruction. The observation of giant platelets trigger consideration of inherited platelet disorders, which are misdiagnosed as ITP.
2. Bleeding time correlates well inversely with platelet count if the count is less than 100×10^9L, but may be normal in patients with mild to moderate thrombocytopenia.
3. The ultrastructure of ITP platelets viewed by electron microscope is similar to normal platelets.
4. Total and differential count of leukocytes are usually normal. Although atypical lymphocytes and eosinophilia may occur in children with ITP, leukocytosis or leukopenia with immature cells are not consistent with the diagnosis of ITP.
5. The presence of anaemia (e.g., resulting from iron deficiency in bleeding patients or association with thalassaemia minor in endemic areas) requires further investigations for evaluation.
6. Acquired Haemolytic Anaemia with a positive Coomb's test and reticulocytosis may accompany with ITP, the association is termed as Evan's syndrome. It includes immune neutropenia. Neither polikilocyte or scistocytes are present in the erythrocyte series.

16.6 MARROW EXAMINATION IS NOT ALWAYS REQUIRED FOR DIAGNOSIS OF ITP

In case of ITP marrow reveals increased number of megakaryocytes, though decreased number does not rule out the possibility. According to ASH guidelines, marrow examination is not mandatory:

1. if the patient is less than 60 years of age
2. if the presentation is typical
3. if there is response to first line of therapy
4. if splenectomy is not considered

16.7 MEASURING PLATELET ANTIBODIES

Various anti-platelet antibody assay methods are in practice but none of these is specific or in widespread clinical use.

(a) Phase I assay- patient's serum is incubated with control platelets and platelet-dependent end points are measured such as aggregation or agglutination, granule release or platelet lysis. These tests are not sensitive or specific for diagnosis of ITP.

(b) Phase II assay- measures IgG type of platelet antibodies that bind to plasma membrane, granules, or canaliculi. This measurement may be abnormal in any other immune thrombocytopenia and also sometimes in healthy people.

(c) Phase III assay- measures platelet glycoprotein specific autoimmune antibodies. Three techniques are used e.g., immunoblotting,immunoprecipitation, and glycoprotein immobilization. Platelet auto-antigens are identified by electrophretic mobility of their bands.

These tests may be useful in distinguishing immune from non-immune thrombocytopenia and monitoring response to treatment. Although they are specific but not sensitive enough to screen ITP.

16.8 DIFFERENTIAL DIAGNOSIS

Diagnosis of ITP is mainly clinical, because no laboratory test can usually diagnose ITP. The ASH guidelines recommend no further investigation in typical cases, bleeding time, platelet survival time, complement. Abdominal ultrasound or computed tomography and PGIgG assays are unnecessary and inappropriate. Additional tests, such as lupus anticoagulant, direct antiglobulin test, reticulocyte count, mean platelet volume, urine analysis, thyroid function tests are indicated when particular clinical condition calls attention to underlying disorder. Anitiplatelet antibodies are seen frequently in patients suffering from ITP. Although some researchers claim that presence of such antibodies have increased the risk of thrombosis, others do not.

16.9 COURSE AND PROGNOSIS

Natural course of ITP is unpredictable, as most patients are stable when treated with glucocorticoids. ITP in adult is essentially a chronic disease with infrequent spontaneous remission in contrast to ITP in children.

An analysis of a big group of adult patients with ITP, mortality rate is found to be 5% predominantly because of intracerebral haemorrhage. With glucocorticoid complete remission is found in 25% of cases. In patients older than 60 years, haemorrhagic complications are more common.

16.10 MODALITIES OF THERAPY

ITP may respond to various agents including glucocorticoids, intravenous immunoglobulin (IVIg), infused Anti-D antibody, Danazol, as well as antineoplastic drugs like Vinicristine, azathioprine, sometimes only to splenectomy.

16.11 NEED OF THERAPY

Because ITP patients are often detected incidentally in routine evaluation, signs and symptoms of bleeding are important in determining whether treatment is necessary or not.

Patients are usually divided into following categories:

1. Patients with *no bleeding* and consistent *platelet counts in excess of* $50 \times 10^9/l$ usually do not require treatment and can be observed clinically.
2. Patients with *platelet counts 30–50* $\times 10^9/l$ usually do not have clinically important bleeding but may have easy bruising. They usually do not require treatment. Careful follow up is necessary. Clinical course is difficult to predict.
3. Patients with *platelet counts between 20 and* $50 \times 10^9/l$ and those with *platelet count below* $20 \times 10^9/l$ or in patients with *significant risk factors* like hypertension, peptic ulcer or vigorous life style careful medical supervision is essential as significant mucosal bleeding may occur or serious life threatening haemorrhage may occur at any moment.

16.12 EMERGENCY TREATMENT

This is required under following situations:

1. Intracranial bleeding 5%
2. Gastrointestinal bleeding
3. Extensive purpura or haemorrhagic bullae
4. Massive haematuria
5. Intestinal haematoma
6. Need of emergent surgical condition.

For emergency treatment patient must be hospitalized with scrupulous care. High dose Methyl prednisolone (1 g/kg/day in divided doses for 2 days) must be administered. [6] Parenteral glucocorticoid in conjunction with intravenous immunoglobulin are recommended to be followed up. Transfused platelets do not elevate platelet count, rather they are destroyed rapidly but may improve formation of platelet plugs and thereby haemostasis.[7] IvIg elevates platelet count in 2 or 3 days and platelet transfusion after IvIg may improve platelet count. Aminocaproic acid which inhibits fibrinolysis, can be used to reduce bleeding and is safe except in cases of haematuria, when it may form thrombi in glomeruli, renal pelvis and ureter. This agent does not affect platelet count or function. Usual dose is 0.01 mg/kg over 30 minutes, then given by continuous IV infusion at 0.5–1mg/hr or an equivalent intermittent dose every 4 hours. Aminocaproic acid may be also administered orally as it is very rapidly absorbed from G.I. tract Vincristine may be used in combination with IvIg treatment.

16.13 DIFFERENT MODALITIES OF TREATMENT: HOW THEY ARE USED?

Glucocorticoids: These are recommended in patients with platelet count less than $20 \times 10^9/l$ or count $20–50 \times 10^9/l$ with significant bleeding. Oral prednisolone in a dose of 1–2 mg/kg/day is usually accepted as initial treatment. Glucocorticoids increase the platelet count through several mechanisms, including (*i*) inhibition of phagocytosis of antibody-coated platelets by macrophages (*ii*) decreases autoantibody production (*iii*) improves marrow platelet production (*iv*) appears to reduce capillary leakage.

Although no consensus exists regarding duration of treatment, treatment should continue till platelet count reaches a safe level. Patients generally respond to initial glucocorticoid therapy within first 3 weeks of treatment. In approximately two-third of patients, platelet counts increase to greater than $50 \times 10^6/l$ within 1 week, but decreases again when the prednisolone dose is tapered. Thus in patients, who respond, the recommendation is to continue glucocorticoid therapy in a dose of 0.1 mg/kg/day for a total of 3 weeks before initiating the taper. The major drawback of glucocorticoid therapy that adverse effect may be worse than the disease itself. Facial swelling, weight gain, folliculitis, hyperglycaemia, hypertension, cataract, osteoporosis, opportunistic infection, and behavioral disturbances are common side effects. A study showed that short course of treatment with high dose glucocorticoids (dexamethasone 40 mg/day, for 4 consecutive days) as initial therapy of ITP Methyl prednisolone or dexamethasone can be used for high dose initial therapy by oral or intravenous route. [8]

Sustained remission with glucocorticoids are infrequent, with reported rates of 5 to 30 p.c. If the patient does not respond to three week therapy with prednisolone, other therapeutic options should be considered.

16.14 SPLENECTOMY

Splenectomy is indicated in adult patients under following conditions:

(*i*) when platelet counts remain less than $10 \times 10^9/l$.

(*ii*) when platelet counts remain less than $30 \times 10^9/l$ and the patients experience excessive bleeding after 4–5 weeks of appropriate medical treatment.

(*iii*) when the patients show transient response to primary treatment and have platelet counts less than $30 \times 10^9/l$ after 3 months of therapy.

(*iv*) when the patients require continuous glucocorticoid therapy to maintain safe platelet count.

At least 2 weeks before splenectomy, patients should be immunized with polyvalent pneumococcal vaccine, haemophilus influenzae Type I vaccine, qudrivalent meningococcal vaccine, because they are susceptible to overwhelming bacterial infections.

Patients with platelet counts less than $50 \times 10^9/l$ and especially those with platelet counts less than $30 \times 10^9/l$ may require glucocorticoid and/or IvIg therapy before the procedure to reach the platelet counts that minimize the risk of surgical bleeding. Platelet transfusion may be required during the perioperative period in severely thrombocytopenic patients.

Result of Splenectomy

Two-thirds of patients who have undergone splenectomy, achieve normal platelet count. Platelet counts only recover transiently and partially and most of these patients relapse within 6 months of splenectomy. Splenectomy can be performed after a long time even after years, the ITP is diagnosed. In most cases, platelet counts recover within 10 days after splenectomy. Patients who attain a normal platelet count after 3 days of splenectomy or platelet counts greater than $500 \times 10^9/l$ by day 10 generally have a long term good response to splenectomy. The mortality associated with splenectomy is very low (< 1%), even in patients with severe thrombocytopenia. Younger patients respond better.

Laparoscopic splenectomy was first introduced in 1991 (because of moderate sized spleen) and is better when spleen is of normal size and of normal vascularity. Splenic irradiation or embolization is used in glucocorticoid resistant ITP, or when surgical splenectomy is contraindicated.

In patients refractory to splenectomy, presence of accessory splenic tissue should be suspected, when blood film shows no evidence i.e., Howell- Jolly bodies, pitting erythrocytes are absent. Such patients should be screened for residual tissue by sensitive nucleotide or magnetic resonance imaging.

16.15 INTRAVENOUS IMMUNOGLOBULIN

Intravenous Immunoglobulin (IVIG) was first shown to be effective in childhood ITP in 1981. IVIG increases the platelet count in 75% of patients with classic ITP and normalizes the platelet count in approximately 50% of cases. The effect of IVIG is similar whether the patient is splenectomized or not and the effect is transient, generally lasting only for 3–4 weeks. The patients become refractory to repeated infusions.

Postulated Mechanisms of Action of IVIG

(*i*) Blockade of macrophage Fc receptor which slows down clearance of antibody-coated platelets

(*ii*) Anti-idiotype neutralization of antiplatelet antibodies

The recommended total dose is 2 g/kg either 0.4 g/kg on 5 consecutive days or 1 g/kg/day on 2 consecutive days. For mainteinance therapy, 0.5 – 1g/kg as a single dose may be used. [9]

Adverse effects are headache, backache, nausea, fever, aseptic meningitis, alloimmune haemolysis, hepatitis, renal failure, pulmonary insufficiency and thrombosis, anaphylactic reactions which can occur in IgA deficient patients. IgA level, therefore, should be measured before this form of therapy. Cost is also prohibitive, so it is recommended in life threatening bleeding.

16.16 ANTI-(Rh) D THERAPY

It is a γ globulin containing high titre of antibodies against the Rh_o D antigen of erythrocytes. It is administered intravenously for treatment of ITP. This antibody binds to Rh_o positive erythocytes and leads to their destruction in spleen. Because splenic Fc receptors are blocked, more antibody-coated platelets survive in the circulation. A positive direct antiglobulin test, increse in serum haptoglobin level, mild and transient haemolysis occurs in all Rh_o positive patients after anti-Rh_oD antibody transfusion. Naturally this therapy is not effective in Rh_o negative patients. Response rate is very low in splenectomized patients. A single dose of 50–100 μg/kg given over 3–5 minutes by intravenous route is usually recommended.[10]

Though this therapy increases the platelet count in 70% of patients with Rh_0 positive erythrocytes and not splenectomized, a randomized controlled trial does not show any difference in the spontaneous remission or need for splenectomy.

16.17 PATIENTS REFRACTORY TO INITIAL THERAPY

One-third of patients do not respond or relapse after a short intrval following splenectomy. Therapeutic options depend upon the clinical status of the patient. Bleeding symptoms rather than platelet count is guide to therapy. Patients with no sign of bleeding but risk factors like peptic ulcer, uncontrolled hypertension should be treated to prevent bleeding.

16.18 SPECIAL MODALITIES OF TREATMENT

Vinca Alkaloids

Both Vincristine and Vinblastine transiently increase the platelet count in 70% of ITP patients within 5 to 21 days but produce sustained remission in 10% of treated patients. The recommended dose is Vincristine 1–2 mg and Vinblastine 0.1 mg/kg to a maximum dose of 10 mg, given by bolus injection at 1 week intervals for maximum 3 courses.

Mechanism of action has been postulated as binding to platelet microtubules, consequent transport to spleen, where the drug inhibits phagocytic action of splenic macrophages. They also stimulate megakaryopoiesis. Peripheral neuropathy, neutropenia, jaw pain, alopecia, constipation are usual side effects.

Cycophosphamide

An alkylating agent may be used 50–200 mg/day by oral or 1–1.5 gm by parenteral route every 4 weeks in refractory ITP patients. It increases platelet counts in 60–80% of ITP cases, 20–40% will remain in remission for 2–3 months of therapy. Its action in increasing platelet counts involves immunosuppression. Major complications are marrow suppression, haemorrhagic cystitis, infertility, alopecia, secondary malignancy.[11]

Azathioprine

It is a purine antagonist which induces sustained normalization of platelet count up to 45% of refractory ITP patients. As with other immunosuppressives, major adverse effects are marrow suppression, secondary malignancy, teratogenesis. Recommended dose is 250 mg/day for 4 months.

Danazol

It is a synthetic androgen with reduced virilizing effect. It is recommended in refractory ITP patients. Recommended dose is 400–800 mg/day. Danazol decreases Fc receptor membranes on phagocytic cells by antagonizing effect of oestrogens. It should not be given to pregnant women, or in patients with liver disease. Common side effects are weight gain, fluid retention, secondary amenorrhoea, vocal change, hepatic toxicity, hirsutism, headache, lethargy, myalgia. Liver function should be evaluated every month.

16.19 OTHER MODALITIES OF TREATMENT ARE

Interferon α, dapsone, immunoadsorption with staphylococcal protein A413, cyclosporin, ascorbic acid, colchicines and plasmapharesis. Several investigators reported rituximab, a monoclonal antibody against CD 20 antigen, which presumably acts by depleting autoreactive B cells clone, in refractory ITP.

16.20 NON-SPECIFIC THERAPY FOR THROMBOCYTOPENIA

This includes platelet transfusion and epsilon-aminocaproic acid.

Platelet transfusions are administered as pooled random donor platelet-concentrates (PC) or as single donor platelets. A random–donor–PC is obtained by centrifugation of routine blood donation and contains an average. $0.7–0.9 \times 10^{11}$ platelets in 50 ml of plasma. I PC should raise the platelet count in an average 70 kg adult by 15,000/ µl. Thus pools of 4–6 PC are administered. Single donor platelets are obtained by platelet-pharesis of an individual donor to obtain approximately 4×10^{11} platelets in 300–500 ml of plasma. Thus, on average, a single donor platelet is equivalent to five random donor PCs. In patients with platelet counts < 20, 000/ µl, spontaneous bleeding is evident and platelet transfusions are mandatory to raise the count to the range of 60,000–80,000/microlitre, at which point prolongation of bleeding time is substantially corrected.

If there is no active bleeding when platelet count is < 20,000/ µl, platelet transfusion is optional. In these cases, prophylactic platelet transfusion is recommended under special situations e.g., sepsis, fever of undetermined cause, high leukaemic blast cell count, associated coagulation abnormality, or drugs inhibiting platelet function are being used. Prophylactic transfusion needs to be repeated every 2 to 3 days.

Difficulties during platelet transfusion- After 2–8 weeks with pooled platelet transfusion, patient may develop alloimmunization to HLA antigens, when there is no increment in platelet count occurs after 10–60 minutes. Moreover, cytomegalovirus may be transmitted by leukocytes. In these cases leukoreduction is to be achieved by filtration either prior to storage or on the bedside before transfusion. Single donor platelet is better in this respect, preferably from HLA-matched donor.

16.21 EPSILON AMINOCAPROIC ACID

The extent of bleeding at any anatomical site depends upon balance between hemostatic factors and fibrinolysis induced by plasmin. This compound inhibits plasmin and often slows thrombocytopenic bleeding at mucosal surfaces where fibrinolytic activity is high, such as nose, mouth, gastrointestinal and urinary tract. So this therapy is begun when thrombocytopenic patients fail to respond to platelet transfusion alone. It is started in a dose of 5 g, followed by 1 g per hour intravenously by continuous infusion. Hemostasis may be maintained at a dosage of 3 g every 6 hours. Adjunctive therapies include agents designed to reduce bleeding without necessarily affecting the platelet count. Aminocaproic acid is such an agent which can therefore be used for preventing excessive menstrual loss in young women. [12]

16.22 THROMBOCYTOPENIA IN SPECIAL SITUATIONS

1. Antiphospholipid Syndrome (APS)

Some investigators suggest that antibodies against platelet glycoprotein, GpIIa-IIIb or Gp IbIX V complexes, rather than APLA, are responsible. These antibodies do not cross react with antibodies against phospholipid or b glycoprotein I. Immuno-suppressive treatment increases the platelet count and reduces titre of anti-Gp antibodies but not the titre of APLA. Platelet antigens in thrombocytopenic patients are different from those in ITP. [13] Another issue of clinical importance in evaluating thrombocytopenia associated with APS is the risk of development of thrombus in future APLA. Patients are divided into three groups according to platelet count:

1. Non-thrombocytopenic — platelet count > $180 \times 10^{9-}$ (40%)
2. Moderately thrombocytopenic — platelet count $50 \times 10^9 - 100 \times 10^9$ (30%)
3. Severely thrombocytopenic— < 50×10^9 (9%)

Risk of thrombosis is indicated in figures within the bracket. Bleeding in APS in moderate thrombocytopenia should trigger evaluation of antithrombin antibodies.

Severe thrombocytopenia should be treated in the same line as in ITP. Glucocorticoids are effective in only 15% of cases. IVIg and cyclophosamide can be used in patients with severe bleeding catastrophes. Splenectomy produces sustained remission in two-third of patients. Because of increased risk of thrombosis, patients should be prophylactically anticoagulated in immediate postoperative period. Cases of thrombocytopenia correction using aspirin, warfarin, antimalarial drugs have been reported.

2. Thrombocytopenia in Patients with SLE

Thrombocytopenia is common in patients with SLE in 20–40% of cases. SLE is an autoimmune disease, commonly affecting women of child-bearing age, may affect any tissue of the body. The diagnostic criteria are based on a classification system proposed by American Society of Rheumatology Patients should fulfil any four of eleven criteria. Its complete discussion is out of scope of this book. However, destruction of platelets by autoantibodies is the major mechanism of thrombocytopenia. Although significant bleeding is uncommon even in severely thrombocytopenic patients, fatal gastrointestinal, cerebral or pulmonary bleeding have been reported. Antiplatelet antibodies are present in 40% of SLE patients.

Besides antiplatelet antibodies antiphospholipid antibodies and immune complexes bind to the platelets non-specifically and accelerate their destruction. Specific antibodies like GpIIB-IIIa have an important role in pathogenesis of SLE thrombocytopenia. [14]

Therapeutic strategies are not well established. Treatment of severe thrombocytopenia is tailored to individual patient The patients with APLA are generally treated with glucocorticoid as first line of therapy, but sustained remission is infrequent. Most patients have nephritis or neurological symptoms for which they receive immunosuppressive therapy, either alone or in combination with glucocorticoids.

16.23 CONDITIONS MIMICKING ITP

Spurious (Pseudo) thrombocytopenia: Incidence is 0.09–0.21p.c. which accounts for 15–30 p.c. of all cases. As a result of platelet clumping ex-vivo, platelet counts reported by automated counters may be much lower than the actual count. [15]

Platelet satellism: Antibodies against Gp IIb-IIIa receptors may react simultaneously with leukocyte FcY receptor III and attach the platelets in the form of a rosette around the periphery of leukocytes. Antibodies are naturally occurring and their presence does not clearly correlate with any specific situation.

Antiphospholipid antibodies: Some antiplatelet antibodies from patients with thrombocytopenia cross react with negatively charged phospholipid and may exhibit anti-cardiolipin antibody activity. Pathogenesis of thrombocytopenia in APLA is not clear. Some investigators suggest that antibodies against platelet glycoprotein GpIIb-Iia or GpIb-IX V complexes, rather than APLA are responsible. Such antibodies do not cross react with antibodies against phospholipids and β glycoprotein. Immunosuppressive treatment increases the platelet count and reduces the anti Gp antibodies but not the titre of APLA. Platelet antigens are different from that of seen in ITP.

Thrombocytopenia has been described in patients with acute coronary syndrome: This has been found in patients treated with GpIIa-IIIb antagonist Abiximib but is seen to be associated with pseudothrombocytopenia also. The mechanism of platelet clumping is unknown. Probably drug itself is not responsible, as it is monovalent. More likely is that other agglutinins bind to GpIIb-IIIa receptors new epitopes being induced by combination of Abiximib binding and Ca channel chelation. Antiplatelet therapy in these cases of unstable angina is frustrating.

16.24 DEFECTIVE PLATELET PRODUCTION

This condition may arise from some hereditary disorders as follows:

1. May-Hegglin anomaly— This is an autosomal dominant disorder. There are macro thrombocytopenia with mutation of 22q 12–13 chromosome in myAE gene.
   There is presence of Double bodies, which are pale blue inclusions in the cytoplasm of granular leukocytes. The protein affected is an important cytoskeletal protein in haemopoietic cells. Patients should be given only platelet transfusion during episode, no IVIg or splenectomy like ITP is required, which may be dangerous. [16]
2. Familial platelet syndrome— There is predisposition to myelogenous leukaemia. Platelets are of normal size and structure but functional defect is present, which is due to genetic mutation of transcription factor Rank I. Stem cell transplantation is the treatment.
3. Wiskott-Aldrich syndrome— This an X-linked recessive disorder in which are found, small platelets on peripheral blood smear, eczema and an increased susceptibility to infection. The thrombocytopenia generally improves after splenectomy but there is life risk from surgery and sepsis and life long penicillin prophylaxis is mandatory.
4. Bernard-Soulier syndrome— Thrombocytopenia is associated giant platelets and a congenital defect in platelet function.
5. Hereditary thrombocytopenia is a group of disorders, which has mostly autosomal dominant inheritance, and moderate thrombocytopenia (30,000–100,000/l). There is markedly decreased or increased size of platelets in peripheral blood smear, or by electronic counter. There is a history in patient dating back from childhood, without spontaneous remission, which is typical of childhood ITP. There is a family history. They rarely have severe bleeding and do not improve on steroid or splenectomy.

6. Autosomal recessive disorder with absent radii syndrome (TAR)— there is marked depletion of megakaryocytes with no associated abnormality of red or white cells.

If the patient survives the first year of life, prognosis is good. Platelet transfusion is rarely needed for surgery.

16.25 IMPAIRED PLATELET PRODUCTION

By definition, there is a bone marrow abnormality reflected by morphological abnormality or decreased count of megakaryocytes. This is rarely seen without abnormalities in the production of white cells and red cells.

1. **Marrow Hypoplasia** is most commonly seen as a response to chemotherapy or radiotherapy in malignancy. It may be also seen as an idiosyncratic reaction to hepatitis or to drugs such as chloramphenicol, phenylbutazone, gold compounds, phenytoin, and sulphonamides or as idiopathic aplastic anaemia. In 2–5% of cases of acquired aplastic anaemia, there is no or only minor abnormalities of white or red cells. Ethanol induced thrombocytopenia: "Binge drinkers" may develop sometimes severe thrombocytopenia with platelet counts in the range of 10,000–20,000 per microlitre because of direct suppression of platelet production and shortening of life span of platelets. Usually the platelet count begins to rise as soon as alcohol is withdrawn.
2. **Malignant Invasion:** Lymphoma, leukaemia, and carcinoma (particularly breast, lung, stomach, kidney and prostate) can produce thrombocytopenia by this mechanism.
3. **Dysmyelopoietic Syndromes:** Megaloblastic anaemia due to deficiency of folic acid or vitamin B_{12} may produce severe thrombocytopenia as a part of general pancytopenia and so also idiopathic dysmyelopoietic syndrome. Normal or increased number of megakaryocytes may be present in this bone marrow due to ineffective erythopoiesis.

16.26 IMMUNOLOGIC REACTION TO DRUGS PRODUCING PICTURE OF ITP

Quinidine and quinine, sulfonamides, gold compounds, and heparin are the major offenders. For the first three rapid improvement occurs after drug withdrawal. In patients with gold induced thrombocytopenia, antibodies cannot be demonstrated. Gold probably induces an autoimmune state that responds to steroid, remission can be maintained by continuing the steroid for 6–12 months. About 1–5% of patients who receive unfractionated heparin develop IgG antibodies against a complex of heparin and platelet factor 4. Patients develop thrombocytopenia in 5–14 days of initiation of therapy. The risk for thrombosis is high. It is recommended that anticoagulation with Hirudin, argatroban or danaparoid, but no warfarin or low molecular weight heparin is to be administered. [17]

Acute thrombocytopenia occurs in 1% of patients treated with humanized monoclonal antibody to GpIIb-IIIa, abiciximab and other such inhibitors. The mechanism is believed to be immunological. Recovery occurs promptly when the drug is discontinued.

16.27 POST-TRANSFUSION PURPURA

It is a common clinical syndrome in which marked thrombocytopenia occurs 5–10 days after routine red cell transfusion. Most patients are women and all of them are transfused previously and have been pregnant. It is generally easy to demonstrate platelet antibody in their serum. In most cases, the antibody is specific for the platelet antigen HPA-Ia (Pl^{ia}) antigen. Recovery is spontaneous in 10 days to 2 months. Because 98% of population is positive for this antigen, it is not known how the alloimmune reaction mediates platelet destruction in patients' antigen negative platelets. Life threatening bleeding occurs with some frequency. Therapy should be begun with intravenous gammaglobulin. Plasmapharesis (exchange of 40 ml/kg of body weight daily) may be added in cases refractory to gammaglobulin. [18]

Post-transfusion purpura may also occur in non-immunologic way.

This is found when massive blood loss is replaced with banked blood, only with red cells and few viable platelets. Platelet transfusion is not routinely indicated, unless thrombocytopenia contributes to continued bleeding.

16.28 OTHER NON-IMMUNOLOGIC DISORDERS THAT MIMIC TRUE ITP

1. **Disseminated Intravascular Coagulation (DIC) and Sepsis:** The condition results from activation of coagulation in the vascular tree. It is differentiated from immune thrombocytopenia by finding prolongation of prothrombin time and thromboplastin time, decreased plasma fibrinogen level,and plasmafibrin-fibrinogen split products.The aetiology of DIC is multi-directional like infections (bacterial, viral, rickettsial or malarial), obstetric catastrophe (abruption placentae, retained dead foetus).
2. **Thrombotic Thrombocytopenic Purpura:** This is a special variety of thrombocytopenia which is caused by microscopic.thrombi produced by endothelial damage of microscopic blood vessels. It has been proposed that antibody-mediated deficiency of vWF-cleaving protease may accumulation of large vWF multimers which facilitate platelet agglutination. [19]

The disease has a subacute or fulminant onset with a combination of various findings, like thrombocytopenia, haemolytic anaemia, presence of polikilocytosis in red cells, burr cells, helmet cells, inperipheral blood smear, elevated serum lactate dehydrogenase, fluctuating central nervous system deficits consistent with intermittent ischaemia, and renal failure. In adults, haemolytic-uraemic syndrome (HUS) and thrombotic thrombocytopenic purpura (TTP) are similar illnesses and former renal failure is predominant feature, the condition may be idiopathic or may be associated with

(*a*) Drugs— quinidine, clopidrogel, mitomycin C, and cyclosporin

(*b*) allogenic bone marrow transplantation

(*c*) HIV infection

(*d*) Pregnancy and post-patrum period

Initial therapy is plasma exchange (removal of 40 ml/kg of BW) and replacement of an equal volume of fresh frozen plasma). This treatment should be continued daily until the platelet count rises to 100,000/microlitre and there is definite fall of LDH, reflecting improvement of haemolysis. Once improvement occurs, frequency of plasma exchange is reduced over 1–2 weeks. The course of the disease is variable, but most of the patients obtain and maintain a remission with treatment.

16.29 THROMBOCYTOPENIA ASSOCIATED WITH PREGNANCY

The condition may arise as:

1. Gestational thrombocytopenia— it is detected in 5–7% of cases, which is a benign disorder, not associated with bleeding. Platelet counts are greater than $70 \times 10^9/l$, return to normal after delivery. Pathogenesis is unknown. Several mechanisms have been suggested as haemodilution, a compensated state of subclinical coagulopathy, platelet consumption by placenta, depression of megakaryocytes in the bone marrow as evident by transient depression and return to normal after delivery.
2. ITP in pregnancy should be suspected by history of repeated epistaxis, episodes before pregnancy, severe thrombocytopenia associated with bleeding. In healthy women, platelet count greater than $75 \times 10^9/l$ in late pregnancy does not require extensive investigations. On the other hand, a patient with platelet count less than $50 \times 10^9/l$ should be discouraged to become pregnant. A patient with platelet count less than $10 \times 10^9/l$ after splenectomy should be explained high risk of pregnancy. ITP may excerbate during pregnancy but generally platelet count settles after delivery. Treatment of ITP during pregnancy is difficult due to teratogenic effects of cytotoxic drug like azathioprine, or effects such as hypertension, osteoporosis, gestational diabetes or psychosis, produced by glucocorticoids which are not teratogenic. [20]
3. Neonatal thrombocytopenia— Circulating antiplatelet antibodies, immunoglobulin G (IgG) is capable of crossing the placenta and producing thrombocytopenia in the neonates. This is more common if the mother is thrombocytopenic during delivery, but if after splenectomy or drug therapy has produced a remission in the mother. Some researchers believe that risk of serious bleeding in these infants is very low. Therefore routine obstetric management should be used. Others hold opinion that an occasional foetus will be severely thrombocytopenic and recommend percutaneous umbilical blood sampling to determine whether caeserean section is indicated to prevent foetal haemorrhage during vaginal delivery. It should be remembered that normal women may develop modest, apparently non-immune thrombocytopenia as pregnancy progresses, and these infants are not at risk of thrombocytopenia. [21]
4. Thrombocytopenia in pregnancy may be seen in presence of a number of clinical conditions, like SLE, antiphospholipid syndrome, viral infections (HIV, CMV, EBV), pre-eclampsia, hypersplenism, marrow dysfunction (leukaemia, aplastic anaemia), or may be drug-induced.

According to ASH guidelines, a patient with $50 \times 10^9/l$ platelet count should not be discouraged to become pregnant. A patient with platelet count $> 10 \times 10^9/l$ should be advised high risk to the foetus. ITP may excerbate during pregnancy but generally platelet settles down to pre-pregnancy level after delivery.

16.30 HIV INFECTION AND THROMBOCYTOPENIA

A number of factors are involved in producing thrombocytopenia:

1. Accelerated platelet destruction results from nonspecific deposition of complement and immune complexes on the platelet surfaces. Antibodies against CD_4 receptor gp 120 have been found in HIV +ve patients. High affinity antibodies against GpIIa have been eluted in thrombocytopenic patients.

2. Decreased platelet production— HIV-1 entry into host cells requires sequential reaction of viral envelope gp120 with CD_4 and co-receptor on the host cell plasma membrane. Defective modulation of HIV infected T lymphocytes can explain impairment of megakaryopoiesis.
3. Increased platelet consumption is another important cause of thrombocytopenia, as incidence of thrombotic thrombocytopenia is much higher and there is risk of developing micro-angiopathies. [22]

Some common clinical causes of thrombocytopenia include haemolytic uraemic syndrome (Thrombotic thrombocytopenic purpura), sepsis, marrow hypoplasia (due to drugs and infections), abnormal platelet pooling (hypersplenism), dilutional thrombocytopenia, related to therapy. Severe thrombocytopenia is rare in such cases and found only in 5% of patients.

REFERENCES

1. Geddis AE, Kashansky K: Inherited thrombocytopenia: *Toward a molecular understanding of disorders of platelet production*: Curr opinion Paed 16:15, (2004).
2. Heyns AD, Lotter MG, Badenhorst PN, Van Reen O, Pieters H, Miener PC: *Kinetics and fate of (iii) Indium-oxide labeled pooled platelets in asplenic subjects*. Thromb Haemostat 44:100, (1980).
3. Lissinger Ca: *Platelet kinetics in immune thrombocytopenic purpura: A qualitative study*. Am J Haematol 12:167, (1982).
4. Berchtold P, Dale GL, Tani P, Mc Millan R. *Inhibition of autoantibody binding to platelet glycoprotein Iib/IIIa by anti idiotypic antibodies in intravenous gammaglobulin*. Blood 74:2414, (1989).
5. Bassel JB: *Fc receptor blockade and immune thrombocytopenic purpura*. Seminar Haematol 37:261, (2000).
6. Narang M, Penner J, Williams D. *Refractory autoimmune thrombocytopenic. purpura: Responses to treatment with recombinant antibody to lymphocyte antigen (CD-20) (rituximab)*. Am J Haematol 74:263, (2003).
7. Rebulla P, Finanzi G, Marangoni A, et al. *The threshold of prophylactic platelet transfusion in adults with acute myeloid leukaemia*. N Engl J Med 337: 1870, (1997).
8. Cheng Y, Wong RS, Soo, Yo, et al. *Initial treatment of immune thrombocytopenic purpura with high dose dexamethasone*. N Engl J Med 349:831, (2003).
9. Bussel JB, Pham LC, Aledort L. *Maintenance treatment of adults with chronic refractory immune thrombocytopenic purpura using repeated infusions of gamma globulin*. Blood 72:121, (1988).
10. George JM, Raksol GE, Vesley SK, et al.: *Initial management of immune thrombocytopenic purpura in adults: A randomized clinical trial comparing intermittent anti-D routine care*. Am J Haematol 74:161, (2003).
11. Riner A, Gerenshimer J, Silcher SJ. *Pulse-Cyclophosphamide therapy for refractory autoimmune thrombocytopenic purpura*. Blood 85: 351, (1995).
12. Mannucci PM. *Haemostatic drugs*. N Engl J Med 339:245-253, (1998).
13. Diz-Kuokkaya R, Hachihanefoglu A, Yeneril H, et al. *Antiphospholipid antibodies and antiphospholipid syndrome in patients presenting with thrombocytopenic purpura: A prospective cohort study*. Blood 98: 1760, (2001).

14. Alacron- Seiria D: *Splenectomy has a limited role in the management of lupus with thrombocytopenia.* J Rheumatol 29:1, (2002).
15. Okder O, Weinstein A, Hoyer LW: *Pseudothrombocytopenia: Clinical comment on 37 cases.* Minerve Med 92:13, (2001).
16. Di Pumpo M, Noris P, Pecci A, et al. *Defective expression of GpIb/ IX/ V complex in platelets with May-Hegglin anomaly and Sebestion syndrome.* Haematologica 87:943, (2002).
17. Aster RH. Drug-induced immune thrombocytopenia: *An overview of pathogenesis.* Semin Haematol 36:2–6, (1999).
18. Mueller- Eckhardt C. *Annotation: post-transfusion purpura.* Brit J Haematol: 64:419, (1986).
19. Rao Ak. *Acquired qualitative platelet defects.* In Colman Rw, Hirsh J, Marder VJ, et al.eds. Haemostasis and thrombosis: basic principles and clinical practice: JB Lippinncott:905-920, (2001).
20. Solanki D, Blackburn BC: *Spurious thrombocytopenia during pregnancy.* Obst Gynaecol. 65: 145, (1985).
21. Roberts I. Review: *Management of thrombocytopenia in neonates.* Brit J Haematol 105:864, (1999).
22. Beirling P, BettrarebA, *Oskenbendler E. Human Immunodeficiency virus-related immune thrombocytopenia.* Semin Thromb Haemostat 21:68–75, (1995).

CHAPTER 17

Thrombocytosis

17.1 INTRODUCTION

The upper limit of the normal platelet count is generally between 350,000/μl (350 × 10^9/l) and 450,000/μl (450 × 10^9). The value varies among different laboratories. In a sample of 10,000 healthy adults aged 18 to 65 years, 99 (1%) had platelet counts greater than 400,000/μl. Among these individuals, thrombocytosis is confirmed in only 8 at repeated examination 6 months to 1 year. [1]

17.2 CLINICO-PATHOLOGICAL CATEGORIES

There are three major categories:

1. Clonal type which includes essential (or primary) thrombocythaemia and other myeloproliferative disorders involving thrombocytes also.
2. Familial type, which includes rare cases of non-clonal myeloproliferation resulting from thrombopoietin mutations.
3. Reactive type, in which thrombocytosis occurs secondary to a variety of non-related acute and chronic clinical conditions.

17.3 ESSENTIAL THROMBOCYTHAEMIA

This condition often remains asymptomatic and is discovered incidentally from blood counts. Its diagnosis comes in the process of exclusion. It is one of a group of myeloproliferative disorders which include polycythaemia, chronic myelogenous leukaemia and myeloid metaplasia with or without myelofibrosis.[2] Major causes of morbidity are bleeding and thromboses, the latter most commonly involving arterial circulation. Reactive thrombocytosis does not cause these complications and does not require treatment.

17.4 REACTIVE THROMBOCYTOSIS

There are several causes of this type of thrombocytosis, the causes belong to different diseases:

1. Transient-arising out of acute blood loss, recovery from thrombocytopenia, acute infection or inflammation, response to exercise.

2. Sustained-arising out of iron deficiency, post-splenectomy/asplenic state, malignancy, chronic infection or inflammation, inflammatory bowel disease, temporal arteritis, tuberculosis, chronic pneumonitis, haemorrhagic anaemia.
3. Thrombocytosis may occur as a part of paraneoplastic syndrome, as a complication of surgery, in Wegner's granulomatosis, in Castleman disease, in rheumatoid disease and in vitamin E deficiency.
4. Primary acquired thrombocytosis may occur in temporal arteritis, Kostman disease, as an autosomal dominant hereditary disorder, benign familial thrombocytosis, and as a part of Blackman-Diamond anaemia.
5. Thrombocytosis may occur as a symptom of poisoning like chronic pesticide poisoning, toxic reaction to the medications e.g. Ceftrizoxime, Cefzox, Ceftazidine, Fortaz, Tazicef.

Transretinoic acid used for treatment of promyelocytic leukaemia produces transcriptional up regulation of thrombopoietin production and thrombocytosis. [3]

Some conditions can lead to high platelet count only for a short time. These are recovery from serious blood loss, recovery from high platelet count caused by excessive alcohol use and lack of vitamin B_{12} or folate, acute infection or inflammation and response to physical activity.

17.5 FAMILIAL THROMBOCYTOSIS

This is a genetically determined heterogenous disorder. There are two main types. Specific mutation in thrombopoietin gene, including single nucleotide deletion in 5′ untranslated region in the gene leading to markedly elevated thrombopoietin level [4]. In another variety a unique dominant activating point mutation developed in c-mpl gene causing autonomous thrombopoietin activation. [5]

17.6 HISTORICAL BACKGROUND

The first description of essential thrombocythaemia was given by De Gugliemo in 1920 [6] and by Epstein and Goedel in 1934 in association with other myeloproliferative disorders. [7]

The separate existence of thrombocytosis as a disease category was first established in 1960. [8]

17.7 PATHOGENESIS

The clonal nature of the disease was established by discovery of a single gene (Gl6-PD) isoenzyme, expressed in all blood cell lines of women with essential thrombocythaemia who were coincidentally heterogenous for two types of Gl-6-PD isoenzymes "A" and "B". This is further confirmed by several approaches using X-linked markers in female patients. Probable explanation for findings of polyclonality include a small population of clonal cells against a polyclonal background, progression of non-clonal essential thrombocythaemia to clonal disease or restriction of clonality in some patients to the megakaryocytic lineage. This explains heterogenous nature of the disease. Despite the origin in multipotential stem cell, dominant phenotypic change involves megakaryocytic lineage. Usually erythopoiesis and granulopoiesis are normal at diagnosis. [9]

Thrombopoietin the ligand for megakaryocytic growth factor receptor c-mpl, is the major humoral regulator of megakaryocytopoiesis and platelet production. Although thrombopoietin supports the entire population of megakaryocyte development at different stages, along with other cytokines (IL-6, IL-

11), in synergy, platelets have an important role in regulating plasma thrombopoietin level, as their receptors (c-mpl) remove it from plasma. As the platelet count drops, increased free plasma thrombopoietin levels stimulate megakaryocytopoiesis. This modulation maintains steady state level of platelet production. Unlike erythropoietin, thrombopoietin levels are normal or elevated in thrombocythaemia. The increased thrombopoietin level may result from abnormal binding and consumption of defective platelets. In support of this, platelet expression of c-mpl is markedly reduced. [10]

The increased number of colony-forming units-megakaryocytes (CFU-Meg) have been cultured from the blood or marrow of patients with essential thrombocythaemia, which are less sensitive to transforming growth factor B_1, an endogenous inhibitor of megakaryocytopoiesis. [11]

Thus, despite the decreased production of thrombopoietin receptors (c-mpl) on megakaryocytes of patients with essential thrombocythaemia, increased megakaryocytic proliferation and production reset for hypersensitivity to stimulator and/or decreased sensitivity to negative regulators of megakaryocytopoiesis.

17.8 MOLECULAR PATHOGENESIS

Jaus Kinase 2 (JAK 2) is a tyrosine kinase inhibitor which functions as an intermediate molecule between cell membrane receptors for haempoietic growth factors and downstream signaling molecules. Mutation involves a valine to phenylallantoin substitution at position 617 in the autoinhibitory domain of the gene controlling JAK 2, thereby promotes uninterrupted cell signaling and increased responsiveness of megakaryocytes to thrombopoietin. Patients who have JAK 2, V 617F mutation, also show a significantly higher rate of complications (fibrosis, bleeding, thrombosis) in clinical practice. [12]

Polycythaemia Rubra Vera-1 (PRV-1) gene is overexpressed on granulocytes in most patients with polycythaemia but also in some patients with essential thrombocythaemia.

Increased risk of thromboembolism is found in patients with monoclonality, PRV-1 overexpression, reduced megakaryocyte c-mpl and low Epo level. [13]

17.9 CLINICAL FEATURES OF THROMBOCYTOSIS

Two out of every three patients have no symptoms at the time of diagnosis. Younger patients may remain symptom-free for years. Enlargement of spleen is detected in 60% of patients with marked thrombocytosis. The liver may also be enlarged. As many as half of patients experience bleeding from the skin, gums or nose and 20–50% have blockage of arteries.

Other symptoms include bloody stool, bruising, dizziness, headache, haemorrhage, prolonged bleeding having surgery or having a tooth pulled, redness or tingling of hands or feet. In rare instances lymph nodes are enlarged.

Highest platelet count shows most severe symptoms. Younger patients especially women may not have symptoms. Complications include stroke, heart attack and formation of blood clots in arms or legs. A doctor should be always informed when bleeding is prolonged or unexplained or if the patient develops chest or leg pain, confusion, numbness, weakness. [14]

In contrast to other myeloproliferative disorder, hypermetabolic symptoms such as fever, sweat, weight loss are highly uncommon in essential thrombocythaemia.

Physical findings usually are limited to mild splenomegaly, which is present in 40% of patients.

Echocardiography may reveal aortic and mitral valvular lesions, including leaflet thickening and vegetations similar to the lesions described in non-bacterial thrombotic endocarditis. The relationship of cardiac valve lesions to thromboembolic complications in essential thrombocythaemia is unclear. [15]

17.10 LABORATORY FEATURES

Untreated patients have elevated **platelet count** ranging from slight elevation to several millions/μl.

Platelet morphology on blood film shows large, pale, blue staining, hypogranular, may have lymphoblastoid appearance, occasional megakaryocytic fragments are seen.

Increased platelet turnover is indicated by increased reticulated platelets (young) in the circulation, which can be detected by flow cytometric analysis of platelets RNA. Although both the percentage and absolute number are elevated, compared to healthy individuals, whether this finding can distinguish it from other forms of thrombocytosis is unclear.

Serum Erythropoietin (Epo) is normal or mildly elevated in clonal form, do not correlate with platelet count. Serum Epo level is also elevated in essential thrombocythaemia so this test can not distinguish between the two. **Plasma level of IL-6 and CRP** are low in essential thrombocythaemia, elevated in secondary thrombocytosis, which often accompanies acute and chronic inflammatory states.

Pseudohyperkalaemia may be found with extreme thrombocytosis. It is diagnosed when serum potassium concentration exceeds plasma potassium concentration. It is caused by release of intracellular potassium during blood clotting.

Marrow pathology reveals increased **cellularity** with megakaryocytic **hyperplasia**. There are frequently **giant megakaryocytes** with increased **ploidy** that occur in **clusters**. Large number of **platelet debris** are seen in marrow samples (platelet drifts). [16]

Most patients have no **cytogenetic abnormality**. However, some **patients may have Philadelphia chromosome. They do not have any feature of CML**. Some patients with essential thrombocythaemia may have **BCR-ABL gene rearrangement** in absence of Philadelphia chromosome. **Deletion of long arm of Chromosome 5(q-)** has been reported.

Clinical tests of haemostasis

Bleeding time is prolonged in fewer than 20 p.c. of cases. Test does not correlate with platelet count or clinical findings, and/or predict reliably bleeding or thrombosis. Platelet aggregation abnormalities are variable. There is reduced platelet response to collagen. Platelet storage pool defect (aspirin-like) is not affected. Epinephrine stimulated defect is abnormal on aggregation. This unusual abnormality is also noted in other myeloproliferative disorder. Some patients have platelet hyperagreegability or spontaneous agreeegation in vitro.

17.11 DIAGNOSTIC CRITERIA FOR ESSENTIAL THROMBOCYTHAEMIA (WHO EXTENDED CRITERIA, 2003)

1. Platelet count > 60,000/μl
2. Haemoglobin 13 g/dl or normal red cell mass (in male > 36 ml/kg, in female > 32 ml/kg)
3. Stainable iron in marrow or failure of iron trial (< 1g/dl rise in Hb after one month of therapy)

4. No Philadelphia chromosome
5. Collagen fibrosis of marrow: (*a*) Absent (*b*) 1/3rd biopsy area without both splenomegaly or leucoerythroblastic reaction
6. No known cause of reactive thrombocytosis
7. Megakaryocytes in clumps

17.12 CLINICAL FEATURES OF CLONAL AND REACTIVE THROMBOCYTOSIS

Features	Clonal Type	Reactive Type
Splenomegaly	Yes in – 40% of cases	No
Platelet Morphology	Giant Platelets	Normal Platelets
Platelet Function	Often abnormal	Normal
Bone Marrow	Increased cellularity with giant, dysplastic platelets having increased ploidy and masses of platelet debris	Increased cellularity with normal morphology
Thrombotic Complications	Digital, cerebrovascular, large vessel arterial or venous	No
Bleeding Complications	Increased risk	No
Underlying Disease	No	Often clinically apparent

17.13 COURSE AND PROGNOSIS

Thrombotic complications in secondary thrombocytosis are often linked to underlying disease like cancer, postoperative state. One exception is splenectomy for haemolytic anaemia, notably thalassaemia, incompletely relieved by surgical procedure. Therapy to reduce platelet count or antiplatelet therapy is not beneficial in secondary thrombocytosis.

Major causes of mortality and morbidity in essential thrombocythaemia are thrombosis and haemorrhage. Although the condition has no potency to revert to acute leukaemia like other myeloproliferative disorder, association is less clear. Treatment with radiophosphorus or alkylating agent increases the potency. A high proportion will develop AML and MDS with hydroxyurea when they have chromosome 17q deletion and other 17p syndrome. Survival study shows no decrease in life expectancy, though significantly worse than that of age and sex-matched controls. [17]

17.14 CLINICAL RISKS OF COMPLICATIONS IN ESSENTIAL THROMBOCYTHAEMIA

Complications are more common if there is previous history of thrombosis, associated risk factors for cerebrovascular accident (e.g. smoking), inadequate control of thrombocytosis in high risk patients.

Use of aspirin and non steroidal anti-inflammatory drugs are highly risky in these patients and risk is very high if platelet count is > 1,50,000/μl.

If there is no associated risk, occurrence of complications depend upon degree of thrombocytosis and prolongation of bleeding time.

17.15 COMPLICATIONS

I. Thrombotic Complications

Although 25% of all thrombotic events are deep vein thrombosis of the lower extremity, the most common site of arterial thrombosis involve cerebrovascular, peripheral vascular and coronary arterial circulation.

Erythromeralgia or digital microvascular ischaemia is characterized by intense burning, throbbing in a patchy distribution in the extremities most proximally involving the feet. The pain is accompanied by warmth, duskiness and mottled edema, sometimes live do reticularis. The pain tends to be excerbated by excertions and dependency.

Erythromeralgia may be confused with Raynaud's syndrome, shoulder hand syndrome or causalgia. Histopathological study shows endothelial swelling, fibromuscular intimal proliferation and vascular occlusion caused by platelet thrombi. Digital microvascular ischaemia may arise independently. Signs of digital microvascular ischaemia primarily involving the toes may develop independent of erythromeralgia. Painful vascular insufficiency may progress to frank gangrene and necrosis of the digits. Arteriographs show major vessels are patent. Erythromeralgia and digital gangrene often respond to aspirin, reduction of elevated platelet count. [18]

Arterial thrombotic complications occur more frequently than venous. Cerebrovascular complications may present as headache, dizziness, decreased mental activity, focal neurodeficit or seizure and ischaemic stroke, retinal artery occlusion. Coronary circulation is also affected. 50% of patients had at least one thrombotic episode in 9 years. Ischaemic stroke often responds to aspirin and platelet reduction. [19] 25% of all thrombotic events are deep vein thrombosis of lower extremities. Hepatic and portal vein thrombosis are more common in polycythaemia vera.

II. Bleeding Complications

Superficial bleeding, mucosal, spontaneous or in response to minimal trauma is most common. Gastrointestinal, genitourinary or cutaneous bleeding may also occur. Some studies indicate that older patients are at markedly increased rate of haemostatic complications, while younger patients are relatively protected from these problems. However, other reports have documented no age related difference.

III. Complications in Pregnancy

Multiple placental infarcts may produce placental insufficiency. This may lead to recurrent spontaneous abortion, foetal growth retardation, premature delivery or abruptio placentae.

This complication may occur in 50% of pregnancy with thrombocytosis. However, successful pregnancy outcome is possible without any form of therapy. To prevent risk of haemorrhage, maternal or neonatal, aspirin should be avoided for at least one week prior to delivery. [20]

17.16 THERAPY FOR THROMBOCYTOSIS

Indications for therapy: This is highly controversial, because of poverty of prospective clinical trials determining the impact of cytoreduction on morbidity and mortality of clonal thrombocythaemia. Although an association of platelet count with thromboses has been suggested, it is not well established. The prophylactic efficacy of platelet lowering agent in asymptomatic low-risk essential thrombocythaemia patients, irrespective of degree of thrombocytosis may result in symptomatic improvement. Indication for prompt cytoreduction is particularly strong in patients with microvascular, digital or cerbrovascular ischaemia syndrome.

17.17 THERAPEUTIC MODALITIES

1. Platepharesis is reserved in selected cases of acute and threatening thrombotic and haemostatic problems. Reduction of platelet count is transient and may be followed by rebound increase in thrombocytosis.
2. Use of Radiophosphorus and Alkylating agents (e.g., mephalan, busulphan) has largely been abandoned because of this leukomogenic potential, except in selected elderly patients who can not tolerate other drugs.
3. Hydroxyurea, a non-alkylating myelosuppressive agent is highly effective as initial therapy for essential thrombocythaemia. Doses required for thrombocytosis control are generally 10–30 mg/kg/day. Blood count should be checked in 7 days of therapy for rapid myelosuppression. Maintainance dose is to be adjusted according to blood count. Daily treatment reduces count appreciably within 8 weeks in 80% of cases. Painful but reversible leg ulceration may occur. Leukomogenic potential is highly controversial, but may occur in essential thrombocythaemia with deletion of 17p chromosome.
4. Anagrelide is effective as alternative first line of therapy. This quinazoline derivative can be given orally and reduces platelet count by inhibiting marrow megakaryocyte maturation. Dose is 0.15 mg q.i.d or 1 mg b.i.d with dose adjustments at weekly interval up to a maximum to 10 mg/day. Dose required to reduce platelet count in average sized adult is 2–3 mg/day. The time of reduction by 50% is average 11 days. It reduces platelet count without altering white blood cell count. About 30% of patients can not tolerate due to positive inotropic action. e.g. fluid retention, palpitation, heart failure, arrhythmia. Side effects diminish over time. Discontinuation gives rise to rapid rise. Important side effects are anorexia, nausea, vomiting, palpitation, edema. Anagrelide is associated with increased risk of arterial thromboses, major bleeding, myelofibrotic transformation but decreased venous thromboses. [21]

   Hydroxyurea should be the first line of therapy in high risk patients.
5. Interferon alpha is also an effective therapy. The drug suppresses the proliferation of abnormal megakaryocytic clone, with decrease in its size and ploidy. Platelet counts are reduced at normal or near normal level within 1 month of starting. An effective therapy is to administer Interferon S.C. at a dose of 3,000,000 units per day initially, doses subsequently adjusted according to individual tolerance and response. Suppression can be maintained for several years, relapse occurs after discontinuation. [22]

Side effects make intolerable in 20% of cases, often accompanied by lowering of white blood cell count but no effect on haematocrit is noted. Although it is non-leukomogenic, toxicity and cost can't make the drug the first line of therapy in low risk patients.

As Hydroxyurea is teratogenic and Anagrelide crosses the placental barrier (with unknown safety), Interferon alpha is the treatment of choice in high risk women patients with essential thrombocythaemia, who are contemplating pregnancy.

6. Haemopoietic Stem Cell Transplantation can be considered for highly selected with younger patients who have complicated advanced disease. Finding of JAK2 V617 F mutation stimulate the targeted therapy against mutant form of kinase. [23]
7. Anti-platelet agents Aspirin (and not warfarin) is highly effective adjunctive therapy in essential thrombocythaemia, in cases of digital or cerebrovascular disease, but can cause prolongation of bleeding time and serious bleeding, improve platelet turn over and clinical symptoms of erythromeralgia. Low dose aspirin (100 mg/day) effectively reduces thrombotic complications. However, its use is still controversial. [25]

REFERENCES

1. Schafer AI: *Thrombocytosis*: New Engl J Med 350:121, (2004).
2. Ruggeri M, Toscetto A, Frezzalo II, Podeghireo F: *The rate of progression to polycythaemia vera or essential thrombocythaemia in patients with erythocytosis or thrombocytosis*. Ann Intern Med 139:470, (2003).
3. Kenjo K, MiyakawaY Uchilide H et al. *All Trans-retinoic acid directly up regulates thrombopoietin transcription in bone marrow stromal cells*. Exp. Haematol 32:45, (2001).
4. Ding J, Kasanatu H, Waika et al. *Familial essential thrombocythaemia associated with one base deletion in the 5' untranslated region of thrombopoietin gene*. Blood 921091, (1998).
5. Weistener A, Schlemper RJ, Van Den Meas APC, Skoda RC: *An activating splice donor mutation in the thrombopoietin gene causing hereditary thrombocytosis*. Nat Genet 18: 49, (1998).
6. De Gugliemo G: *Erithileukaemia e piastinemia*. Folie Med 1:36, (1920).
7. Epstein E, Goedel A: *Haemorrhagischie Thromboerythaemic bie Vaskutaner SchrumptmilzVirchows*: Arch Pathol Anat Physiol Klin Med 292:233, (1934).
8. Ozer Fl, Truax WE, Miesch DC, Levin WC: *Primary haemorrhagic thrombocythaemia*. Am J Med 28:807, (1960).
9. Fiaklow PJ, Faguet GB, Jacoben RJ et al. *Evidence that essential thrombocythaemia is a clonal disorder with origin in a multipotent stem cell*. Blood 58:916, (1987).
10. Teofilli L, Pierconti F, Difebo A et al. *The expression pattern of c-mpl in megakaryocytes correlates with thrombotic risk in essential thrombocythaemia*. Blood 100:714, (2002).
11. Lier E, Jelinek J, Pastore Yd et al. *Discrimination of polycythaemia and thrombocytosis by novel, simple, accurate clonality assays and comparision with PRV-1 expression and BFU-E response to erythropoietin*. Blood 101:3294, (2003).
12. Ogawa M, *Cellular Mchanisms of myeloproliferative syndrome*. Brit J Haematol 58:563, (1964).

13. Johansen P, Rick Stein A, Wennstormt et al. *Increased risk for vascular complications in PRV-1 positive patients with essential thrombocythaemia*. Brit J Haematol 123:513, (2003).

14. Hoaguland Hc, Silverstein MN: *Primary thrombocythaemia in the young patient*. Mayo clinic Proc. 53: 578, (1978).

15. Reisner SA, Rinerich D, Markiurez W, et al. *Cardiac involvement in patients with myeloproliferative disorders*. Am J Med 93:498, (1992).

16. George TI, Arber DA: *WHO Extended Criteria to bone marrow findings: Pathology of myeloproliferative diseases*. Haematol Oncol Clin North Med 17: 1101, (2003).

17. Finazzi G, Ruggeri M, Rodeghireo F, Barbni T: *Efficacy and safety of long term use of hydroxyurea in young patients with essential thrombocythaemia and a high risk of thrombosis*. Blood 101:3749, (2003).

18. Michiells JJ: *Erythromeralgia and vascular complications in polycythaemia vera*. Semin Thromb Haemostat 23:441, (1997).

19. Kesler A, Ellis MH, Manor Y et al. *Neurological complications of essential thrombocythaemia (ET)*. Acta Neurol Scand 105:299, (2000).

20. Vantroyen B, Vanstaclen D: *Management of essential thrombocythaemia during pregnancy with aspirin, interferon alpha and no treatment. A comparative analysis of the literature*. Acta Haemato 1107:156, (2002).

21. Thiele J, Krasmicka Hm, Fuchs N et al. *Anagrelide induced bone marrow changes during therapy of chronic myeloproliferative disorders with thrombocytosis: An immunohistochemical and morphometric study of sequential. Trephine biopsies*. Haematologica 88:1130, (2003).

22. Ludwig AH, Linkesh W, Gisslinger Het al. *Interferon alpha corrects thrombocytosis in patients with myeloproliferative disorders*. Cancer Immunol Immunother 25:206, (1987).

23. Jurado m, Deeg H, Goody M et al. *Haemopoietic stem cell transplantation for advanced polycythaemia vera and essential thrombocythaemia*. Brit J Haematol 112:392, (2001).

Part VI

Miscellaneous

CHAPTER

18 Transfusion Medicine

18.1 HISTORY

The transfusion therapy began as early as 1665 when the first transfusion was effected from dog-to-dog. In 1667, first transfusion was done by Jean Dennus in Paris, using lamb blood and curiously enough the transfusion was free from any adverse effect. Unfortunately, the fourth patient, transfused in this way, experienced a reaction and died after 2 years. Though, ultimately, the death, being investigated by a court of law, was declared to be due to arsenic poisoning by his wife, the transfusion fell into disrepute and was disapproved by law.

The modern medicine of transfusion started in 1818, when Landsteiner discovered the blood group ABO system. The idea of modern Blood Bank was born in 1914 when Hustin discovered citrate as anticoagulant, and when in 1915 Weisley introduced the use of refrigerated blood. The knowledge of transfusion went into a footstep further with the discovery of Blood Group Rho system, by Landsteiner and Weiner, in 1940. Blood component therapy began with plasma transfusion by Strumula and McGraw in 1941. The Modern Blood Bank was born in 1943 when Loulit and Mollison introduced ACD as a preservative.

18.2 ETHICAL ASPECTS

Consideration of blood transfusion from ethical point of view must be done as blood is a component of human body, as it is a limited resource, and as blood transfusion is associated with several intrinsic hazards that are being increasingly recognized. During the Second World War, the growing need of blood transfusion became well established. After the war was over, several guidelines have been formulated.

18.3 SAFE BLOOD TRANSFUSION

Recent advancements in blood transfusion are due to improved method of donor selection, screening for infectious diseases by modern tests, and separation of different components of blood, which are safer than whole blood transfusion. [1] Blood bank regulations impose collection of blood from 'safe' donors who are free from risk of adverse medical events. For this purpose haemoglobin percentage of the donor should be equal to or above 11 gm%, and the donor must be free from hepatitis, HIV infection, human T-lymphocytic virus (HTLV-1; HTLV-2) infection. Blood Bank procedures require testing for hepatitis B surface antigen, core antigen, and test for syphilis [2]. A new research test, nucleic acid test (NAT) is now being performed, on all blood donations, for hepatitis C and HIV. This test shortens the period between onset of infection and positive test.

18.4 TYPES OF BLOOD DONATION

I. Autologous Blood Donation

It involves collection and subsequent re-infusion of a patient's own blood. This can be done in three ways. [3]

(a) Preoperative blood transfusion

Preoperative blood collection should begin at least 2 weeks before a scheduled surgical procedure and can be repeated every 3 days provided the patient's haemoglobin level remains above 11 gm%.

(b) Perioperative blood salvage

This procedure involves blood collected at the time of surgery. The blood is then anti-coagulated, washed using semi-automated equipment and re-infused to the patient. Cell salvage is not done if operative field is likely to be contaminated with tumor or bacteria. Post-operative cell salvage involves collection of defibrinated blood through catheter inserted into joint spaces, the mediastinum, and filtration of the same followed by transfusion of the blood to the same patient, from whom it is collected.

(c) Normovolaemic haemodilution

Blood is removed immediately before surgery with simultaneous infusion of crystalloid or colloid solutions to replenish intravascular volume. Following surgery, the removed blood is re-infused. This procedure is of growing need and soon has to be combined with infusion of blood substitute.

II. Directed or Designated Blood Donation

It involves donation by patient's relative or friend according to his choice. These are no safer than those provided by motivated volunteer donor.

III. Apheresis Donation

By this process more than one type of products are collected from one donation process, using blood cell seperator. Certain donors can donate 2U of RBC by Apheresis technique and then donation can be deferred for 16 weeks instead of normal 8 weeks.

Apheresis technique is useful in the sense that:

1. The technique allows the collection of a red cell and a platelet product at the same donation.
2. It produces collection of plasma as a single separate product or in combination with a red cell or a platelet product.
3. One greatest advantage of this Apheresis technique is the collection of a platelet concentrate containing a therapeutic dose of platelets obtained from a single donor. These platelets are transfused as platepheresis or single donor's platelets (SDP). If donor's human leukocyte antigen (HLA) type is similar to the patient, the SDP is considered to be HLA matched.

4. Cell separators are also of use to collect granulocytes for transfusion by leukopheresis technique and can be used for collection of peripheral blood stem cells for autologous transplant. There is also growing need of the technique in allogenic transplant.

After collection of blood it is subjected to following tests:

1. ABO and RH typing.
2. Patient's serum is tested for alloantibody; the corresponding antibody screening is done in the blood cells to be transfused.
3. Test for screening of viruses, such as HBV, HCV, HIV, as well as spirochetes and malaria parasites should be done according to necessity.
4. Haemoglobin in gm% as well as, serum SGPT level should be estimated.

18.5 STORAGE OF BLOOD AND BLOOD COMPONENTS

The anticoagulant preservative solution for storage of whole blood comprises of citrate, phosphate, dextrose (CPD). Citrate acts as the anticoagulant and the phosphate-dextrose as the preservative. Depending on the type of solution used, red cells may be stored for 21, 35 or 42 days at 1–6 °C, whole blood may be stored for 21 – 35 days.

Anticoagulant-preservative solution that contains dextrose, mannitol, adenine in 100 ml of saline can reduce the haematocrit of red cells by 55% while improving the flow characteristics similar to whole blood. Red cells or whole blood that is subjected to gamma irradiation to prevent post-transfusion graft-versus-host disease has a limited half-life of 28 days after irradiation but no longer than the originally assigned expiration date.

Depending upon the plastic container used to store platelet concentrates, the dating period of room temperature-stored random platelets varies between 72 hours to 5 days.

Granulocyte concentrates are generally stored at room temperature for up to 24 hours. FFP and cryoprecipitate are stored at 18 °C or colder for 1 year.

Three types of preservatives are used as follows:

1. Acid-Citrate-Dextrose (ACD-A) 330 ml
2. Citrate-Phosphate-Dextrose (CPD) 130 ml
3. Mannitol-Adenine-Phosphate (MAP) 200 ml

TABLE 18.1: Storage Temperature of Different Blood Components

Blood: Whole blood/Blood component	Temperature
Whole Blood/RBC	4 – 6° C
Fresh Frozen Plasma	–20° C
Platelets (Should be kept being stirred and shaken)	20 – 24 °C (at room temperature) (Should be transfused as soon as possible)

Storage Period

Depending on the type of anticoagulant-preservative solution, the blood may be preserved for 21, 35, 42 days at 1–6 °C.

18.6 EFFECT OF STORAGE ON BLOOD COMPONENTS

During the storage of RBC, the Ph, adenosine diphosphates (ATP), 2,3 disphospoglycerate (2,3 DPG) levels fall. Plasma potassium levels increase, so that at the end of expiration, there is approximately a total of 8–10 mEq of potassium in each red cell. Plasma haemoglobin levels also increase slightly during storage but do not give plasma a pinkish tinge. Posttransfusional haemoglobinuria does not occur as a result of haemolysis during storage. Irradiated RBCs have plasma potassium levels that are approximately 1.5–2 times higher than non-irradiated units. 2,3 DPG levels decrease significantly during storage falling to 50% of initial level by 7 days. Restoration of 2,3 DPG levels occur within 7 hours of transfusion. The most significant impact on platelets stored for 5 days is a slight increased risk of bacterial contamination as bacteria proliferate during storage. FFP has approximately normal levels of all coagulation factors, including the labile factor V and VII.

18.7 DETERMINATION OF COMPATIBILITY

This is the essential preliminary step for blood transfusion. Compatibility test is done for whole blood and RBC transfusions but not for FFP, cryoprecipitate, or platelet transfusion. In general, platelet concentrates should be ABO compatible, although it is not possible to provide the product in this way. Granulocyte concentrates contain red cells and require compatibility testing.

Procedure

1. ABO and Rh type is determined on both the patient's blood sample and the donor unit.
2. Compatibility testing involves donor and recipient ABO and Rh types, performing the "antibody screen" for unexpected red cell alloantibodies.
3. An actual cross match between recipient serum and donor RBC is done. Antibody screen is important because it may cause haemolytic transfusion reaction.
4. If unexpected alloantibodies are present, RBCs are selected that lack the antigen. In a "STAT" administration situation, a fully cross matched sample of blood can be ready to send to the floor in approximately 45 minutes from the time blood samples are received to the blood bank. As a general rule, approximately 1% of hospitalized patients and 10% of multiple transfused patients have alloantibodies.

If blood is needed in an acute emergency, type O red cells (universal donor), usually Rh negative, may be used prior to determining patient's ABO type. Type specific RBC may be provided after ABO and Rh type of the patient are determined on a concurrent blood sample. The physician ordering emergency blood must consider the possible benefit of blood transfusion against the risk of infusion of potentially incompatible blood. Proper identification of attended patient and verification of written information on the container are essential to prevent potential hazards of major haemolytic blood transfusion reaction.

18.8 SOME PRACTICAL HINTS FOR BLOOD TRANSFUSION

Equipment

Blood and its components must be infused through a 19-gauge or larger needle and through a 23-gauge needle for paediatric patients to ensure free flow and to prevent haemolysis. All components must pass through a filter that should have a pore size of 170 micro m. The same blood filter should not be used for more than 4 hours.

Warmer

Blood warmers are indicated to prevent cardiac arrhythmia and cardiac arrest. Warmers should have visual and audible alarm system. Warmers are specially indicated during massive transfusion, exchange transfusion or in patients with cold agglutinin disease. Blood bags should not be held under tap water or immersed in unmonitored water bath or heated in microwave oven. Blood that has been warmed but not used should be discarded.

Infusion rate

The infusion rate must be 5 ml/min for first 15 minutes. Serious reactions frequently occur during first 50 ml of transfusion. If no complications occur during this period the flow may be increased, depending on the clinical situation. Routinely one unit of red cells should be infused within 2 to 3 hours but not over 4 hours. If patient's condition is such that it needs more hours then one unit should be subdivided into aliquots. This is needed when circulatory overload is a concern. Granulocytes should be infused within 4 hours. Cryoprecipitate must be infused within 6 hours of thawing or within 4 hours if the units are pooled.

Addition of drugs and solutions

Drugs or medications should not be added to blood. Only normal saline may be added, however.

18.9 GUIDELINES FOR BLOOD TRANSFUSION

1. *Identification of the blood* bottle must be done, by the attending physician and the ward sister separately by comparing the expiry date, blood group, batch number, noted on the label of the container, on the cross-match slip.
2. *Physical examination of the blood, to be transfused give some important clues* e.g. pinkish tinge is evidence of haemolysis, or clot formation indicates inappropriate preservation.
3. *Inspection of the container* for any leak is mandatory before transfusion.
4. *Identification of the patient,* by interrogating the relatives or attendants, especially if he/she is comatose or anaesthetized.
5. *Record of the particulars of patient and blood bag must be done* on the bed head ticket.
6. In cases of *identical or similar names*, other parameters (date of birth, ID number) should be noted.
7. Only one blood transfusion should be dealt with at a time.

Stored blood must be kept for several minutes at room temperature before transfusion. Ideally a blood warmer with alarm system should be used to bring the blood to room temp. This is to prevent cardiac arrest or cardiac arrhythmia due to cold blood transfusion.

18.10 OBSERVATIONS DURING AND AFTER BLOOD TRANSFUSION

1. **During first 5 minutes**

   The patient should be observed for appearance of chest pain, abdominal pain, or pain at the injection site, any discomfort or respiratory distress. Transfusion of red blood cells must be slow. Rapid transfusion may be needed for emergency patients. Accordingly signs of haemolysis such as change of urine colour or bleeding from the operation field should be noted at frequent intervals, along with cardiovascular or respiratory status.
2. **During next 15 minutes**

   Signs of anaphylactic or allergic reaction such as fever or urticaria should be noted.
3. The patient's blood specimen in the pilot tube should be preserved at 4°C for at least 1–2 weeks or for 2–3 months if possible, so that investigations can be done in cases of adverse reactions.

18.11 INDICATIONS OF BLOOD TRANSFUSION

1. **Objectives**
   (i) To supply sufficient oxygen to the peripheral circulation and to the vital organs.
   (ii) To maintain circulating blood volume.
2. **Goal**
   (i) To achieve Haemoglobin (Hb) level of about 7 gm/dl.
3. **Immediate indications**
   (i) Acute and chronic bleeding specially from G.I. tract and genitourinary tract.
   (ii) Rapid correction of anemia in aplastic, myelodysplastic, or malignant transformation of haemopoietic system.

Monitoring

1. Clinical improvement is the guide of effectiveness of blood transfusion.
2. Rise of Haemoglobin level above 10 gm/dl is undesirable and unnecessary.
3. Too frequent administration of blood may produce iron overload in chronic anemia.
4. Longest feasible interval should be allowed in such cases.
5. Blood transfusion should be withheld when the condition is likely to respond to Iron, Vitamin B_{12}, or Erythropoietin and should not be done until the effect of the drug is fully exerted. [4]
6. Transfusion should be continued to maintain the systolic B. P. 90 mm Hg or above and mean B.P. 60–70 mm Hg or above and urine output 0.5–1 ml/kg/hour, in cases of hypo-volaemic shock. [4]
7. It is recommended to keep Haemoglobin level below 10 gm/dl in patients with cardiopulmonary or cerebrovascular disease. Sufficient oxygen supply is usually possible when haemoglobin level is 7–8 gm/dl in patients without serious cardiopulmonary disease. [4]

Amount of Transfusion Required

This should be judged on

(i) age of the patient,

(ii) body weight,

(iii) presence of active bleeding,

(iv) patient's cardiopulmonary function and the underlying disease process (benign or malignant).

18.12 EFFECTIVE BLOOD FUNCTION

Haemoglobin level elevation is determined by the following formula:

Predicted elevation of Hb level (gm/dl) = Hb content of volume administered (gm) / Circulating Blood Volume (dl), CBV being = BW (kg) × 70 ml /kg /100.

Haematocrit (Hct) should increase by 3% and haemoglobin level should increase by 1 gm/dl after 1 unit of blood transfusion.

18.13 BLOOD COMPONENTS

Blood transfusion may be given in the following forms:

1. Whole Blood
2. RBC
3. Fresh Frozen Plasma
4. Platelets
5. Granulocytes
6. Coagulation Factors

Each one has its own indications, merits and hazards. The following few paragraphs will describe them one by one.

Whole Blood

Composition

Whole blood contains red cells, plasma proteins, stable clotting factors (reduced factor V and VII) and 70 ml of anticoagulant preservative solution. The haematocrit is approximately 35 to 40%. Platelets and granulocytes are non-viable. The period of expiration is 21–35 days, depending on the anti-coagulant preservative solution.

Indications

Whole blood is indicated when replenishment of both of oxygen carrying capacity and blood volume are needed. Specific indications are massive transfusion required for trauma, major surgical procedure involving massive blood loss, exchange transfusion and organ like liver transplantation.

Dose and infusion rate

It depends on the clinical situation to stabilize the haemodynamic status.

Expected outcome: Symptoms of decreased intravascular volume and anaemia are expected to resolve. The haemoglobin and haematocrit values tend to fluctuate in relationship to fluid shift. In non-bleeding patients, 1 unit of whole blood should increase the haematocrit by 3% and the haemoglobin by 1 g per decilitre.

Red Blood Cells

The vast majority of red cells are prepared by centrifugation of whole blood and supplementation with an additive solution of 100 ml of normal saline, additional dextrose and adenine. The final haematocrit is about 55% and the storage period is 42 days. The volume of red cells with additive solution is approximately 300–350 ml (55–64 gm. of haemoglobin). The red cells may be also collected in CPD or CPDA-1 anticoagulant preservative solutions that give them a 21 to 35 days expiration period. These products can have an approximate 250 ml volume and a haematocrit between 65% and 80% (55–64 gm. of haemoglobin).

Leukocyte reduced red blood cell

Filtration is the most efficient method of removing leukocytes from red cells. Adhesion on third generation leukocyte reduction filters removes at least 99.9% of leukocytes from red cell preparations. Storage shortly after blood collection is the growing method of producing leukocyte reduced red cells. Less efficient methods are centrifugation, washing, or freezing and subsequently washing them. Leukocyte reduced red cells should contain at least 85% of original red cells and should have a leukocyte content of less than 5×10^6 WBC. [5]

Washed red cells

Washed red cells are produced by adding normal saline to red cells and by using semi-automated machine to wash cells with saline and remove almost all the plasma. 90–99% of leukocytes are removed by this process. The RBC volume is approximately 250 ml with a residual haematocrit of approximately 65–80% (55–64 gm of haemoglobin) with the product being suspended in saline rather than plasma.

Frozen red cells

In the presence of a cryoprotective agent, red cells may be stored in the frozen state for up to 10 years at a temperature of at least –65°C. Following thawing the cryoprotective agent is removed by saline washing and the product is suspended in normal saline.

Irradiated red cells

Red cells and other cellular components are subjected to a minimum of 2500 cGy gamma irradiation. The cells may be stored up to 28 days after irradiation but no longer than the original expiration date.

Indications

In general red cell transfusion is indicated when the need for increasing oxygen carrying capacity of blood exists in presence of severe anaemia but there is no need for volume expansion, which my rather produce more harmful effect like volume expansion and consequent heart failure. In earlier time clinicians preset haemoglobin level as 'transfusion trigger'. Currently symptoms and signs of anaemia (like tachycardia, anginal pain, fatigue, syncope, signs of cerebral hypoxia) in conjunction with low haemoglobin- haematocrit level, are gaining importance in determining requirement of transfusion. In other words, while searching for the cause of anaemia, transfusion is deferred till compensatory mechanism becomes insufficient to ameliorate symptoms and signs of anaemia. Most patients can tolerate haemoglobin concentration of 7–9 gm per decilitre without the need for transfusion. In patients with significant cardiovascular disease or pulmonary disease or in elderly patients with cerebrovascular insufficiency symptoms and signs may develop at higher haemoglobin level of 4–6 gm per decilitre. Patients with diseases that would respond to iron, Vitamin B_{12}, folic acid, or Erythropoietin, these should be prescribed in adequate dose before transfusion is attempted (unless patient's condition warrants so.)

Leukocyte reduced red cells

Leukocyte reduced red cells are required in three different clinical conditions. These are:

1. In patients receiving multiple transfusions to reduce allo-immunization against HLA-antigen. This is especially required in patients with acute leukaemia or aplastic anaemia, where bone marrow transplant may be required.
2. Prevention of non-haemolytic febrile transfusion reaction.
3. Prevention of post-transfusion Cytomegalovirus (CMV) infection, which may reside in leukocytes. There is a growing trend toward universal pre-storage leukocyte reduction.

Washed red cells

Their use is indicated to reduce the incidence of anaphylactic and allergic reaction, as the process removes the plasma protein including Immunoglobulin A which is implicated in these reactions.

Irradiated red cells

These are required in significantly immunosuppressed patients, who are at risk for graft versus host disease following transfusion. Such patients include bone marrow transplant patients, both allogenic and autologous; Patients treated with high dose chemotherapy, patients with Hodgkin and non-Hodgkin lymphoma, congenital immunodeficiency disorders, low birth weight neonates, and those receiving intrauterine transfusion. Because of rare occurrence of GVH disease, when a blood relative donates as a directed donation, such units are also irradiated. Once the decision of irradiation is made, all cellular components should be irradiated.

Dose and infusion rate

In a stable clinical condition, 1 unit of blood is transfused over 2–4 hours.

Expected outcome

Symptoms of anaemia should resolve following transfusion. The haematocrit should increase by 3% and the haemoglobin by 1 gm per decilitre in non-bleeding adult patient for each unit of blood transfused.

Platelets are available in thee forms:

Random donor platelets (RDP)

Platelet concentrates are prepared by separating platelets from a single unit of whole blood so that a minimum 5.5×10^{10} platelets are suspended in approximately 50 ml of plasma (I.U.). Platelets should be separated from whole blood within 8 hours of collection. Depending on the container in which RDP are stored, the shelf life varies from 3–5 days when stored at room temperature.

Pheresis-Apheresis platelets or single donor platelets (SDPs)

Platelets collected by Apheresis technique from a single donor, using blood cell seperator, contain a minimum of 3.5×10^{11} platelets suspended in 200–400 ml of plasma. Apheresis platelets have a shelf life ranging from 24 hours to 5 days and are stored at room temperature.

HLA- matched platelet-concentrates

If the donor of an Apheresis platelet concentrate is selected because the donor's HLA type is matched to the recipient's HLA type, the Apheresis platelet product is considered to be HLA-matched platelet component.

Indications of platelet transfusion

1. To prevent or to control bleeding, when the platelet count is deficient or their functions are defective.

   Platelets are used in haematological malignancy, when the platelet count is 10,000 to 20,000 per micro litre, in the course of the disease or as an effect of chemotherapy. [6]
2. Patients who are undergoing minor surgical procedure or having a line replacement may require the platelet count to be greater than 50,000 per micro litre before the procedure.
3. Patients who are undergoing major surgical procedure may require platelet count greater than 75, 000 per micro litre.
4. Patients, who are undergoing neurological or ophthalmological procedure may require 100,000 per micro litre of platelets before the procedure.
5. There is a growing trend of reducing the prophylactic platelet transfusion to counts as low as 5000 – 10000 per micro litre in asymptomatic patients.

As demonstrated in a recent multi-institutional national trial, the incidence of refractoriness is similar when RDP or SDP are used. Leucocyte reduction decreases the occurrence of allo-immunization. [7]

HLA-matched platelets are used when an immunological basis for refractoriness to platelet transfusion is suspected on clinical ground as in autoimmune disease but not indicated when refractoriness is due to some other pathological processes e.g. sepsis, endotoxic shock, disseminated intravascular coagulation [8].

Dose and Infusion Rate of Platelet Transfusion

The platelet units are usually pooled into one bag by the transfusion service prior to infusion. They should be transfused within 4 hours at a rate that depends on patient's ability to tolerate the volume. RDP may be 'volume reduced' by centrifugation of pooled platelets from the platelet poor plasma. Excess platelet poor plasma is discarded and therapeutic dose is then concentrated to 100 ml. Volume reduced platelet can be transfused more rapidly than normo-volaemic platelets and should be transfused within 4 hours of pooling. The average adult platelet concentrate dose is one unit of RDP per 12 kilogram of body weigh. One SDP concentrate is equivalent to 6 units of RDP. Dose and infusion rate of HLA-matched platelet are similar to those of SDP.

Follow-up after platelet transfusion:

As a general rule, platelet count should be done 18 to 24 hours post-infusion. An average sized adult who receives 1 unit of RDP per 12 kg of BW or one SDP dose should have a post-infusion platelet increment of 30,000 to 50,000 per micro litre. [9] Patients who have smaller or no increment at 18 to24 hours, should have platelet count done at 10–60 minutes after next platelet infusion. If

10–50 minutes platelet count is minimal or not increased at all, the possibility of refractoriness caused by allo-immunization should be entertained. The patient should then be considered for HLA-matched platelet transfusion. Patients who have life threatening haemorrhage or who have bleeding after a major surgical procedure in association with thrombocytopenia, may require larger platelet dose. Whether extra large dose platelet infusion is better than repetitive small dose infusion is under recent randomized controlled study.

Relative merits and demerits of platelet infusion

The underlying cause of thrombocytopenia is important in this respect.

1. Thrombocytopenia secondary to bone marrow failure: The patients are most likely to be benefited from platelet transfusion if they suffer from bone marrow suppression due to chemotherapy, radiotherapy, or myelodysplastic diseases.
2. Thrombocytopenia due to platelet destruction: Patients who are thrombocytopenic due to platelet destruction or consumption are not much benefited by platelet transfusion. They should not be given platelet transfusion unless there is life threatening haemorrhage. Such conditions are idiopathic thrombocytopenic purpura, drug induced immune thrombocytopenia, thrombotic thrombocytopenic purpura, and post-transfusion purpura. The recovery and survival of infused platelets are diminished in these conditions. Some consider the use of platelet transfusion in the setting of thrombotic thrombocytopenic purpura may be hazardous and is therefore, a relative contraindication of platelet transfusion.
3. Thrombocytopenia due to splenomegaly and hypersplenism may not improve with platelet transfusion, as infused platelets may be sequestered and destroyed in the spleen.
4. Dilutional thrombocytopenia: Patients who receive massive transfusion develop thrombocytopenia as platelets are lost with haemorrhage. This does not improve with infusion of concentrated RBC or whole blood transfusion, which is devoid of viable platelets. In these patients platelet transfusion is essential to maintain platelet count and haemostasis thereby.

Compatibility of platelets

A and B antigens are expressed on platelet surface. So testing for ABO compatibility of donor and recipient is essential before platelet transfusion. When ABO compatible platelets are not available, the post transfusion platelet increment may be lower due to use of ABO incompatible platelets. If plasma is ABO incompatible with the patient, volume reduced platelet transfusion should be considered because haemolytic reactions have been reported infrequently, when blood group A or B patients have received group O platelets containing Anti-A or Anti-B antibody in the plasma.

Rh antigens are not present on platelet surface but are present in trace amounts on red cells that contaminate platelet concentrates. For this reason Rh-compatible platelets are essential for girls or women of child bearing age. Administration of Rh immunoglobulin should be considered for Rh negative patients who receive platelets from Rh-positive donors, especially for female children or women of child bearing age.

Fresh Frozen Plasma

Fresh frozen plasma (FFP) is the plasma which is separated from whole blood within 8 hours of collection and has normal levels of all coagulation factors and anticoagulants. Three different forms of FFP are available for transfusion, which are as follows:

1. **Donor retested FFP**

   It is the plasma that is donated, frozen and stored for 112 days. The donor then returns and if tests for all infectious diseases are still negative, the original unit is then released to inventory. This type of plasma has the value of closing the window period for the infectious diseases that are currently tested for Hepatitis B, HIV, and Hepatitis C.

2. **Pooled solvent detergent-treated plasma**

   It is frozen and sent for the special treatment which will prevent transmission of envelope viruses *i.e.*, HIV, HCV viruses. It is a pooled product and recipients are exposed to1500–2500 donors with each transfusion of a unit of frozen plasma.

   Indications of fresh frozen plasma transfusion

3. The first and foremost requirement of FFP is the replacement of clotting factors in patients with demonstrable deficiency of coagulation factors (*e.g.*, prothrombin time greater than 1.5 times of normal and INR > 1.6) Most common use is acquired coagulopathy as in liver disease, DIC, or warfarin treated patients who are actively bleeding or undergoing an emergency surgery, as vitamin K takes 12 hours to be effective.

4. FFP is the preferred replacement fluid for patients undergoing therapeutic plasma exchange for thrombotic thrombocytopenic purpura. Recent evidence suggests that FFP supplies a metalloproteinase that is deficient in these patients. Cryo-poor plasma is a FFP variant in which cryoprecipitate fraction containing von Willebrand fraction is removed. This plasma is also used in the treatment of thrombotic thrombocytopenic purpura.

5. FFP is also indicated when plasma albumin is deficient as in cirrhosis of liver. In this condition it replenishes the albumin, restores the plasma oncotic pressure, and reduces the burden of ascites and oedema, though human albumin is also available, but it is more expensive than FFP.

   Dose and infusion rate

   The average adult dose is determined by the underlying disease process and clinical situation.

   It is reasonable to administer plasma at a dose of 10–15 ml per kg of BW (2–4 units of FFP) followed by laboratory evaluation to determine responsiveness and to decide the interval between the doses. The infusion rate is determined by patient's clinical need and haemodynamics status. [10]

ABO compatibility

Plasma does not contain red cells therefore, transfusion doesn't need cross matching. The ABO type of the donor should be compatible with the recipient, however. FFP is thawed at 37C and must be transfused within 24 hours of thawing, if coagulation factors are to be supplied. Plasma can be thawed and maintained in the refrigerated state for 5 days but there is some loss of factor V and a greater decrease of factor VII.

Expected outcome

Clinical improvement as well as improvement of deficient factor, as assessed by laboratory tests, is found within few days.

Cryoprecipitate

It is the concentrate of plasma containing some specific coagulation factors. Each bag of cryoprecipitate is prepared from 1 unit of whole blood, the volume varying from 5–20 ml per bag.

Each bag contains more than 80 units of factor VII, vWF, more than 150 mg of fibrinogen, small amounts of factor XIII and fibronectin.

Indications

1. Cryoprecipitate is the only available source of fibrinogen in a concentrated form.
2. The other significant use of cryoprecipitate is as fibrin sealant in major surgical procedure.
3. Use of cryoprecipitate in Haemophilia and Von Willebrand disease, is now superseded by new and safer factor VIII concentrates, as these are freed from viral load by inactivation procedure.

Dose and infusion rate

The dose is calculated on the basis of plasma volume. Most patients with fibrinogen levels of more than 125 mg per decilitre, have an adequate amount of fibrinogen to form clot In general, 12 bags of cryoprecipitate should result in an increment of 100 mg per decilitre of fibrinogen in a 70 kg adult. Patient's toleration usually determines the rate of infusion, which is as high as possible.

ABO compatibility

The test is not essential as no RBC is present and only a small volume of plasma is present. Cryoprecipitate should be transfused within 6 hours of thawing.

Follow-up

Fibrinogen level should be determined before and after transfusion to determine the effectiveness of therapy and the need and timing of further transfusion.

Coagulation Factors

The following coagulation factors are in current use:

(1) Factor VIII (2) Factor IX (3) Antithrombin III (AT III) (4) Factor VIIa.

Factor VIII concentrate

Factor VIII concentrates are prepared from human plasma, inactivated for virus like hepatitis B, C or HIV. Such treatment does not inactivate Hepatitis A or parvovirus. Recently recombinant factor VIII concentrates have come into the market and replaced human derived factor VIII. All newly detected patients of Haemophilia are subjected to recombinant products rather than human derived products because of safety from infectious agent. Several human derived factor concentrate also contain von Willebrand factor to treat patients with von Willebrand disease. This product contains a relatively normal distribution of factor VIII of high molecular weight. The number of units of factor VIII contained in each vial of factor VIII concentrates is stated on the product label. This is also so for the products which are used to treat von Willebrand disease. [11]

Dose and infusion rate

The amount required depends on whether the treatment is prophylactic or for active bleeding or bleeding has occurred, the extent and site of the bleeding. Approximately 30–40% of factor VIII levels are recommended to treat haemorrhage in the joints, and approximately 100% factor VIII levels are appropriate for patients undergoing major surgery or suffering central nervous system injury. Infusion of 1 gm of factor VIII increases its level by 2%. The infusion should occur at a rate as fast as tolerated and should be repeated every 12 hours to maintain adequate concentration for haemostasis. The duration of therapy depends on the clinical setting.

Expected outcome

Haemostasis should occur and as a result of increased level of factor VIII or von Willebrand factor. Laboratory response should be done to determine the adequacy of response and to calculate the timing of the next dose.

Factor IX concentrate

Factor IX concentrare is now available as a recombinant factor IX product. The amount is stated on product label. Factor IX is also available, as a product of intermediate purity, which is a prothrombin complex concentrate. Recombinant factor IX is the product of choice for newly diagnosed patients of Haemophilia B. Activated prothrombin complex concentrate (FEIBA and AUTOPLEX) are available to treat haemophilic patients with inhibitors of factor VIII. This use is gradually declining, as recombinant factor VIIIa is now available for such treatment. The amount of factor IX contained in the concentrate is stated on the product label.

Dose and infusion rate

In general, infusion of 1 unit of factor IX per kg of BW increases the factor IX level by 1%.

The infusion rate should be as fast as tolerated. A slightly higher dose is needed when recombinant factor IX is infused.

Expected outcome

Haemostasis should occur and laboratory testing should be performed as and when required. It helps in determining time and dose of next transfusion.

Antithrombin III concentrates (AT-III)

Heat-treated and lypholised preparation of human derived AT-III, are available.

Indications

This product is used in congenital AT-III deficiency in connection with surgical or obstetric procedure, for therapeutic control of thromboembolic events because it serves as an important antithrombotic plasma protein. The product is also used in acquired AT III deficiency as in DIC or resistance to heparin therapy from AT III deficiency. The efficacy of this product in these conditions has not been firmly established. [12]

Dose and infusion rate

The dose is calculated on the basis of the site of the bleeding and underlying clinical condition. The dose is designed to have post-transfusion AT III level of approximately 120%. Subsequent dose should maintain the level of 80% to 120% and will need to be determined by measuring AT III levels at periodic intervals.

Prevention of occurrence and recurrence of thrombosis is expected after infusion of this product.

Factor VIIIa concentrate

Haemophilia A and B are treatable with plasma derived as well as recombinant factor VIII and factor IX. Recombinant factors are free from human blood derived diseases. However, a life threatening complication is development of neutralizing antibodies against the missing factor. Up to 25% of patients develop inhibitor of factor VIII and 3–5% of patients develop antibodies to factor IX. Some of the therapeutic options are use of large amount of factor VIII, plasmapheresis with or without adsorption of antibody, use of activated and non-activated prothrombin complex. All these interventions are prohibitive due to high cost, unpredictability of response and transmission of blood derived diseases.

Recombinant factor VII (rFVIIa) is a potential solution to this problem for treating haemophilic patients with inhibitors. Moreover, this product may be a valuable general haemostatic agent for non-haemophilic bleeding episode.

Although the mechanism is not clear, some studies indicate that thrombin generation on activated platelets due to high level of rF VIIa binding to platelet surface. It acts by enhancing natural coagulation pathway by activating formation of prothrombinase complex and has a local action only in areas where tissue factor and/ or phospholipids are exposed. At pharmacological doses, rFVIIa by passes conventional steps in coagulation cascade and directly generates a thrombin burst on the activated platelets at the site of injury, leading to generation of a stabilized fibrin plug. This has the advantage of limiting the extent of its activity to areas of injury and thus minimizing the thromboembolic phenomena. [13]

Indications

1. Recently rFVIIa has been used successfully to control bleeding in association with surgical procedure, in critically ill trauma patients, who have to undergo major operation. In these cases hypothermia, anaesthesia, and metabolic acidosis produce a perpetuating vicious cycle of coagulopathy. Failure may be due to overwhelming shock. [14]
2. There are some reports demonstrating the efficacy of rFVII in controlling intra-abdominal bleeding during liver surgery or liver transplantation, in which blood loss is more than in any other type of surgery. [15]
3. Spontaneous intracerebral haemorrhage is a condition in which morbidity and mortality depend on the volume of blood lost in the brain parenchyma or ventricle. Recently, one medical intervention ICH group has reported encouraging results that early administration of this factor is associated with reduced haematoma size, improved clinical condition with marginal thromboembolic phenomena. [16]
4. Glanzman's thrombasthenia: It is a rare inherited bleeding disorder due to deficiency or dysfunction of glycoprotein GPIIb-IIIa on platelets. An efficacious alternative regime, than frequent platelet transfusion, which may generate antibodies, is the transfusion of rFVIIa. [17] Practically rFVIIa is licensed for treatment of haemophilia with inhibitor only. Its use in all other indications are under clinical trial.

Dose and infusion rate

This varies with the clinical condition.

1. Average recommended dose in Haemophilia with inhibitor is 90 mcg kg IV bolus every 2 hours or until clinical haemostasis is achieved. The recommended dose in factor VII deficiency is 15–30 mcg/kg every 4–6 hours until haemostasis is achieved.
2. In Glanzman's thrombasthenia, the recommended dose is 15–30 mcg/kg every 4–6 hours until haemostasis is achieved.
3. In critically ill haemorrhagic trauma patients, rFVII dose, administered in various studies, varies from 40–120 mcg/kg to arrest bleeding.
4. In controlling intraoperative bleeding in liver transplant, 70 mcg/kg of rFVIIa has been successfully used.
5. In spontaneous cerebral haemorrhage, reduction of volume of haematoma is found to be proportionately more with increase of dose from 40 mcg/kg to160 mcg/kg.

In general, 90 mcg/kg dose is effective in minor and major bleeding episodes.

Drawbacks of rFVII

Though the clot formation is initiated locally, in two conditions, widespread thrombosis is possible. When tissue factor is up-regulated on surface of circulating monocytes as in endotoxic septicaemia resulting in DIC or when the lipid core of atherosclerotic plaque is exposed at the fissure, the probability of acute thrombus formation or thromboembolic phenomena is, at least theoretically possible. Fortunately such cases are not reported in significant number.

Factor VII is prepared from baby hamster kidney cell line cultured in bovine albumin and is purified with the use of mouse monoclonal antibody, hence should not be used in patients with hypersensitivity to mouse, hamster, or bovine proteins.

Follow-up

The measurement of Factor VII in haemophilic patients with inhibitor related bleeding has led to the recommendation of a minimum level of 6–10 IU/ml and peak level of 30–50 IU/ml of FVII when IV bolus is given.

Immune Globulins

Intravenous and intramuscular preparations of Immune globulins are available. They should contain at least 90% of Immunoglobulin G (IgG) with subclasses in physiological ratio. This maintains biologic activity and fixes complement

Indications

1. Passive immune protection against a number of infectious agents
2. Treatment of hypogammaglobulinaemia

   In these conditions intramuscular preparations are generally used.
3. Immune mediated disorders:
   (a) Gullain-Barre syndrome
   (b) Immune thrombocytopenic purpura
   (c) Post transfusion purpura
   (d) Neonatal alloimmune thrombocytopenic purpura
   (e) Pure red cell aplasia caused by parvo virus infection
4. To rduce the incidence of CMV in patients undergoing various forms of transplantation.
5. In acquired immune deficiency syndrome.

Dose and infusion rate

The dose depends on the underlying clinical condition. In immune thrombocytopenic purpura intravenous immunoglobulin is administered at doses of 2 g per kg of BW in divided doses over 2–5 days. [18]

Expected outcome

The outcome depends on the underlying clinical condition. Adverse effects of this form of therapy include anaphylactic reactions, pyrogenic reactions, like flushing, headache, myalgia, chills, nausea, hypotension, and tachycardia. Several intravenous preparations are reported to be associated with development of renal failure.

Chapter 18

Rh Immunoglobulin

It is a human plasma derived product containing anti-D antibodies against the major antigenic determinant of the Rh system.

Indications

1. It is used as prophylactic measure against anti-D mediated haemolytic disease of newborn.
2. The immunoglobulin is used for prevention against iso-immunisation associated with transfusion of red cells from Rh positive donor to Rh negative recipient.
3. For similar reason, it is used when platelet concentrates are transfused from Rh positive donor to Rh negative recipient.
4. Rh immunoglobulin has been used in idiopathic thrombocytopenic purpura, in patients who are Rh positive. This preparation is not effective in those who are Rh negative, as well as in previously splenectomized patients.

Dose and infusion rate

One vial of intramuscular immunoglobulin is given to prevent iso-immunisation from exposure up to 15 ml of RBCs. It is standard to treat Rh negative pregnant women with Rh immunoglobulin at 28 weeks and following delivery of Rh negative infant. The standard dose at this time is 300. Rh immunoglobulin is also used in miscarriage or bleeding associated with pregnancy when there is concern that there is fetal or neonatal haemorrhage.

Expected outcome

The outcome depends on the condition for which treatment is given. Outstanding records of Rh immunoglobulin are available in prevention of allo-immunization to D antigen.

Fibrin sealants

A recent new fibrin sealant called Tissel has been approved to help control bleeding in certain surgical situations. Tissel is a pooled human plasma product whose active ingredient is fibrinogen. IT is used as a fibrin glue to stop bleeding from small blood vessels during surgery. The product comes as a freeze dried preparation and is applied locally at the site of haemorrhage. [19]

Plasma derived volume expanders (Albumin and plasma protein fraction)

Albumin is available in 5% and 25% solution. In both solutions 98% of total protein is albumin. Plasma protein fraction is available in a 5% solution, of which at least 83% of the protein is albumin and. Not more than17% is globulin. Both of these products are heated for at least 10 hours at 60° C to inactivate contaminated viruses.

Indications

Albumin and plasma protein fractions are infused

1. To meet the demand of urgent restoration of intravascular volume, as in cases of thermal injury within 24 hours, or following large volume paracentesis.
2. For inducing diuresis in patients with nephrotic syndrome, cirrhosis of liver.
3. For patients undergoing therapeutic plasma exchange procedure,
4. For replenishment of body protein as in severe malnutrition, or when total parenteral nutrition is indicated in critically ill patients.

Dose and infusion rate

The volume of crystalloid is two to three times that of a 5% albumin solution to provide equal haemodynamics improvement. The average adult dose depends on the clinical situation. The infusion rate can be more rapid if volume expansion is urgently required. Compatibility testing is not required. Sterile water should not be used to dilute 25% albumin, as haemolysis may occur. [20]

Granulocyte Transfusion

Granulocyte transfusions are obtained by Apheresis technique and should contain a minimum of 1×10^9 granulocytes. Recently by using steroid or Granulocyte-colony-stimulating factor (G-CSF) to stimulate the donor prior to Apheresis technique has resulted in ability to collect 3 to 5 times the number of granulocytes previously obtained by Apheresis technique only. This has allowed for a significant rise in granulocyte count following transfusion and possible greater survival of the granulocytes. Granulocyte concentrate also contain lymphocytes and RBC. The presence of RBCs necessitates that granulocyte transfusion red cell cross matching prior to transfusion. The volume ranges from 200–4000 ml [21].

Indications

Granulocyte transfusions are used infrequently because antibiotic therapy or G-CSF and Granulocyte-macrophage-colony-stimulating factor (GM-CSF) are effective in treating or preventing infectious complications associated with neutropenia. In general granulocyte transfusions should be restricted to patients who have an absolute neutrophil count of less than 500 per micro litre, documented sepsis, or serious infection that is not responding to antibiotic therapy, and is expected to have a long period of neutropenia. The recent collection of high dose granulocytes by using steroid or G-CSF have significant promise, but no large randomized controlled trials have been done to demonstrate their effectiveness.

Dose and infusion rate

Granulocyte transfusions prepared by Apheresis technique, should be infused daily, until no longer needed. Granulocyte transfusion should be infused slowly over 1–4 hours. Premedications with antihistaminics, acetaminophen, corticosteroid or meperidine may be needed to prevent adverse reaction. If the patient is immunologically refractory to platelet transfusion, consideration should be given to obtaining granulocytes from HLA-matched donors. Because of a perceived adverse interaction between the infusion of granulocytes and amphotericin B therapy (acute pulmonary distress), granulocyte transfusion should be separated by a minimum 4 hours from the amphotericin therapy.

Expected outcome

With the higher dose of granulocyte concentrate, the WBC count will increase following granulocyte transfusion in adult. The clinical endpoint is improvement or resolution of the infections. In patients who respond to granulocyte concentrates, transfusion should be continued until resolution of infection has occurred or restoration of the patient's own granulocyte production occurs.

18.14 NEW BLOOD DERIVATIVES UNDER CLINICAL TRIAL

Several new blood derivatives are now in process of development. The cellular products like lymphocytes and natural killer cells (NK-cells) are being tried in the treatment of malignancy *e.g.*, solid tumor or haematological malignancy and in certain viral illness.

Several oxygen carrying blood substitutes are currently being tried in clinical situations like orthopaedic surgery, cardiac surgery, or preoperative haemodilution. Such products are stroma-free haemoglobin solution, or a compound called per-fluorocarbons. All such products are not yet licensed, but within the next few years, it will become important to know their indications, limitations, and adverse reactions which will become evident with more and more clinical use.

TABLE 18.2: Blood Components and Plasma Derivatives

Component /Product	Composition	Volume	Indications
Whole blood	RBC (40%), plasma deficient in labile coagulation factors, WBC, platelets non-functioning	500 ml	Increase both red cell mass and plasma volume (WBCs and platelets not functional; plasma deficient in labile clotting Factors V and VIII)
Red blood cells	RBC (Hct 75%), reduced WBC, plasma, platelet	250 ml	Increase red cell mass, WBC, platelets not functional
Red blood cells, Adenine saline added	RBC (approx. Hct 60%); reduced plasma, WBCs, and platelets; 100 mL of additive solution	330 ml	Increase red cell mass in symptomatic anemia (WBCs and platelets not functional)
RBCs Leukocyte reduced (prepared by filtration)	> 85% original volume of RBC; $< 5 \times 10^6$ WBC; few platelets; minimal plasma	225 ml	Increase red cell mass; $< 5 \times 10^6$ WBCs to decrease the likelihood of febrile reactions, immunization to leukocytes (HLA antigens) or CMV transmission
RBCs (Washed)	RBCs (Hct 75%), $> 5\times10^8$ WBC, no plasma	180 ml	Increase red cell mass; reduce risk of allergic reactions to plasma proteins

18.15 ADVERSE REACTIONS ASSOCIATED WITH TRANSFUSION

The knowledge of Transfusion Medicine can never be complete without the awareness of its possible hazards, some of which may be life threatening. The adverse reactions may be immediate or delayed, may be immune-mediated or simple acquirement of some infections. The physicians' responsibility is to prevent these adverse events and to explain to the patient's relatives about their prognosis.

Immediate transfusion reactions may be classified as: (1) Acute haemolytic reactions (2) Febrile non-haemolytic reactions (3) Allergic reactions (4) Consequences of Hypervolaemia.

18.16 ACUTE HAEMOLYTIC REACTIONS

This complication is most common and most life threatening complication, which may occur in 1 in 600 cases of transfusion and 1 in 25,000 components infused. Death associated with acute haemolytic reaction is most commonly due to ABO incompatibility.

Pathogenesis

Antibodies such as anti-A, anti-B, anti-Kell, anti-Duffy, anti-Fy^3 are associated with intravascular haemolysis by having the ability to activate the complement through C9. Antibodies against Rh system such as anti-D and anti-E do not activate complement and are associated with extravascular haemolysis, both of which may occur within the same episode of transfusion reaction. Fever with or without chill and rigor is the most common symptom. Nausea, vomiting, tachycardia, hypotension, wheezing, dyspnoea, back-pain, restlessness, discomfort around infusion site are other symptoms. The most serious consequences are renal failure and disseminated intravascular coagulation. In unconscious patient bleeding at surgical incision site or haemoglobinuria may be the only signs of acute haemolytic reaction. Cytokine generation is thought to play an important role in pathogenesis of haemolytic reaction.

In case of haemolytic reaction the following measures must be taken immediately as follows:

1. There should be a thorough clerical check to ensure that proper unit of blood has been transfused and this must be verified by transfusion service.
2. ABO compatibility of transfused blood must be checked and colour of the serum or plasma of pre-transfusion and post-transfusion blood must be noted. The presence of pink or red colour in the post sample compared to pre sample is the evidence of haemolysis.
3. A direct anti-globulin test is performed to determine whether transfused red cells have become coated with immunoglobulin. A urine sample should be also tested for presence of haemoglobin.
4. If following all these tests haemolytic reaction can not be confirmed, additional testing should be done. These tests include repeating the cross match and additional blood work, such as plasma-free haemoglobin, serum haptoglobin, bilirubin, and lactate dehydrogenase level.
5. Transfusion must be stopped. The intravenous line should be kept open with 0.9% of normal saline.
6. A diuretic like furosemide 40–120 mg is administered intravenously Urine output must be maintained at 100 ml per hour or more.
7. Blood bag and administration set must be sent to Blood Bank.
8. Transfusion reaction must be recorded on patient's bedside record.

18.17 FEBRILE NON-HAEMOLYTIC REACTIONS

Clinical Presentation

These reactions are characterised by symptoms beginning to develop at the end of transfusion or shortly after transfusion is over. There is a rise of diastolic blood pressure, headache, chill and rigor, followed by a rapid rise of temperature. Similar reactions may occur in cases of platelet transfusion when chill and rigor occur without or less rise of temperature. These reactions are caused by allo-antibodies against granulocytes, lymphocytes, or platelets. Febrile reactions usually respond to symptomatic therapy.

Diagnosis

When a red cell product is associated with these symptoms the most important intervention is to stop the transfusion, and to rule out a haemolytic transfusion, in which fever is the most common symptom. In cases of platelet transfusion, reaction is due to increase of various cytokines during storage of platelets. In general, diagnosis is made on the basis of absence of evidence of haemolysis and additional tests are not done to determine presence of WBC antibodies. These reactions occur with a frequency of 0.5% or more per component transfused.

Prevention

Prevention of febrile reactions is accomplished by removing the WBC from the blood product because many of the reactions are associated with antibodies against transfused leukocytes. This is best achieved by providing with pre-storage leukocyte-reduced blood products. At present random donor platelet concentrates are not leukocyte reduced, and so they may have the ability of developing increased levels of cytokines associated with febrile reactions. Pheresis platelets are usually leukocyte reduced and, therefore are usually not associated with febrile reactions.

18.18 TRANSFUSION RELATED ACUTE LUNG INJURY

The condition is characterised by development of non-cardiogenic pulmonary oedema. It is thought to be due to passively transferred donor's antibody that reacts against recipient's leukocyte antigen.

Clinical Presentation

Patients manifest fever, substernal chest pain, dyspnoea, cyanosis, cough, blood stained sputum and hypoxaemia 1 to 4 hours after transfusion of whole blood, FFP, platelet concentrate, or even cryoprecipitate. The heart size is normal but bilateral diffuse pulmonary infiltrate is seen on chest radiograph. Left atrial and pulmonary wedge pressures are within normal limit.

Treatment and Prevention

Patient may require respiratory support and mechanical ventilation. Recovery usually occurs within 48 hours. Rarely pulmonary oedema is sufficient to result in hypovolaemia and hypotension. If this occurs patient will require volume replacement. Recurrence is prevented by identifying the donor with antibodies leading to this complication and restricting future use of their blood. [22]

18.19 ALLERGIC REACTIONS

These reactions are characterised by development of urticaria, pruritus, or severe anaphylactic reactions. Mild reactions may occur in as many as 1% to 3% of transfused patients, and severe reactions occur at a rate of approximately 1 in 150,000 components transfused. Urticaria may occur without fever as a result of a reaction between a protein in donor plasma and corresponding antibodies in the recipient.

Because urticaria is not a sign of haemolysis routine investigations for transfusion reaction is not necessary. It is important, however, that such reactions be reported to blood bank, so that recurrence of such may require changes in blood product.

Treatment and Prevention

Hives are treated with anti-histaminics. Patients with severe or recurrent urticarial reactions should receive blood components that have been saline washed to remove plasma.

Anaphylactic transfusion reactions occur predominantly among patients who are IgA deficient and are extremely rare event with an estimate of 1 in 150,000 components transfused.

The general signs and symptoms of anaphylaxis are present and may include apprehension, a feeling of doom, chest or lumbar pain, facial or upper body flushing, generalized urticaria with Pruritus, laryngeal or facial oedema, bronchospasm, wheezing, hypotension, loss of consciousness, vomiting, diarrhoea.

No diagnostic testing is helpful prior to transfusion. Patients who suffer an anaphylactic reaction should be tested for IgA level and for presence of antibodies directed against IgA.

Treatment should be initiated promptly with epinephrine and careful clinical monitoring. If subsequent transfusions are required, red cells and platelets are washed to remove plasma or should be obtained from an IgA deficient donor if that is the cause. Plasma should be also obtained from IgA deficient donors.

18.20 HYPERVOLAEMIA

One of the most unrecognized complications of blood transfusion is hypervolaemia. Patients should be evaluated carefully prior to transfusion for their cardiac status and state of hydration. Patients who are at risk of hypervolaemia should have their blood transfused slowly over as long as 4 hours for 1U of blood. It is important to note that the blood contains a significant amount of sodium, with whole blood containing approximately 56 mEq sodium and packed red cells with additive solutions having 24–30 m Eq of sodium per unit.

18.21 NON-IMMUNE HAEMOLYSIS

Rupture of transfused red cells may occur because of mechanical stress or osmotic stress if solutions other than normal saline or other approved solutions are added to blood or red cells, if overheating occurs as a result of a malfunctioning blood warmer or if an infusion pump injures red cells. When haemolysis is suspected in a patient, these possibilities should be always considered, in addition to immune mediated haemolysis.

18.22 COMPLICATIONS OF MASSIVE TRANSFUSION

These include haemostatic defect, metabolic abnormalities, hypothermia. Patients receiving massive transfusion often experience hypotension, and shock. Massive transfusion which is given as an urgent measure, always an added risk of clerical error.

Clinical Presentations and Pathogenesis

1. **Bleeding complications:** Microvascular bleeding associated with thrombocytopenia, haemodilutional or consumptive coagulopathy is a frequent complication in these patients, especially those who are associated with packed red cells or crystalloids or albumin-containing solutions or who have prolonged hypotension.
2. **Hypocalcaemia:** Blood products contain citrate as anticoagulant, and some patients transfused with massive amount of blood can develop hypocalcaemia. Such patients should be monitored for the presence of impairment of cardiac function Hypothermia and acidosis potentiate hypocalcaemic symptoms.
3. **Hypokalaemia:** Massive transfusion usually is associated with hypokalaemia rather than hyperkalaemia.
4. **pH abnormalities:** Acidosis associated with hypoperfusion and tissue oxygen deprivation is usually reversed by transfusion and volume repletion. Citrate metabolism in stored blood generates bicarbonate with resultant alkalosis rather than acidosis in patients who do not have prolonged hypotension.
5. **Hypothermia:** Infusion of cold blood leads to hypothermia and potentiates myocardial depressant effect of hypocalcaemia and hypokalaemia, if they are present.
6. **Adult respiratory distress syndrome:** Although adult respiratory distress syndrome has been reported in the setting of massive transfusion, pulmonary insufficiency is more likely to be the consequence of injury to the upper abdomen or thorax rather than as a result of infused micro-aggregates contained in the stored blood.

Laboratory Testing

Laboratory testing of the haemostatic state is mandatory during massive transfusion. These include platelet count, prothrombin time (INR), partial thromboplastin time and fibrinogen level. Blood gas and electrolyte determination should be also performed.

Treatment

Treatment of thrombocytopenia and coagulopathy due to dilutional effect should include replacement of platelets, coagulation factors, and fibrinogen through transfusion of platelets, FFP and cryoprecipitate respectively. The need for these components should be based on results of laboratory tests and should not be given on an empirical basis or according to predetermined algorithms. Metabolic abnormalities should be treated appropriately when recognized. Blood warmers should be used in any patient undergoing transfusion in order to prevent hypothermia.

18.23 BACTERIAL SEPSIS

Although transfusion related sepsis occurs infrequently, it is an extremely important complication of blood transfusion and has received increased attention for this reason. Both RBC and platelet concentrates have been associated with bacterial contamination.

Clinical Presentation

Chills and rigors often associated with nausea, vomiting, lethargy and fever occur after infusion of 50 to 70 ml of blood. Fever and hypotension subsequently develop and may progress to shock and disseminated intravascular coagulation.

Laboratory Testing

Because such reaction may not be totally distinguishable from a haemolytic transfusion reaction, the patient should be evaluated as previously described for haemolytic transfusion reaction. In addition, blood transfusion should be immediately stopped, and an aliquot obtained from the remaining component should be examined for bacteria by gram stain and a bacterial culture should be performed. A negative Gram stain does not rule out the possibility of bacterial infection of the blood product. Reaction caused by Gram negative bacteria often are exacerbated by the presence of endotoxin contained in the contaminated compound.

Treatment

The symptom complex of chill shortly after the onset of a transfusion should raise clinical suspicion of transfusion-related sepsis. The blood transfusion should be immediately stopped. Gram stain and bacterial culture should be immediately performed. Broad spectrum antibiotics should be started. Supportive measures should be instituted for maintaining blood pressure. [23]

18.24 DELAYED HAEMOLYTIC TRANSFUSION REACTIONS

These reactions are the result of alloantibody-mediated red cell destruction by antibodies that are not detected at the time of pre-transfusion testing is performed. The alloantibodyes are generally secondary to amnestic responses that manifest several days to 2 weeks after transfusion. Clinical reactions occur with a frequency of 1 per 1,500 to 8000 units transfused approximately, and are usually mild. [24]

Clinical Presentation

A delayed haemolytic transfusion reaction should be suspected when unexpected anaemia develops in a patient with a history of recent transfusion. Besides anaemia, fever is the most common symptom. (75%) Jaundice (67%) and oliguria (17%) may occur. Most of these symptoms occur approximately 1 week after transfusion.

Laboratory Testing

Patient should be evaluated with a both direct and indirect antiglobulin test. Implicated antibodies usually include Rh antibodies as well as antibodies directed against Kell, Kidd, Duffy antigens. Delayed haemolytic transfusion reactions should be suspected in patients, who have unexpected fall in haematocrit following a blood transfusion and in particular, in a patient who develops fever or clinical and laboratory evidence of haemolysis.

Treatment

Significant clinical consequences other than anaemia and fever occur infrequently. Supportive therapy is indicated if serious complication such as oliguria occurs.

18.25 POST-TRANSFUSION GROWTH-VERSUS-HOST DISEASE

This rare complication is considered a result of infused viable lymphocytes present in a blood product that recognizes and reacts against host tissues. The condition occurs when a blood product with viable lymphocytes is given to a patient who is immunosuppressed. As previously noted, rare incidence has occurred when family members have directed their blood transfusion to another family member. The donor lymphocytes detect immunological difference in the recipient, proliferate, and mount a cellular response against host tissue. Graft-versus-host disease has been reported after transfusion of whole blood, red cells, platelet concentrates, granulocyte transfusion, and fresh plasma. [25]

Clinical Presentation

Transfusion-related Growth-versus-host disease occurs 4 to 30 days after transfusion. It resembles the condition associated with bone marrow transplantation. Patients develop fever, erythema, diarrhoea, liver function abnormalities, bone marrow suppression marked by pancytopenia.

Laboratory Testing

The diagnosis is made by performing a biopsy of the skin or gastrointestinal tract. In addition DNA testing may be performed, to determine whether the circulating lymphocytes show non-patient type, presumably those of the blood donor.

Treatment and Prevention

Treatment is usually unsuccessful and mortality approaches 90%. Prevention is the most effective therapy. Gamma irradiation of blood products (2500Gy) prevents lymphocyte proliferation, but results in no or minimal damage to other cells.

18.26 IRON OVERLOAD

The complication occurs in adult patients who receive 60 to 210 (mean 120) units of blood. In such cases endocrine, liver, and cardiac dysfunction occurs. Iron chelation therapy is effective in decreasing and slowing the onset of organ dysfunction associated with iron overload.

18.27 POST-TRANSFUSION PURPURA

This uncommon syndrome is manifested by profound thrombocytopenia that develops approximately 5 to 9 days after a blood transfusion. The exact pathogenesis is not known. Other causes of thrombocytopenia *e.g.*, drug-induced, heparin-induced, and DIC must be excluded. Patients with this disorder develop an antibody to a platelet antigen that is not on their own platelets. The most common platelet antigen against which antibody develops is the Pl^{A1} antigen. Treatment modalities include use of intravenous gamma-globulin or therapeutic plasma exchange. Transfusion Pl^{A1}negative platelets to patients who are positive for this antibody is not successful.

18.28 IMMUNOSUPPRESSIVE EFFECT OF BLOOD TRANSFUSION

Blood transfusion causes down-regulation of immune system. There is controversy whether this produces any adverse effect. There are a large number of publications, both pro and con, revealing whether there is increased frequency of tumor recurrence after resection or increased frequency of pot operative infections, in cases of blood transfusion, but the issue has not been settled. Removal of leukocytes might be beneficial to this potential complication.

TABLE 18.3: Hazards of Blood Transfusion

Complications	Pathogenesis	Symptoms	Remedies
Haemolytic Reactions	Antibodies to ABO system activate complement through C9 produce I.V. Haemolysis, Renal failure, DIC	Nausea, chest pain, abdominal pain, breathlessness, oliguria, bleeding at injection or operation site	Stoppage of transfusion, I. V. Furosemide, Mannitol to maintain urine volume, Management of renal failure and DIC
Febrile Non Haemolytic Reactions	Alloantibodies against lymphocytes, granulocytes, platelet and various cytokines accumulating during storage are responsible.	Rapid rise of temperature with chill and rigor and leukocytosis at the end of transfusion	Stoppage of transfusion and symptomatic treatments are mainstay. Prevention is by use of leukocytes- free blood products.
Delayed Haemolytic Reactions (several days to 2 weeks)	Alloantibodies which are not detected by pretransfusion tests	Unexplained Anemia, fever, oliguria	Same as in haemolytic reactions
Anaphylactic reactions	Antibody to IgA present in donor's plasma (in IgA deficient patients)	Apprehension, chest pain, lumbar pain, flushing, bronchospasm	Treatment by epinephrine and antihistaminic.
Allergic Reactions	Antigen antibody reaction of donor's plasma protein and recipient's tissues	Urticaria, pruritus, fever	Use of saline washed blood products.
Transfusion related lung injury	Donor's antibody acts against recipient's leukocyte antigen.	Pulmonary infiltrate, non-cardiac pulmonary edema	Mechanical ventilation, respiratory support, use of leucocyte free blood products
Non-immune haemolysis	Rupture of transfused cells due to osmotic or mechanical stress		Avoidance of solutions other than normal saline in the transfusion line, infusion pump

Complications	Pathogenesis	Symptoms	Remedies
Transmission of infections	In elderly or immunocompromised patients usually	Hepatitis B or C, CMV, HIV, malaria, trypanosomiasis, J-C disease	Proper screening and treatment of the blood with a solvent detergent that destroys envelope viruses
Post transfusion Purpura (5-9 days)	Antibody to platelet antigen		I V Gammaglobulin, plasma exchange
GVH disease (After 4-30 days)	Infused viable lymphocytes which react with host tissues, especially when family member donates the blood and the subject is immunosuppressed		Gamma irradiation prevents lymphocyte proliferation
Bacterial sepsis	Contamination which is common in platelet transfusion	Fever, hypotension associated with DIC, if persists long	Culture and sensitivity of aliquots of blood transfused and treatment accordingly
Massive transfusion	Dilutional coagulopathy, hypocalcaemia, cardiac overload, iron overload	Bleeding from multiple sites, CCF, cardiac, renal, hepatic dysfunction	Proper assessment before transfusion

18.29 TRANSFUSION TRANSMITTED DISEASES

Viral Infections

(1) **Hepatitis:** About 10% of patients, infected with hepatitis C, acquire infection during blood transfusion. At present, the estimated risk of post-transfusion hepatitis C, is 1 in 263,000 components transfused. Donor screening and testing procedures have reduced the risk of post-transfusion hepatitis B to approximately 1 in 63,000 from 1 per 233,000 components transfused.

(2) **HIV infection:** More than 8000 persons develop HIV infection from blood transfusion prior to development of testing in 1985. Since implementation of testing for HIV infectivity in blood donor units, only 47 cases have been reported. Blood donors have to undergo testing for antibodies against HIV-1, HIV-2, p24Ag and now a new research testing evolves i.e., nucleic acid test for HIV in an attempt to shorten the window period. The current risk of acquiring HIV infection through blood product transfusion is approximately1 per 1,000,000 units transfused.

(3) **Other retroviral infections:** HTLV-I and HTLV-II infections are transmitted by blood, but only by cell containing components and not via FFP or cryoprecipitate. Tests should be done on all blood donations and hence the risk of these infections is extremely low.

(4) **Cytomegalovirus (CMV) infection:** Certain patients receiving blood transfusion are extremely vulnerable to this infection. Such patients are foetuses who receive intrauterine transfusion, premature infants smaller than 1200 gm of BW born to CMV sera-negative mother, CMV sera-negative pregnant women, who may place the foetuses at increased risk, CMV sera-negative recipients of kidney, liver, lung or bone marrow transplants. Post-transfusion infection is prevented by providing blood products, produced by providing blood products which are freed from leukocytes by using third generation leukocyte filter. [26]

Non-Viral Infections

(1) **Spirochaete infection:** Syphilis is an unusual complication of blood transfusion, because donors are tested and spirochaetes are not viable after 24–36 hours at 4°C storage.

(2) **Parasitic infections:** Transfusion transmitted malaria occurs infrequently. Transfusion associated babesiosis is a potentially fatal complication when occurs in immunocompromised, splenectomised, or elderly patients. Chagas' disease (Trypanosoma cruzi) is associated with blood transfusion. Chagas' disease is named after Carlos Chagas, a Brazilian who in 1910 discovered this parasite in the vector. (Thus, the correct name is Chagas' disease, not Chaga's disease.) The parasite is found throughout much of central and northerns America, South America, Central America, and Mexico. In the human host, Chagas' disease affects primarily the nervous system and heart. Chronic infections result in various neurological disorders, including dementia, megacolon, and megaesophagus, and damage to the heart muscle. Left untreated, Chagas' disease is often fatal.

Slow Virus Infections

Creutzfeldt – Jacob Disease

Though not a single case has been reported to be transmitted by blood transfusion, it is mandatory to exclude this disease or its variant in the donor and in his family.

Conclusion

All over the world, researches are going on and on to evolve methods of testing blood products to provide safe blood transfusion. At the same time attempts are being made to separate the blood components in such a way that sterilization and storage of blood products do not make the different components nonviable. Probably, in near future, absolutely safe 'blood' can be supplied, which will meet the exact demand of the particular clinical situation.

REFERENCES

1. American Society of Anaesthesiologists Task Force on Blood Component Therapy. *Practice guidelines for blood component therapy*. Anaesthesiology (1996); 84 : 732–747.
2. Hebert PC, Wells G, Blajchman MA, et al., *A multicentre, randomized, controlled clinical trial of transfusion requirements in critical care*. N Engl J Med (1999); 340 : 409–417.
3. Wallace EL, Churchill WH, Surgenor DM et al., *Collection and Transfusion of blood and blood components in the United States*, (1994). Transfusion (1998); 38 : 625–635.

4. Welch HG, Meehan KR, Goodnough LT. *Prudent strategies for elective red blood cell transfusion.* Ann Intern Med (1992); 116: 393–402.
5. Dzik D, Aubuchou J, Jeffries L, et al., *Leukocyte reduction of blood components: public policy and new technology*. Transfus Med Rev. (2000); 14: 34–52.
6. Beutler E. *Platelet transfusions: the 20,000/microL trigger*. Blood (1993); 81: 1411–1413.
7. The Trial to reduce Alloimmunization to Platelets Study Group. *Leukocyte reduction and ultraviolet B irradiation of platelets to prevent alloimmunization and refractioriness to platelet transfusions*. N Engl J Med (1997); 337: 1861–1869.
8. Friedberh RC,et al., *Clinical and blood bank factors in the management of refractionariness and alloimmunization*. Blood (1993); 81: 3428-3434.
9. Norol F, et al., *Platelet transfusion: a dose response study*. Blood (1998); 92: 1448–1453.
10. Contreras M and the British Committee for Standards in Haematology, Working Party of the Blood Transfusion Task Force. *Guidelines for the use of fresh-frozen plasma*. Transfus Med (1992); 2: 57–63.
11. Alving B, ed. *Blood components and pharmacologic agents in the treatment of congenital and acquired bleeding disorders*. Bethesd, MD, AABB Press, (2000).
12. Menache D, Grossman BJ, Jackson CM. *Antithrombin III: physiology, deficiency, replacement therapy. Transfusion* (1992); 32: 580–588.
13. Lindlay CM, SwayerWT, Maick BJ Lusher J, Harrison JF, Baird –Cox K, et al., *Pharmacokinetics and pharmacodynamics of recombinant factor VIIa*. Clin Pharmacol Ther (1994); 55:638–48.
14. Mauricio L, Jeroukhimov L, Klein Y, Martinowitz U. *Updates in the management of severe coagulopathy in trauma patients*. Intensive Care Med (2002); 28: 5241–5247.
15. Hendriks HG, Meijer K, de Wolf JT, et al., *Reduced transfusion requirements by recombinant factor VIIa in orthoptics liver transplantation: a pilot study*. Transplantation (2001); 71: 402–405.
16. Mayer SA,Brun NC,Begtrup KBroderick J, et al., *Recombinant Activated factor VII for Acute Intracerebral haemorrhage*. NEJM (2005); 352: 777–785.
17. D'Oiron R, Menart C, Trzeciak MC, et al., *Use of rVIIa in 3 patients with inherited type I Glanzman thromboasthenia undergoing invasive procedures*. Thromb Haematol (2000); 83: 644–647.
18. Ratko TA, Burnett DA, Toulke GE, et al., *Recommendations for off-label use of intravenously administered immunoglobulin preparations*. JAMA (1995); 273: 1865–1870.
19. Radosevich M, Goubran DA, Bournouf T. *Fibrin sealant: scientific rationale, production methods, properties, and current clinical use*. Vox Sang (1997); 92: 133–143.
20 Erstad B, Gales BJ, Rappaport WD. *The use of albumin in clinical practice*. Arch Intern Med (1991); 151: 901–911.
21. Dale DC, Liles WC, Price TH. *Renewed interest in granulocyte transfusion therapy*. Br. J Haematol (1997); 98: 497–501.
22. Popavsky MA, Chaplin HC, Moore SB. *Transfusion-related acute lung injury: a neglected serious complication of Haemotherapy*. Transfusion (1992); 32: 589–592.
23. Tripple MA, et al., *Sepsis associated with transfusion of red cells contaminated with Yersinia enterocolitis*. Transfusion (1990); 30: 207–210.
24. Nees PM, et al., *The differentiation of delayed serologic and delayed haemolytic transfusion reactions: incidence, long-term serologic findings, clinical significance*. Transfusion (1990); 30: 688–693.
25. Shivdasoaric RA, Anderson KC. Graft-versus-host disease. In Petz et al., eds., *Clinical Practice of transfusion medicine*, 3rd ed. New York. Churchil Livingston, (1998); 1998: 931–946.
26. Bowden RA, Slichter SJ, Sayers M, et al., *A comparison of filtered leukocyte reduced and cytomegalovirus (CMV) seronegative blood products for the prevention of transfusion associated CMV infection after marrow transplant*. Blood (1995); 86: 3598–3603.

Index

D

E

F

G

H

I

J

K

L

M

N

O

P

R

S

T

U

V

W

Z